The Hippocampus - Cognitive Functions and Disorders

Edited by Maurice Ptito and Daniel-Robert Chebat

Published in London, United Kingdom

The Hippocampus - Cognitive Functions and Disorders
http://dx.doi.org/10.5772/intechopen.1004674
Edited by Maurice Ptito and Daniel-Robert Chebat

Contributors
Alexandra Haddad, Amari Eubanks, Annalia Burke-Carreno, Anthony Okeh, Ashim Pandey, Banuja Munasinghe, Constantin Tsarouchas, Daniel-Robert Chebat, Dipesh Shrestha, Fabien C. Schneider, Fereshteh Azedi, Frédéric Bernard, Gaël Malleret, Julia Malone, Maria Sneed, Mark W. Burke, Maurice Ptito, Maxime Bleau, Mohammad Taghi Joghataei, Nicholas Tsarouchas, Nick Tsarouchas, Prateek Mehra, Roberta Palmour, Serdar Ercan, Shawn Malone, Sujaya Neupane

First published in London, United Kingdom, 2026 by IntechOpen
IntechOpen is the global imprint of INTECHOPEN LIMITED, registered in England and Wales, registration number: 11086078, 167-169 Great Portland Street, London, W1W 5PF, United Kingdom

For EU product safety concerns: IN TECH d.o.o., Prolaz Marije Krucifikse Kozulić 3, 51000 Rijeka, Croatia, info@intechopen.com or visit our website at intechopen.com.

British Library Cataloguing-in-Publication Data
A catalogue record for this book is available from the British Library

The Hippocampus - Cognitive Functions and Disorders
Edited by Maurice Ptito and Daniel-Robert Chebat
p. cm.
Print ISBN 978-0-85014-960-9
Online ISBN 978-0-85014-959-3
eBook (PDF) ISBN 978-0-85014-961-6

Meet the editors

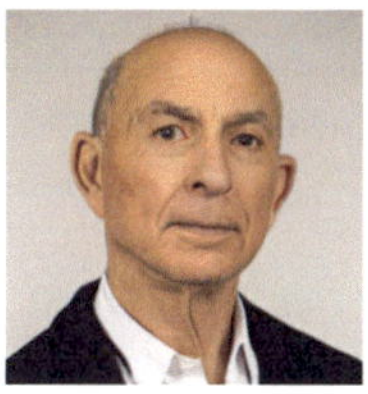

Dr. Maurice Ptito is a Professor of Visual Neuroscience at the School of Optometry (Université de Montréal). He is an internationally recognized neuroscientist whose work has significantly shaped contemporary understanding of neuroplasticity, sensory substitution, and visual system reorganization, particularly in the context of congenital and acquired blindness. He holds a doctorate in Medicine and a Ph.D. in Neuropsychology. He also holds the H. Sanders Research Chair in Visual Science. Dr. Ptito's research integrates psychophysical, neuroanatomical, and neuroimaging methods to examine how the brain processes sensory information in the absence of primary sensory modalities. A core focus of his work has been the recruitment and repurposing of visual cortical areas in blind individuals, in which he has demonstrated the occipital cortex's capacity to process tactile and auditory inputs via sensory substitution devices. His work has helped establish the concept of supra-modal processing and contributed to the development of functional frameworks for understanding cross-modal cortical reorganization. He has also made notable contributions to the study of the hippocampus, especially regarding its role in spatial memory and navigation under conditions of visual deprivation. His findings suggest that hippocampal function is maintained and may even adapt via alternative sensory pathways, with implications for both cognitive neuroscience and rehabilitative approaches. Dr. Ptito has received several awards and was recently appointed a Knight of the National Order of Quebec.

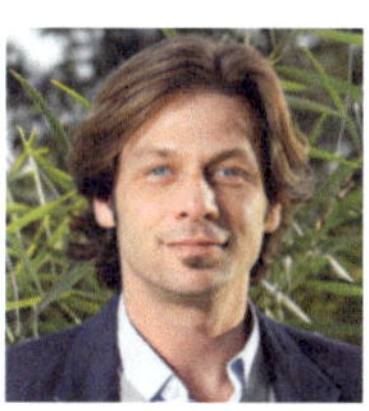

Dr. Daniel-Robert Chebat is a cognitive neuroscientist whose work has advanced contemporary understanding of brain plasticity, multisensory integration, and spatial cognition in blindness. He is a Senior Lecturer at Ariel University and Director of the Visual and Cognitive Neuroscience Laboratory. Dr. Chebat's research integrates sensory substitution technologies, real and virtual Hebb–Williams mazes, human-scale obstacle courses, and advanced neuroimaging to examine how spatial knowledge is acquired and represented in the brain in the absence of vision. Dr. Chebat is the recipient of fellowships from CIHR, the Azrieli Foundation, and the Edmond & Lily Safra Center for Brain Sciences.

Contents

Preface

The hippocampus (**Figure 1**), a brain structure located within the temporal lobe, has long interested neuroscientists and clinicians alike. Believed to be the locus of memory formation and spatial navigation, this small yet intricately connected region is essential for cognitive and emotional processes. A large body of studies spanning decades has unveiled its complex roles and its susceptibility to dysfunction. This book, *The Hippocampus – Cognitive Functions and Disorders*, offers a comprehensive exploration of one of the brain's most intricate and vital structures. Edited by Maurice Ptito and Daniel R. Chebat, it brings together a diverse array of chapters authored by experts in neuroscience, neuropsychology, and clinical research. Covering both the fundamental neuroscience of the hippocampus and its implications for various disorders, the volume provides valuable insights for students, researchers, clinicians, and anyone interested in understanding the multifaceted roles of this critical brain region. Through its interdisciplinary approach, the book highlights the hippocampus's significance in cognition, emotional regulation, neuroplasticity, and pathology, inspiring further research and clinical innovation.

The first collection of chapters, entitled *Hippocampal-based Behaviors*, offers a comprehensive overview of the hippocampus's pivotal role in cognition and neural plasticity. Ashim Pandey, Dipesh Shrestha, and Sujaya Neupane discuss how perceptual-cognitive training harnesses brain plasticity to improve visual and mnemonic functions, particularly in cortical blindness, and emphasizes integrated perception and navigation strategies. Frédéric Bernard examines the expanding understanding of the hippocampus beyond memory, proposing its involvement in reading processes such as word decoding and comprehension, and advocating for its inclusion in the reading network. Gaël Malleret explores the active role of the hippocampus in adaptive forgetting through synaptic depression mechanisms, such as LTD, which are essential for cognitive efficiency and overload

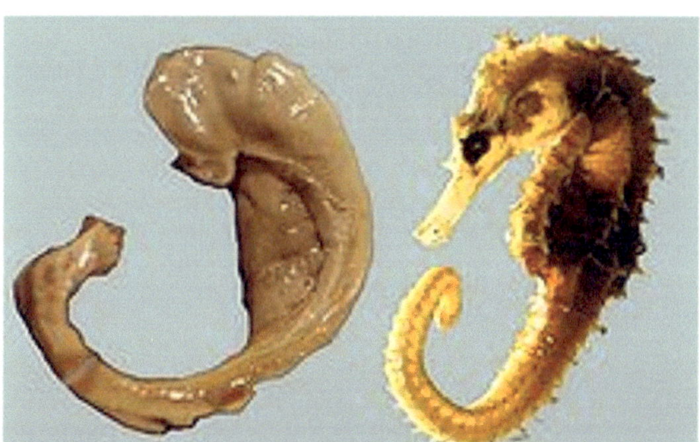

Figure 1.
A: the human hippocampus dissected out and B: the Seahorse it was named after.

prevention. Maxime Bleau, Daniel-Robert Chebat, Fabien C. Schneider, and Maurice Ptito demonstrate how the hippocampus and navigation networks adapt in congenital blindness, supporting non-visual navigation through cross-modal plasticity and highlighting the brain's remarkable capacity for functional reorganization. Lastly, Nick Tsarouchas, Nicholas Tsarouchas and Constantin Tsarouchas, in a perspective chapter, focus on the role of hippocampus-centered limbocortical networks in emotional regulation and functional neurological disorders, modeling how dynamic interactions among default-mode, salience, and executive networks generate complex emotional states, and how their dysregulation leads to distorted self-representation, maladaptive predictions, and functional symptoms.

The following collection of chapters, on *Hippocampal Dysfunctions*, highlights the diverse and critical roles of the hippocampus in brain health and disease. Mohammad Taghi Joghataei and Fereshteh Azedi explore how hippocampal vascularization patterns influence vascular impairment, impacting cognitive and emotional functions. Emerging evidence from Prateek Mehra, Julia Malone, and Shawn Malone underscores the importance of minimizing hippocampal damage during radiotherapy to preserve cognition. Haddad et al. demonstrate how prenatal alcohol exposure causes structural deficits in the hippocampus, linked to impaired cognitive development, exemplifying its vulnerability during critical periods. Serdar Ercan provides a detailed account of anterior temporal lobectomy for medically refractory temporal lobe epilepsy, outlining indications, patient selection, surgical anatomy, and technique, and showing how resection of hippocampal and mesial temporal structures can achieve high rates of seizure control while carrying specific cognitive, visual, and psychiatric risks. In a broad clinical neurophysiology perspective, Nick Tsarouchas, Nicholas Tsarouchas, and Constantin Tsarouchas characterize hippocampal and limbocortical "oscillopathies" across dementia, schizophrenia, mood and anxiety disorders, autism, ADHD, PTSD, functional neurological syndromes, movement disorders, and epilepsies, framing these conditions as disturbances of large-scale network oscillations that support memory, navigation, affect, and behavior. Collectively, these chapters underline the hippocampus's central role across a range of neurovascular, neuropsychiatric, and functional disorders, and inform strategies for diagnosis and prevention.

By bringing together contributions from these leading experts in the field, *The Hippocampus – Cognitive Functions and Disorders* aspires not only to educate but also to inspire future research. We certainly hope this collection highlights the lasting importance of the hippocampus in advancing our understanding of brain function and dysfunction. New research can pave the way for innovative strategies to reduce the impact of hippocampal disorders.

Maurice Ptito, DMSc, Ph.D., FRSC, OQ
School of Optometry,
Université de Montreal,
Montreal, (Qc) Canada

Daniel R. Chebat, Ph.D.
Department of Psychology,
Ariel University,
Ariel, Israel

Section 1

Hippocampal-based Behaviors

Chapter 1

Perceptual-Cognitive Training Paradigms for Understanding Cognition and Cortical Visual Impairments

Ashim Pandey, Dipesh Shrestha and Sujaya Neupane

Abstract

Brain plasticity and behavioral compensation after neurological injury offer promising clinical potential for targeted functional neurorehabilitation. An active area of research in neurorehabilitation is vision restoration *via* perceptual learning. Despite exciting success stories, vision rehabilitation strategies have faced limitations of achieving longevity and generalization beyond the training parameters. In this chapter, we propose that perceptual learning involves more than just sensory brain regions, suggesting that the search for neural mechanisms of visual learning should expand beyond the visual system. We hypothesize that engaging cognitive circuits with a navigation paradigm that involves visual encoding promotes plasticity in the visual system, a key input to the brain's navigation networks. Under this hypothesis, we propose an integrated approach for neurorehabilitation where perceptual and cognitive systems are dynamically interacting. Furthermore, we argue that studying cognitive functions in the context of navigation necessitates controlled omission of sensory input in experimental paradigms, and such studies have implications for designing effective rehabilitative training for patients with cortical blindness. We review animal studies on the neural mechanisms of navigation without sensory input, focusing on the hippocampal formation and posterior parietal cortex-brain regions thought to subserve spatial navigation. Finally, we explore potential perceptual-cognitive training tasks for vision restoration and their hypothetical neural mechanisms to address the limitations of existing vision training paradigms. Overall, we identify a promising research direction for developing innovative tools to rehabilitate visual function in individuals with cortical blindness.

Keywords: neurorehabilitation, perceptual learning, brain plasticity, navigation circuits, cortical blindness

1. Introduction

A remarkable property of the brain is its capacity to change. When facing adverse conditions such as a stroke, the brain's propensity toward adaptation and plasticity offers a powerful potential to restore lost functions. Although post-stroke adaptation often occurs spontaneously, the recovery is seldom complete. For example, after cortical visual impairment (CVI), in which a lesion in the visual cortex causes blindness in the contralateral visual field, the chances of spontaneous visual recovery are around 50% during 1 month, reduce to 20% after 6 months, and go to zero after 12 months [1]. A perennial challenge for clinicians and neuroscientists is to design interventional paradigms to augment spontaneous recovery and achieve a fuller restoration of lost perceptual, cognitive, or motor functions after brain damage [2–4].

One way to achieve plasticity beyond spontaneous recovery is by designing training paradigms targeted at the lost function. The logic of this approach is as follows: Since there are redundant and flexible connections between brain areas [5–7], an appropriate rehabilitative training paradigm will leverage the intentionality of a patient with brain damage and unmask the residual anatomical pathways leading to functional restoration [3, 4, 8]. Supporting evidence for this approach comes from the observation that congenitally blinds patients naturally repurpose their brain structures to gain visual function [6, 9]. Researchers have designed interventional tools with this approach and successfully restored lost function to a certain extent. For example, there is a rich literature on perceptual training to regain vision in partially blind subjects with visual cortical damage [4, 10–14]. Despite its success in restoring lost function beyond spontaneous recovery, a consistent limitation of the domain-specific training approach is that the functional restoration is often restricted to training parameters and period [12]. What alternative approaches could promote longevity and generalization after rehabilitative behavioral training?

We propose an integrated approach for neurorehabilitation where perceptual and cognitive systems are dynamically interacting. Such an approach can offer several advantages to overcome the specificity and poor retention of vision recovery. First, generalization and flexibility are hallmarks of cognition, and as such, this approach can leverage the cognitive functions attributed to domain-general brain areas [6]. Second, targeting higher brain areas with behavioral training can induce plasticity in the feedback connectivity along the sensory hierarchy, opening the possibility of achieving functional generalization while stimulating specific sensory areas of interest [8, 15]. Finally, an integrated approach using multiple tasks and continual learning is more natural than a trial-based task. The brain evolved to perform goal-directed tasks and solve problems in its umwelt by recruiting its various neural circuits in coordination, for example, to detect food or threats, rapidly and flexibly make plans, and control its actions for enacting those plans [16]. Therefore, although neuroscientists use reduced experimental setups to probe these systems in isolation, a naturalistic alternative where the multiple systems work in unison would be more appropriate for rehabilitating a lost natural function [17].

A natural link to study perceptual and cognitive circuits as interactive systems is spatial navigation. Navigation behavior is ubiquitous across animal species and is thought to rely on multiple brain regions, including the hippocampal formation (HF). Navigation combines sensory information like self-motion with mnemonic information like a mental map [18–20]. While inferring self-motion relies on processing sensory information such as the optic flow in visual areas [21], navigation involves making flexible decisions based on both sensory and mnemonic information, often attributed to cognitive regions such as frontoparietal cortices and the HF [19, 20]. More specifically, in primates with an evolved fovea-based visual system, the HF and posterior parietal cortex (PPC) are implicated in the perception of visual scenes for informing appropriate navigational decisions [22]. Such evolutionary perspective and commensurate findings [23–25] suggest that the hippocampal cognitive functions are coopted in primates for perceptual function, thus making our integrative approach more compelling. Furthermore, neurons in PPC encode self-motion [26, 27] and are implicated in spatial navigation, complementing the function of HF [28–30]. PPC and HF appear to be complementary neural circuits connecting perception and cognition. Indeed, by studying blind patients, researchers have shown that navigation training can induce plasticity in the parietal visual areas [31–33]. Therefore, navigation is a promising behavior to study which can inform task design for neurorehabiliative training.

In this chapter, we focus on vision restoration in cortical blindness and the neurophysiological studies of two brain areas—PPC and HF. They are the crucial hubs in the primate brain underlying perceptual-cognitive behavior and thus capable of inducing top-down plasticity for vision restoration. In what follows, we first review the literature on visual perceptual learning in cortical visual impairment (CVI) patients. We then review the hippocampal studies that employed behavioral assays in which sensory information was absent or impoverished. We will subsequently review the literature on PPC and its complementary role in navigation and visual processing. With this knowledge, we will describe our integrated framework for neurorehabilitation with potential experiments and hypothetical neural mechanisms. In brief, our integrated approach aims to leverage three ways of inducing more effective neural plasticity that can cause long-lasting improvement and generalization: (1) continual tasks to mimic naturalistic behavior and go beyond trial-based training, (2) stimulate top-down feedback connections to visual areas from higher areas, including PPC and HF, and (3) transfer generalizability of cognitive behavior to perceptual learning [3, 4, 8, 10, 12, 34–36].

2. Perceptual learning: Merits and limitations

Perceptual learning is a well-studied phenomenon in humans and animals in which improvement in sense perception is observed after repeated training or exposure. A refined palate's capacity to distinguish variations in a cuisine, a radiologist's capability to read X-ray images, and a field biologist's ability to recognize baboon faces are all attributed to perceptual learning. While other reviews exist on the topic, we focus on visual perceptual learning to outline its benefits as a neurorehabilitation tool, point out its limitations, and propose integrated approaches to tackle them.

Perceptual learning as a neurorehabilitation tool is most successfully used in cases of CVI [4, 10, 35]. CVI results from a lesion in the visual cortex past the optic chiasm, which causes blindness in the contralateral visual field. There are very few clinical interventions available for these patients, and most of them live their lives with partial blindness. More recently, insights from visual perceptual learning have been used to develop vision training protocols to ameliorate CVI by maximizing residual functional vision. One way to do this is to place a visual stimulus on the blind field of a CVI patient and ask them to respond to queries made on the features of the stimulus. Although the subjects cannot directly see the stimulus, they can respond to it, a phenomenon termed "blindsight" [37]. This approach utilizes the patient's intentionality and appears to activate the residual visual pathways for re-routing visual information to bypass the lesioned brain tissue [4, 10, 37]. In computational terms, perceptual discrimination of stimulus features presented in the blind field is made possible by gradually reweighting the readout of visual information—weakening the readout from the lesioned area and strengthening it from an intact area [34, 38]. By using visual stimuli with complex features typically processed in higher visual areas, vision scientists have achieved greater generalization in both healthy subjects and CVI patients [10–12, 39–41].

Early CVI studies leveraged the known neural selectivity in primary visual cortex (V1) to design perceptual training paradigms after its partial damage. Patients were trained to detect vertical grating presented on their blind field in a two-alternative forced-choice task. They showed improved contrast sensitivity limited to trained stimuli and location within the blind field [42], as was expected from perceptual learning studies that focused on lower visual areas [43]. Subsequent studies used visual stimuli that would allow for generalization to untrained stimuli. Huxlin and colleagues [44] used motion discrimination training to induce targeted plasticity in the extrastriate visual cortex. The perceptual improvements they observed transferred to untrained stimulus and task but were retained only at the training location [10, 44]. To overcome the location specificity, Pack and colleagues used a discrimination task on complex motion stimuli such as optic flow or rotating clouds of dots. Such complex motion is known to stimulate neurons in the medial superior temporal (MST) area [45]. Since MST receives converging inputs from neurons in the upstream motion-sensitive areas, MST neurons have large response fields straddling the midline [46, 47]. In healthy individuals and CVI patients, they used optic flow stimuli and an "in/out" binary discrimination task and monitored their perceptual learning. This approach showed generalization of learning across stimulus features as well as spatial locations [11, 12, 34], but the spatial transfer did not last beyond the training period [12].

Visual perceptual learning studies have primarily focused on understanding neural plasticity across different cortical regions of the visual system [48]. While this approach has seen limited success in restoring vision in CVI patients, the retinotopic organization of visual areas puts a fundamental limit on location transfer, even though the extent of transfer can be expanded by targeting higher visual areas with relatively less spatial specificity [12, 34, 43]. Therefore, there is a need to design training paradigms that are not bound by retinotopic constraints.

One way to achieve this is to take an integrative approach of combining perception with cognitive behavior. The potential of cognitive training to enhance perceptual experiences has been explored with navigation tasks in blind subjects who exhibit enhanced activity in their visual cortex after navigational behavioral training [31, 32]. To get a more detailed characterization of the underlying neural circuits of navigation and assess its utility in vision rehabilitation training, we review the neural mechanisms of navigation behavior in the next two sections.

3. Navigation without sensory input

Everyday navigation is a multi-sensory integration process that relies on internal and external information. When the destination is visible, navigation becomes a process of calibrating one's bearing to the goal location. In most cases, however, navigation involves traveling to a place not immediately visible and often entails taking novel routes to new destinations. Such flexible navigation relies on a learned mental map, which is viewpoint independent and readily accessible to the agent. Over many decades, various neural and behavioral studies have supported the notion that animals encode and use such an internal *cognitive map* to plan and execute routes [18–20].

The evidence for the neural representation of the hypothetical cognitive map first came with the landmark discovery of *place cells* in the hippocampal formation of rodents [49]. *Place cell* gets its name from its functional property, namely its characteristic encoding of an animal's particular location within an arena, irrespective of its orientation or speed. Unlike the response field of sensory and motor neurons, which encode space relative to eye, head, or body position, place cells encode space with respect to objects external to the animal. The discovery of such an allocentric spatial code inspired a significant interest in the potential existence of a viewpoint independent, generalizable cognitive map in the brain. Naturally, it spawned a new subfield of neuroscience that focused on characterizing the nature of this spatial representation in the brain [50–53]. Experimental verification of the usage of an internal map, however, requires behavioral paradigms in which subjects must make inferences over the map without access to external input [19]. Numerous experiments were conducted toward this goal, as reviewed below, albeit with limitations [54, 55].

When the hippocampal place cell was discovered, researchers established its generality by varying the external cues in both light and darkness [56, 57]. In the first systematic probing of place cells by O'Keefe, he tested them in the dark, reporting no change in their spatial code but only if rats were pre-exposed to the maze with lights on [58]. However, removing both visual and tactile cues caused the place fields to destabilize. This finding was later confirmed in a more extensive study [59], suggesting that place cells encode a memory of the local spatial environment.

Further support for the mnemonic spatial code in the hippocampus came with interventional studies in which blind and deaf rats navigated an open arena [60]. The authors found that only a minority of hippocampal place fields remained stable in blind and deaf rats [60]. In contrast, when Save et al. recorded activity from the hippocampus of blind rats, they found stable place cells. There was one crucial difference between the two studies—while in the earlier study, the rats were pre-exposed to the foraging box before sensory deprivation; in the latter study, rats were made blind shortly after birth, precluding any prior visual exposure to any environment. These studies suggest that the hippocampal place cell system uses multisensory input to map the spatial environment, and the stability of the place system is disrupted if the relational structure of the environment initially used for cognitive mapping is altered [61, 62]. In other words, the place cell system is disrupted if there is a mismatch between the learned map and the spatial environment, as reported two decades earlier by O'Keefe [58]. The destabilization of the place cell system does not mean the hippocampal function is disrupted. Instead, the apparent disruption is popularly known as *remapping* of what the animal perceives as a new environment [63].

A major caveat for testing endogenous recruitment of a cognitive map in a dark environment is access to olfactory information. Indeed, the studies that robustly controlled for olfactory input showed that olfactory cues are enough to maintain place cell firing in the dark [59, 61]. For example, Save et al. thoroughly cleaned the experimental box to remove any olfactory cues before turning the lights off. Under this tightly controlled setup, place code stability was abolished in most previously identified place cells [64]. This suggests that the hippocampal place representation underwent remapping. The rodents perceived the environment as new without any previously experienced sensory cues. The result of this particular study is striking because when most sensory inputs were removed, including olfactory cues, it became clear that the idiothetic information alone was insufficient for place cell stability [62], suggesting that external and internal information must be in constant coordination for the stability of a cognitive map.

The above studies observed rats in their natural behavior—free foraging—and their hippocampal place cells in light and dark conditions [65–67], shedding light on the mnemonic nature of hippocampal spatial representation. However, they do not address how a mental map is recruited endogenously to drive behavior. A lack of behavioral readout in those studies makes it difficult to link neural phenomenology to the intentional use of a cognitive map.

Following a productive decade of investigating the nature of place cells in freely foraging rodents, new studies employed hypothesis-driven experimental tasks to find the link between the hippocampal circuits and navigation behavior. In one such experiment, researchers systematically displaced the animal's home box immediately after the animal had left it to retrieve food from a fixed target location [68, 69]. They found that the place representation near the box remained anchored to the box even when displaced by different distances on each trial. Far from the box, however, the place representation was anchored to the running track, regardless of the home box location. The animal used internal monitoring of self-motion to keep track of its location to a certain point on its outbound journey from the box to the food. By assessing whether the place representation was anchored to the box at different points along the animal's journey, researchers quantified where, along the journey, the animal's internal monitoring system switched to the external cue-based system for updating self-location. Crucially, when this experiment was repeated in the dark, the switch point was significantly further along the journey, suggesting that the behavioral demand led to a greater reliance on the internal self-localization system [69]. Other experiments analyzed the homing behavior and used lesioning techniques to show that besides the hippocampus, the entorhinal cortex and posterior parietal cortex played a significant role in the internal monitoring of self-location [70–72]—also known as path integration [73]. What was still lacking was a mechanistic account of how neural dynamics in these brain areas could give rise to internal monitoring of self-motion or endogenous navigation over a cognitive map in the absence of sensory input.

About 25 years after the discovery of place cells, the landmark discovery of *grid cells* in rodent medial entorhinal cortex (MEC) steered the field toward a mechanistic understanding of the hippocampal formation and cognitive map-based navigation behavior [74, 75]. Grid cells, like place cells, represent an allocentric spatial code but differently—each grid cell is active at multiple spatial locations; the active locations form an interconnected tessellation of equilateral triangles, giving the connectivity pattern of active sites a hexagonal structure. In the initial studies, the authors characterized the phenomenal grid cells in dark conditions and verified that grid cells were light-invariant, similar to the hippocampal place cells [74–76]. Studies in mice, in contrast, have reported the disruption of entorhinal grid fields while running in darkness [77]. These apparent disparate findings were likely due to a lack of exposure to the dark testing environment, similar to what was repeatedly observed in the early studies of place cells. In their supplementary figures, Chen et al. (2016) reported partial rescue of the gridness structure when mice gained experience running in a dark environment. What could such a precisely patterned spatial grid code in the brain mean for navigation behavior? The modeling work that followed the discovery of grid cells uncovered a crucial insight.

The hexagonal pattern of grid fields emerges in a network of neurons on a planar sheet locally connected with a strong enough inhibitory connection. At steady state, all phases of the network are equally stable, making the network pattern a continuous attractor. When such a network is driven by velocity input, the magnitude and direction of the input are coupled to the translation of the activity pattern on the neural sheet. The network activity is thus continuously updating the current location, essentially performing path integration [78, 79]. Two critical predictions of this model were subsequently verified experimentally—that the entorhinal grid cell system is a continuous attractor network [80–82] and it plays a role in path integration [83–85].

Recent studies have shown that when the internal information (path integration) and external information (visual cue or optic flow) are in conflict, both the entorhinal grid cells and hippocampal place cells show commensurate changes in their spatial representation [84, 86, 87]. These studies quantified and perturbed the latent variables, which are undoubtedly the right approach for robustly linking neurobiology to cognitive processes. However, such approaches must be combined with goal-directed behavior to link latent variables to the deliberate usage of a cognitive map. Two new studies have made significant progress in this direction by training animals to "mentally" navigate a previously learned map of an environment.

In the first study, Lai and colleagues [88] exploited the known place code of the hippocampal CA1 neurons in rodents. They built a brain-machine-interface (BMI) to probe the animals' ability to use their cognitive map volitionally. The authors collected neural recordings from hippocampal CA1 neurons as the animals ran on a treadmill that controlled a virtual reality display. Randomly located navigation goal locations were visually cued to the animal. A nonlinear decoder was trained to learn the spatial code from the recorded hippocampal firing patterns. After building the decoder, the animal's movement on the treadmill was disconnected from the display. The animal had to generate appropriate activity patterns in its CA1 to reach the goal location so the decoder could transform these activities into virtual movement on the display. Remarkably, the animals learned to perform the BMI task by controlling their hippocampal pattern, which controlled the decoder that controlled the animals' "avatar," providing compelling evidence that they used the hippocampal spatial code.

Next, the authors fixed the animals at the center of the arena. They trained them to generate a new pattern of neural activity that could control the movement of an external object to a goal location. They repeated the method to build a decoder to control the object's movement. The animals again successfully exhibited voluntary control of their hippocampal pattern, which caused the decoder to move the object to the goal locations. Since the discovery of hippocampal place cells, this is the first direct demonstration of animals using its place cell pattern to control self- and object movement. Although the BMI task is a powerful demonstration of how hippocampal place cells control navigation behavior, the animal is exposed to continuous sensory feedback in this task. The animal also makes motor movements in most of the trials. Therefore, it is unclear if the animals employ a map-based strategy or calibrate their bearing to the goal location as they approach it. The latter strategy could have been picked up by a sophisticated decoder for the successful completion of the task. Regardless, the hippocampus-dependent cognitive BMI offers a crucial test for volitional access and use of cognitive maps.

In the second study, we addressed the above shortcomings with a different approach. We developed a navigation task paradigm in which monkeys virtually travel between two cued positions on a linear sequence of landmarks [89]. Crucially, sensory feedback was removed during mental navigation—neither optic flow nor interleaving landmarks were visible. The task demand compelled the animals to rely entirely on their memory of the map and mentally keep track of the distance traversed to solve the task accurately. In other words, the animals relied solely on internal information to navigate between cued landmarks. Generalization tests and behavioral modeling further confirmed that the animals used their cognitive map to solve the task. More specifically, we found that the animals' timing variability was captured by a dynamic process punctuated by landmark-induced reset events, except that these landmark events were mnemonic and not perceptual. We then recorded activity from the entorhinal cortex (EC) and found a subregion where neurons exhibited a periodicity that matched the inter-landmark interval. To establish a more robust link between the periodic neural activity and behavior, we tested if the variability in the phase of periodic activity bumps could predict the animals' timing variability across trials. We found that animals consistently undershot if the periodic bumps occurred earlier and vice versa. Together, our newly discovered neural dynamics in primate EC provide compelling evidence for computation over an internal cognitive map to support mental navigation behavior.

The above two studies have opened new avenues for studying the neural mechanisms of cognitive behavior that demand endogenous recruitment of cognitive maps. The first study offers a proof-of-principle for using the BMI framework in the HF to investigate cognitive control mechanisms. The second study provides a promising paradigm for developing tasks, enabling the study of how the perceptual system coordinates with the cognitive system in the brain. The rest of the chapter focuses on the latter.

4. Perceptual-cognitive system interactions: PPC and HF

The importance of coordination between the perceptual and cognitive systems in navigation behavior has been emphasized long before [90]. Spatial navigation is a naturalistic cognitive task that relies on both optic flow input and a cognitive map of the local environment. As we move through the environment, the apparent motion of objects, surfaces, and textures in our visual field generate optical flow patterns and visual cues that teach us about our movement. The pattern of optic flow radiates outward from the direction we are traveling, which enables us to determine our heading direction and traveling speed [91, 92]. However, optic flow alone is insufficient to plan a route to a goal that is not immediately visible. Taking the first step in the correct direction requires a decision based on the goal location and an internal model of the external environment. Such cognitive decisions require computations over the internal model and continuous integration of optic flow visual input to keep track of one's heading and speed to infer one's position and distance traveled. In contrast, two alternative forced-choice visual perceptual tasks require a simple binary readout of, for instance, an optic flow visual stimulus. Therefore, a navigation-based task design, besides being more naturalistic, demands richer computations and coordination of perceptual-cognitive systems.

Besides the hippocampal formation, the posterior parietal cortex has been implicated in its unique contribution to navigation behavior. PPC is an associative brain region located in the dorsal visual pathway of the primate brain. PPC is thought to underlie a range of functions at the intersection of perception, cognition, and action. Within the PPC, primate area 7a is particularly relevant as it is implicated in abstract spatial reasoning and mental simulation [93–95]. More importantly, area 7a is sensitive to navigational signals such as the speed of optic flow stimulus [26, 27, 96, 97] and allocentric spatial code [98–100]. Anatomically, area 7a has monosynaptic connections to HC [101], vestibular nucleus [102], and sensorimotor areas [103], suggesting that this area might be a hub of neural computations that complement the navigational function of HF.

The functional relationship between PPC and HF was first demonstrated by observing the impact of PPC lesions on hippocampal place cells. Place cells are known to represent allocentric spatial code as their activities are anchored to the configuration of spatial cues in the local environment. However, when PPC was lesioned, the rotation of a previously learned set of landmark objects did not rotate the place fields [71, 104], suggesting that PPC is an essential node in the neural circuit for learning mental maps of the environment. Other studies provide further clues as to the function of PPC in coordinate transformation—first to transform egocentric visual and vestibular input to allocentric spatial code and then to transform allocentric mnemonic code into body-centric action sequence plans [28–30]. Area 7a of PPC in monkeys is particularly implicated in coordinate transformation [100]. Finally, PPC neurons showed a first-person route mapping function in monkeys trained to use a joystick to navigate a virtual house [105]. A similar observation about human PPC was made in a neuroimaging study [106].

These studies provide compelling initial evidence that motivates the design of perceptual-cognitive training paradigms for inducing plasticity in PPC and HF. Such task designs can go beyond a binary task and target brain areas outside the canonical visual hierarchy for training-induced plasticity. In the next section, we will describe new training paradigms and outline hypothetical mechanisms of neural plasticity they can potentially induce for vision restoration.

4.1 Perceptual-cognitive training for neurorehabilitation

Our overarching hypothesis is that cognitive task demand can induce plasticity in brain regions that process visual inputs, leading to a long-lasting improvement in visual perception. In a network of dynamical systems, connectivities exist in a given circuit at its input, its output, and within its local interaction. Plasticity can occur in any one of these subspaces. A naturalistic cognitive task that offers continual learning can activate the entire circuit, inducing richer plasticity and resulting in longer-lasting and more general learning. We expand on this hypothesis with three inter-related mechanisms for linking cognitive-perceptual training to neural plasticity for vision recovery: (1) continual tasks to mimic naturalistic behavior, (2) top-down feedback connections to visual areas from upstream regions including PPC and HF, and (3) transfer generalizability of cognitive behavior to perceptual learning.

One way to adopt continual learning in a naturalistic task in vision restoration programs for CVI is to motivate task design by the specific behavioral loss patients experience after visual deficits. Most patients lose their driving license after suffering CVI. A simple cognitive task for vision training, then, is a *steering task*. In this task, a continuous dynamic optic flow pattern that radiates outward from the central focus of expansion (FoE) is presented to the subject. The stimulus gives the perception of moving forward on a straight path, like driving a car. The FoE drifts randomly to either left or right for a random duration. The task is to correct the course by compensating for the drift and keeping a straight heading. Although the behavioral report is still impoverished since it is binary, the behavior is continuous in time, and more importantly, the action is in close-loop with optic flow presentation [107]. The naturalistic task should engage not only the dorsal visual areas for motion perception but also PPC and premotor circuits for continuous action output. By placing the optic flow stimulus inside the blind field, one can test whether the steering task can induce visual plasticity and restoration with higher generalization.

How could continual learning tasks induce more effective recovery? One valuable insight generated from trial-based visual training is that double training confers superior outcomes in vision recovery [10, 41]. Double training entails incorporating two locations or stimulus features in the rehabilitation training protocol. The double-training effect can be boosted with a continuous paradigm where each instant of time in the perception-action loop can act as a trial. By using stimuli that change location or feature, we can utilize the double-training effect at a larger scale.

A task that extends the driving task with a higher cognitive demand task is the *time-to-memorized-landmark* task. By placing an invisible target location in the optic flow field, subjects now have a memory demand besides keeping track of the heading. The invisible target determines the stopping time obtained by accurate path integration over the perceived speed. A similar *time-to-contact* task has previously been studied with neural modulation in area 7a of primate PPC [27, 108–110].

Similarly, another cognitive task that leverages the memory of landmarks is the mental navigation task [89], known to modulate both PPC and HF [111]. To induce perceptual learning, the mental navigation task can be modified by introducing a visible optic flow field that cues the required speed of navigation over memorized landmarks. In this task, the computational demand is twofold: first, spatiotemporal integration of the perceived optic flow stimulus to infer velocity, and second, temporal integration over the inferred velocity for accurate mental navigation. Although these tasks appear computationally demanding, they approximate the natural navigation behavior in which we have continuous access to optic flow stimuli, but no direct visual access to the destination or the map of the environment. We believe such tasks are more conducive to stimulating residual anatomical pathways in neurological damage [112].

What neural mechanism could potentially induce plasticity for vision restoration *via* cognitive training? Several interrelated neural mechanisms have been proposed for perceptual learning. One mechanism of perceptual learning is through the adjustment of readout weights such that behavioral-relevant visual representations are weighted more heavily by the downstream decision circuit [113, 114]. By designing visual stimuli with higher complexity, higher visual areas with less location specificity can be targeted for neural plasticity [10–12]. Complementary to reweighting, perceptual learning in attentional tasks is thought to exert influence *via* feedback projections along the visual hierarchy [8, 15, 115]. We extend this reverse hierarchical framework of visual learning to include the hippocampal formation, given its specialization in perceptual and attentional function [22–25]. Specifically, accurately perceiving the optic flow field will leverage the aforementioned visual plasticity mechanisms in PPC and other visual areas sensitive to motion. The cognitive demand of using the perceived flow information for solving navigation tasks will engage HF and its connection with the visual system. By using navigation-based perceptual-cognitive tasks that are known to modulate HF and PPC, we expand both the task space and the range of neural plasticity they might exert in the visual system.

The tasks mentioned above demand an accurate estimate of elapsed time. A behavioral feature in goal-directed navigation tasks is time estimation [89]. Estimation of time intervals is a task that is, by definition, internally controlled. Therefore, it has been used as a valuable tool to study neural mechanisms of cognitive behavior [116, 117]. One feature of temporal learning is particularly relevant to the generalization of visual perceptual learning. While visual perceptual learning is usually limited to training location but generalizes to visual features, temporal learning generalizes to new spatial locations but remains specific to the trained time interval [118]. Therefore, training on our tasks should confer generalization of temporal learning across space, as shown in Ref. [118]. Exploiting the features of temporal learning thus adds another dimension to overcoming the specificity of vision restoration.

Lastly, our proposed integrated perceptual-cognitive paradigms are not limited to visual function. They can induce plasticity in neural circuits responsible for cognitive functions [86, 119]. As a result, the flavor of navigation paradigms we highlight here can also restore cognitive deficits. The extent to which we can control plasticity for cognitive functions through targeted brain training is an exciting area of research that remains to be explored.

5. Conclusion

We started by highlighting the capacity of the brain to change and pointing out the limitations in the field of vision neurorehabilitation to leverage this capacity for targeted improvement of lost function after brain damage. We identified navigation as one of the most ubiquitous, naturalistic behaviors in which perceptual and cognitive systems continually interact. We described how navigation-based training paradigms could potentially induce long-lasting and generalizable plasticity in neural circuits for vision restoration by exploiting naturalistic task design, feedback connections from navigation circuits to visual areas, and the generalizability of cognitive functions. We reviewed a specific literature of the hippocampal formation in which researchers studied the neurobiology of spatial navigation in the absence of sensory input. Based on this literature and recent new studies, we proposed various perceptual-cognitive experimental paradigms to test the role of cognitive tasks on perceptual learning and its hypothetical neural mechanisms.

Author details

Ashim Pandey[1,2†], Dipesh Shrestha[3,2†] and Sujaya Neupane[2,4*]

1 McGill University, Montreal, Canada

2 Coherent Research Collective, Montreal, Canada

3 Independent Researcher, Kathmandu, Nepal

4 York University, Toronto, Canada

*Address all correspondence to: sujay@yorku.ca

†Equal authorship

References

[1] Zhang X, Kedar S, Lynn MJ, Newman NJ, Biousse V. Natural history of homonymous hemianopia. Neurology. 2006;**66**(6):901-905. DOI: 10.1212/01.wnl.0000203338.54323.22

[2] Zeiler SR, Krakauer JW. The interaction between training and plasticity in the poststroke brain. Current Opinion in Neurology. 2013;**26**(6):609-616. DOI: 10.1097/WCO.0000000000000025

[3] Makin TR, Krakauer JW. Against cortical reorganisation. eLife. 2023;**12**:e84716. DOI: 10.7554/eLife.84716

[4] Sabel BA, Henrich-Noack P, Fedorov A, Gall C. Vision restoration after brain and retina damage: The 'residual vision activation theory'. Progress in Brain Research. 2011;**192**:199-262. DOI: 10.1016/B978-0-444-53355-5.00013-0

[5] Sharma J, Angelucci A, Sur M. Induction of visual orientation modules in auditory cortex. Nature. 2000;**404**(6780):841-847. DOI: 10.1038/35009043

[6] Hauptman M, Liu Y-F, Bedny M. Built to adapt: Mechanisms of cognitive flexibility in the human brain. Annual Review of Developmental Psychology. Dec 2024;**6**(1):133-162. DOI: 10.1146/annurev-devpsych-120621-042108

[7] Wiesel TN, Hubel D. Single-cell responses in striate cortex of kittens deprived of vision in one eye. Journal of Neurophysiology. 1963;**26**:1003-1017. [Online]. Available from: https://www.ncbi.nlm.nih.gov/pubmed/14084161

[8] Ahissar M, Hochstein S. The reverse hierarchy theory of visual perceptual learning. Trends in Cognitive Sciences. 2004;**8**(10):457-464. DOI: 10.1016/j.tics.2004.08.011

[9] Siuda-Krzywicka K et al. Massive cortical reorganization in sighted braille readers. eLife. 2016;**5**:e10762. DOI: 10.7554/eLife.10762

[10] Das A, Tadin D, Huxlin KR. Beyond blindsight: Properties of visual relearning in cortically blind fields. The Journal of Neuroscience. 2014;**34**(35):11652-11664. DOI: 10.1523/JNEUROSCI.1076-14.2014

[11] Awada A, Bakhtiari S, Legault C, Odier C, Pack CC. Training with optic flow stimuli promotes recovery in cortical blindness. Restorative Neurology and Neuroscience. 2022;**40**(1):1-16. DOI: 10.3233/RNN-211223

[12] Pandey A, Neupane S, Adhikary S, Vaidya K, Pack CC. Cortical visual impairment at birth can be improved rapidly by vision training in adulthood: A case study. Restorative Neurology and Neuroscience. 2022;**40**(4-6):261-270. DOI: 10.22541/au.167935463.38022632

[13] Bergsma DP, Elshout JA, van den Berg AV. Segregation of spontaneous and training induced recovery from visual field defects in subacute stroke patients. Frontiers in Neurology. 2017;**8**:681. DOI: 10.3389/fneur.2017.00681

[14] Ajina S, Kennard C, Rees G, Bridge H. Motion area V5/MT+ response to global motion in the absence of V1 resembles early visual cortex. Brain. 2015;**138**(Pt 1):164-178. DOI: 10.1093/brain/awu328

[15] Buffalo EA, Fries P, Landman R, Liang H, Desimone R. A backward progression of attentional effects in

the ventral stream. Proceedings of the National Academy of Sciences of the United States of America. 2010;**107**(1):361-365. DOI: 10.1073/pnas.0907658106

[16] Cisek P. Resynthesizing behavior through phylogenetic refinement. Attention, Perception, & Psychophysics. Oct 2019;**81**(7):2265-2287. DOI: 10.3758/s13414-019-01760-1

[17] Cisek P, Green AM. Toward a neuroscience of natural behavior. Current Opinion in Neurobiology. 2024;**86**(102859):102859. DOI: 10.1016/j.conb.2024.102859

[18] Tolman EC. Cognitive maps in rats and men. Psychological Review. 1948;**55**(4):189-208. DOI: 10.1037/h0061626

[19] O'Keefe J, Nadel L. The Hippocampus as a Cognitive Map. London, England: Oxford University Press; 1978. p. 296

[20] Ekstrom AD, Spiers HJ, Bohbot VD, Rosenbaum RS. Human Spatial Navigation. Princeton, NJ: Princeton University Press; 2018. [Online]. Available from: https://press.princeton.edu/books/hardcover/9780691171746/human-spatial-navigation

[21] Redlick FP, Jenkin M, Harris LR. Humans can use optic flow to estimate distance of travel. Vision Research. 2001;**41**(2):213-219. DOI: 10.1016/s0042-6989(00)00243-1

[22] Murray EA, Wise SP, Graham KS. Representational specializations of the hippocampus in phylogenetic perspective. Neuroscience Letters. 2018;**680**:4-12. DOI: 10.1016/j.neulet.2017.04.065

[23] Killian NJ, Jutras MJ, Buffalo EA. A map of visual space in the primate entorhinal cortex. Nature. 2012;**491**(7426):761-764. DOI: 10.1038/nature11587

[24] Wilming N, König P, König S, Buffalo EA. Entorhinal cortex receptive fields are modulated by spatial attention, even without movement. eLife. 2018;**7**:1-16. DOI: 10.7554/elife.31745

[25] Lee ACH et al. Perceptual deficits in amnesia: Challenging the medial temporal lobe 'mnemonic' view. Neuropsychologia. 2005;**43**(1):1-11. DOI: 10.1016/j.neuropsychologia.2004.07.017

[26] Phinney RE, Siegel RM. Speed selectivity for optic flow in area 7a of the behaving macaque. Cerebral Cortex. 2000;**10**(4):413-421. DOI: 10.1093/cercor/10.4.413

[27] Avila E, Lakshminarasimhan KJ, DeAngelis GC, Angelaki DE. Visual and vestibular selectivity for self-motion in macaque posterior parietal area 7a. Cerebral Cortex. 2019;**29**(9):3932-3947. DOI: 10.1093/cercor/bhy272

[28] Whitlock JR, Pfuhl G, Dagslott N, Moser M-B, Moser EI. Functional split between parietal and entorhinal cortices in the rat. Neuron. 2012;**73**(4):789-802. DOI: 10.1016/j.neuron.2011.12.028

[29] Whitlock JR, Sutherland RJ, Witter MP, Moser MB, Moser EI. Navigating from hippocampus to parietal cortex. Proceedings of the National Academy of Sciences of the United States of America. 2008;**105**(39):14755-14762. DOI: 10.1073/pnas.0804216105

[30] Whitlock JR. Posterior parietal cortex. Current Biology. 2017;**27**(14):R691-R695. DOI: 10.1016/j.cub.2017.06.007

[31] Aggius-Vella E, Chebat D-R, Maidenbaum S, Amedi A. Activation

of human visual area V6 during egocentric navigation with and without visual experience. Current Biology. 2023;**33**(7):1211-1219.e5. DOI: 10.1016/j.cub.2023.02.025

[32] Amedi A, Shelly S, Saporta N, Catalogna M. Perceptual learning and neural correlates of virtual navigation in subjective cognitive decline: A pilot study. iScience. 2024;**27**(12):111411. DOI: 10.1016/j.isci.2024.111411

[33] Merabet LB, Rizzo JF, Amedi A, Somers DC, Pascual-Leone A. What blindness can tell us about seeing again: Merging neuroplasticity and neuroprostheses. Nature Reviews Neuroscience. 2005;**6**(1):71-77, [Online]. Available from: https://scholar.google.com/citations?view_op=view_citation&hl=en&citation_for_view=WADV6B4AAAAJ:zYLM7Y9cAGgC

[34] Bakhtiari S, Awada A, Pack CC. Influence of stimulus complexity on the specificity of visual perceptual learning. Journal of Vision. 2020;**20**(6):13. DOI: 10.1167/jov.20.6.13

[35] Ajina S, Pestilli F, Rokem A, Kennard C, Bridge H. Human blindsight is mediated by an intact geniculo-extrastriate pathway. eLife. 2015;**4**. DOI: 10.7554/eLife.08935

[36] Elshout JA et al. Improvement in activities of daily living after visual training in patients with homonymous visual field defects using goal attainment scaling. Restorative Neurology and Neuroscience. 2018;**36**(1):1-12. DOI: 10.3233/RNN-170719

[37] Weiskrantz L, Warrington EK, Sanders MD, Marshall J. Visual capacity in the hemianopic field following a restricted occipital ablation. Brain. 1974;**97**(4):709-728. DOI: 10.1093/brain/97.1.709

[38] Dosher BA, Jeter P, Liu J, Lu Z-L. An integrated reweighting theory of perceptual learning. Proceedings of the National Academy of Sciences of the United States of America. 2013;**110**(33):13678-13683. DOI: 10.1073/pnas.1312552110

[39] Cavanaugh MR, Huxlin KR. Visual discrimination training improves Humphrey perimetry in chronic cortically induced blindness. Neurology. 2017;**88**(19):1856-1864. DOI: 10.1212/WNL.0000000000003921

[40] Jobke S, Kasten E, Sabel BA. Vision restoration through extrastriate stimulation in patients with visual field defects: A double-blind and randomized experimental study. Neurorehabilitation and Neural Repair. 2009;**23**(3):246-255. DOI: 10.1177/1545968308324221

[41] Xiao L-Q, Zhang J-Y, Wang R, Klein SA, Levi DM, Yu C. Complete transfer of perceptual learning across retinal locations enabled by double training. Current Biology. 2008;**18**(24):1922-1926. DOI: 10.1016/j.cub.2008.10.030

[42] Sahraie A, Trevethan CT, MacLeod MJ, Murray AD, Olson JA, Weiskrantz L. Increased sensitivity after repeated stimulation of residual spatial channels in blindsight. Proceedings of the National Academy of Sciences of the United States of America. 2006;**103**(40):14971-14976. DOI: 10.1073/pnas.0607073103

[43] Sinha P, Poggio T. High-level learning of early visual tasks. In: Perceptual Learning. Cambridge, Massachusetts: The MIT Press; 2002. pp. 273-298. DOI: 10.7551/mitpress/5295.003.0019

[44] Huxlin KR et al. Perceptual relearning of complex visual motion after V1 damage in humans. The Journal

of Neuroscience. 2009;**29**(13):3981-3991. DOI: 10.1523/JNEUROSCI.4882-08.2009

[45] Duffy CJ, Wurtz RH. Sensitivity of MST neurons to optic flow stimuli. I. A continuum of response selectivity to large-field stimuli. Journal of Neurophysiology. 1991;**65**(6):1329-1345. DOI: 10.1152/jn.1991.65.6.1329

[46] Mineault PJ, Khawaja FA, Butts DA, Pack CC. Hierarchical processing of complex motion along the primate dorsal visual pathway. Proceedings of the National Academy of Sciences of the United States of America. 2012;**109**(16):E972-E980. DOI: 10.1073/pnas.1115685109

[47] Duffy CJ, Wurtz RH. Sensitivity of MST neurons to optic flow stimuli. II. Mechanisms of response selectivity revealed by small-field stimuli. Journal of Neurophysiology. 1991;**65**(6):1346-1359. DOI: 10.1152/jn.1991.65.6.1346

[48] Watanabe T, Sasaki Y. Perceptual learning: Toward a comprehensive theory. Annual Review of Psychology. 2015;**66**:197-221. DOI: 10.1146/annurev-psych-010814-015214

[49] O'Keefe J, Dostrovsky J. The hippocampus as a spatial map. Preliminary evidence from unit activity in the freely-moving rat. Brain Research. 1971;**34**(1):171-175, [Online]. Available from: https://www.ncbi.nlm.nih.gov/pubmed/5124915

[50] Taube JS, Muller RU, Ranck JB Jr. Head-direction cells recorded from the postsubiculum in freely moving rats. I. Description and quantitative analysis. The Journal of Neuroscience. 1990;**10**(2):420-435. DOI: 10.1523/jneurosci.10-02-00420.1990

[51] Lever C, Burton S, Jeewajee A, O'Keefe J, Burgess N. Boundary vector cells in the subiculum of the hippocampal formation. The Journal of Neuroscience. 2009;**29**(31):9771-9777. DOI: 10.1523/JNEUROSCI.1319-09.2009

[52] Wood ER, Dudchenko PA, Robitsek RJ, Eichenbaum H. Hippocampal neurons encode information about different types of memory episodes occurring in the same location. Neuron. 2000;**27**(3):623-633. DOI: 10.1016/s0896-6273(00)00071-4

[53] Frank LM, Brown EN, Wilson M. Trajectory encoding in the hippocampus and entorhinal cortex. Neuron. 2000;**27**(1):169-178. DOI: 10.1016/s0896-6273(00)00018-0

[54] O'Keefe J, Krupic J. Do hippocampal pyramidal cells respond to nonspatial stimuli? Physiological Reviews. 2021;**101**(3):1427-1456. DOI: 10.1152/physrev.00014.2020

[55] Duvelle É, Grieves RM, van der Meer MAA. Temporal context and latent state inference in the hippocampal splitter signal. eLife. 2023;**12**. DOI: 10.7554/eLife.82357

[56] O'Keefe J, Conway DH. Hippocampal place units in the freely moving rat: Why they fire where they fire. Experimental Brain Research. 1978;**31**(4):573-590. DOI: 10.1007/BF00239813

[57] O'Keefe J, Speakman A. Single unit activity in the rat hippocampus during a spatial memory task. Experimental Brain Research. 1987;**68**(1):1-27. DOI: 10.1007/BF00255230

[58] O'Keefe J. Place units in the hippocampus of the freely moving rat. Experimental Neurology. 1976;**51**(1):78-109. DOI: 10.1016/0014-4886(76)90055-8

[59] Quirk GJ, Muller RU, Kubie JL. The firing of hippocampal place cells

in the dark depends on the rat's recent experience. The Journal of Neuroscience. 1990;**10**(6):2008-2017, [Online]. Available from: https://www.ncbi.nlm.nih.gov/pubmed/2355262

[60] Hill AJ, Best PJ. Effects of deafness and blindness on the spatial correlates of hippocampal unit activity in the rat. Experimental Neurology. 1981;**74**(1):204-217. DOI: 10.1016/0014-4886(81)90159-x

[61] Save E, Cressant A, Thinus-Blanc C, Poucet B. Spatial firing of hippocampal place cells in blind rats. The Journal of Neuroscience. 1998;**18**(5):1818-1826. DOI: 10.1523/JNEUROSCI.18-05-01818.1998

[62] Poucet B, Save E, Lenck-Santini P. Sensory and memory properties of hippocampal place cells. Reviews in the Neurosciences. 2000;**11**:112-195. DOI: 10.1515/REVNEURO.2000.11.2-3.95

[63] Fenton AA. Remapping revisited: How the hippocampus represents different spaces. Nature Reviews. Neuroscience. Jun 2024;**25**(6):428-448. DOI: 10.1038/s41583-024-00817-x

[64] Save E, Nerad L, Poucet B. Contribution of multiple sensory information to place field stability in hippocampal place cells. Hippocampus. 2000;**10**(1):64-76. DOI: 10.1002/(SICI)1098-1063(2000)10:1<64::AID-HIPO7>3.0.CO;2-Y

[65] Cooper BG, Mizumori SJ. Temporary inactivation of the retrosplenial cortex causes a transient reorganization of spatial coding in the hippocampus. The Journal of Neuroscience. 2001;**21**(11):3986-4001. DOI: 10.1523/jneurosci.21-11-03986.2001

[66] Mizumori SJ, Ragozzino KE, Cooper BG, Leutgeb S. Hippocampal representational organization and spatial context. Hippocampus. 1999;**9**(4):444-451. DOI: 10.1002/(SICI)1098-1063(1999)9:4<444::AID-HIPO10>3.0.CO;2-Z

[67] Markus EJ, Barnes CA, McNaughton BL, Gladden VL, Skaggs WE. Spatial information content and reliability of hippocampal CA1 neurons: Effects of visual input. Hippocampus. 1994;**4**(4):410-421. DOI: 10.1002/hipo.450040404

[68] Gothard KM, Skaggs WE, Moore KM, McNaughton BL. Binding of hippocampal CA1 neural activity to multiple reference frames in a landmark-based navigation task. The Journal of Neuroscience. 1996;**16**(2):823-835. DOI: 10.1523/jneurosci.16-02-00823.1996

[69] Gothard KM, Hoffman KL, Battaglia FP, McNaughton BL. Dentate gyrus and ca1 ensemble activity during spatial reference frame shifts in the presence and absence of visual input. The Journal of Neuroscience. 2001;**21**(18):7284-7292. DOI: 10.1523/jneurosci.21-18-07284.2001

[70] Save E, Guazzelli A, Poucet B. Dissociation of the effects of bilateral lesions of the dorsal hippocampus and parietal cortex on path integration in the rat. Behavioral Neuroscience. 2001;**115**(6):1212-1223. DOI: 10.1037//0735-7044.115.6.1212

[71] Parron C, Save E. Evidence for entorhinal and parietal cortices involvement in path integration in the rat. Experimental Brain Research. 2004;**159**(3):349-359. DOI: 10.1007/s00221-004-1960-8

[72] Miller VM, Best PJ. Spatial correlates of hippocampal unit activity are altered by lesions of the fornix and endorhinal cortex. Brain Research. 1980;**194**(2):311-323. DOI: 10.1016/0006-8993(80)91214-7

[73] Gallistel CR. The Organization of Learning. Cambridge, Massachusetts: The MIT Press; 1990

[74] Hafting T, Fyhn M, Molden S, Moser M-B, Moser EI. Microstructure of a spatial map in the entorhinal cortex. Nature. 2005;**436**(7052):801-806. DOI: 10.1038/nature03721

[75] Fyhn M, Molden S, Witter MP, Moser EI, Moser MB. Spatial representation in the entorhinal cortex. Science. 2004;**305**(5688):1258-1264. DOI: 10.1126/science.1099901

[76] Barry C, Ginzberg LL, O'Keefe J, Burgess N. Grid cell firing patterns signal environmental novelty by expansion. Proceedings of the National Academy of Sciences of the United States of America. 2012;**109**(43):17687-17692. DOI: 10.1073/pnas.1209918109

[77] Chen G, Manson D, Cacucci F, Wills TJ. Absence of visual input results in the disruption of grid cell firing in the mouse. Current Biology. 2016;**26**(17):2335-2342. DOI: 10.1016/j.cub.2016.06.043

[78] Burak Y, Fiete IR. Accurate path integration in continuous attractor network models of grid cells. PLoS Computational Biology. 2009;**5**(2):e1000291. DOI: 10.1371/journal.pcbi.1000291

[79] Fuhs MC, Touretzky DS. A spin glass model of path integration in rat medial entorhinal cortex. Journal of Neuroscience. 2006;**26**(16):4266-4276. DOI: 10.1523/JNEUROSCI.4353-05.2006

[80] Trettel SG, Trimper JB, Hwaun E, Fiete IR, Colgin LL. Grid cell co-activity patterns during sleep reflect spatial overlap of grid fields during active behaviors. Nature Neuroscience. 2019;**22**(4):609-617. DOI: 10.1038/s41593-019-0359-6

[81] Gardner RJ, Lu L, Wernle T, Moser M-B, Moser EI. Correlation structure of grid cells is preserved during sleep. Nature Neuroscience. 2019;**22**(4):598-608. DOI: 10.1038/s41593-019-0360-0

[82] Gardner RJ et al. Toroidal topology of population activity in grid cells. Nature. 2022;**602**:123-128. DOI: 10.1038/s41586-021-04268-7

[83] Jacob PY, Capitano F, Poucet B, Save E, Sargolini F. Path integration maintains spatial periodicity of grid cell firing in a 1D circular track. Nature Communications. 2019;**10**(1):1-13. DOI: 10.1038/s41467-019-08795-w

[84] Campbell MG, Ocko SA, Mallory CS, Low IIC, Ganguli S, Giocomo LM. Principles governing the integration of landmark and self-motion cues in entorhinal cortical codes for navigation. Nature Neuroscience. 2018;**21**(8):1096-1106. DOI: 10.1038/s41593-018-0189-y

[85] Campbell MG, Attinger A, Ocko SA, Ganguli S, Giocomo LM. Distance-tuned neurons drive specialized path integration calculations in medial entorhinal cortex. Cell Reports. 2021;**36**(10):109669. DOI: 10.1016/j.celrep.2021.109669

[86] Jayakumar RP, Madhav MS, Savelli F, Blair HT, Cowan NJ, Knierim JJ. Recalibration of path integration in hippocampal place cells. Nature. 2019;**566**(7745):533-537. DOI: 10.1038/s41586-019-0939-3

[87] Madhav MS et al. Control and recalibration of path integration in place cells using optic flow. Nature Neuroscience. 2024;**27**(8):1599-1608. DOI: 10.1038/s41593-024-01681-9

[88] Lai C, Tanaka S, Harris TD, Lee AK. Volitional activation of remote place

representations with a hippocampal brain-machine interface. Science. 2023;**382**(6670):566-573. DOI: 10.1126/science.adh5206

[89] Neupane S, Fiete I, Jazayeri M. Mental navigation in the primate entorhinal cortex. Nature. 2024;**630**(8017):704-711. DOI: 10.1038/s41586-024-07557-z

[90] Strelow ER. What is needed for a theory of mobility: Direct perceptions and cognitive maps—Lessons from the blind. Psychological Review. 1985;**92**(2):226-248. DOI: 10.1037/0033-295x.92.2.226

[91] Gibson JJ. The Perception of the Visual World, Xii. Vol. 242. Boston, MA: Houghton Mifflin; 1950, [Online]. Available from: https://psycnet.apa.org/record/1951-04286-000

[92] Warren WH Jr, Kay BA, Zosh WD, Duchon AP, Sahuc S. Optic flow is used to control human walking. Nature Neuroscience. 2001;**4**(2):213-216. DOI: 10.1038/84054

[93] Crowe DA, Averbeck BB, Chafee MV, Georgopoulos AP. Dynamics of parietal neural activity during spatial cognitive processing. Neuron. 2005;**47**(6):885-891. DOI: 10.1016/j.neuron.2005.08.005

[94] Crowe DA, Averbeck BB, Chafee MV, Anderson JH, Georgopoulos AP. Mental maze solving. Journal of Cognitive Neuroscience. 2000;**12**(5):813-827. DOI: 10.1162/089892900562426

[95] Crowe DA, Chafee MV, Averbeck BB, Georgopoulos AP. Neural activity in primate parietal area 7a related to spatial analysis of visual mazes. Cerebral Cortex. 2004;**14**(1):23-34. DOI: 10.1093/cercor/bhg088

[96] Siegel RM, Read HL. Analysis of optic flow in the monkey parietal area 7a. Cerebral Cortex. 1997;**7**(4):327-346. DOI: 10.1093/cercor/7.4.327

[97] Read HL, Siegel RM. Modulation of responses to optic flow in area 7a by retinotopic and oculomotor cues in monkey. Cerebral Cortex. 1997;**7**(7):647-661. DOI: 10.1093/cercor/7.7.647

[98] Andersen RA, Mountcastle VB. The influence of the angle of gaze upon the excitability of the light-sensitive neurons of the posterior parietal cortex. The Journal of Neuroscience. 1983;**3**(3):532-548, [Online]. Available from: https://www.ncbi.nlm.nih.gov/pubmed/6827308

[99] Andersen RA, Essick GK, Siegel RM. Encoding of spatial location by posterior parietal neurons. Science. 1985;**230**(4724):456-458. DOI: 10.1126/science.4048942

[100] Zipser D, Andersen RA. A back-propagation programmed network that simulates response properties of a subset of posterior parietal neurons. Nature. 1988;**331**(6158):679-684. DOI: 10.1038/331679a0

[101] Rockland KS, Van Hoesen GW. Some temporal and parietal cortical connections converge in CA1 of the primate hippocampus. Cerebral Cortex. 1999;**9**(3):232-237. DOI: 10.1093/cercor/9.3.232

[102] Faugier-Grimaud S, Ventre J. Anatomic connections of inferior parietal cortex (area 7) with subcortical structures related to vestibulo-ocular function in a monkey (*Macaca fascicularis*). The Journal of Comparative Neurology. 1989;**280**(1):1-14. DOI: 10.1002/cne.902800102

[103] Rozzi S et al. Cortical connections of the inferior parietal cortical convexity of the macaque monkey. Cerebral Cortex. 2006;**16**(10):1389-1417. DOI: 10.1093/cercor/bhj076

[104] Save E, Poucet B. Role of the parietal cortex in long-term representation of spatial information in the rat. Neurobiology of Learning and Memory. 2009;**91**(2):172-178. DOI: 10.1016/j.nlm.2008.08.005

[105] Sato N, Sakata H, Tanaka YL, Taira M. Navigation-associated medial parietal neurons in monkeys. Proceedings of the National Academy of Sciences of the United States of America. 2006;**103**(45):17001-17006. DOI: 10.1073/pnas.0604277103

[106] Maguire EA, Burgess N, Donnett JG, Frackowiak RS, Frith CD, O'Keefe J. Knowing where and getting there: A human navigation network. Science. 1998;**280**(5365):921-924. DOI: 10.1126/science.280.5365.921

[107] Bonnen K, Burge J, Yates J, Pillow J, Cormack LK. Continuous psychophysics: Target-tracking to measure visual sensitivity. Journal of Vision. Mar 2015;**15**(3):14. DOI: 10.1167/15.3.14

[108] Lakshminarasimhan KJ, Petsalis M, Park H, DeAngelis GC, Pitkow X, Angelaki DE. A dynamic Bayesian observer model reveals origins of bias in visual path integration. Neuron. 2018;**99**(1):194-206.e5. DOI: 10.1016/j.neuron.2018.05.040

[109] Lakshminarasimhan KJ, Avila E, Neyhart E, DeAngelis GC, Pitkow X, Angelaki DE. Tracking the Mind's eye: Primate gaze behavior during virtual Visuomotor navigation reflects belief dynamics. Neuron. 2020;**106**(4):662-674.e5. DOI: 10.1016/j.neuron.2020.02.023

[110] Chang C-J, Jazayeri M. Integration of speed and time for estimating time to contact. Proceedings of the National Academy of Sciences. 2018;**115**:E2879-E2887. DOI: 10.1073/pnas.1713316115

[111] Neupane S, Fiete I, Jazayeri M. Generalizable relational inference with cognitive maps in a hippocampal model and primates. In: Presented at the Society for Neuroscience. Washington DC: Society for Neuroscience; 2023. [Online]. Available from: https://www.abstractsonline.com/pp8/#!/10892/presentation/20196

[112] Lu Z-L, Lin Z, Dosher BA. Translating perceptual learning from the laboratory to applications. Trends in Cognitive Sciences. 2016;**20**(8):561-563. DOI: 10.1016/j.tics.2016.05.007

[113] Lu ZL, Dosher BA. External noise distinguishes attention mechanisms. Vision Research. 1998;**38**(9):1183-1198. DOI: 10.1016/s0042-6989(97)00273-3

[114] Dosher BA, Lu ZL. Mechanisms of perceptual learning. Vision Research. 1999;**39**(19):3197-3221. DOI: 10.1016/s0042-6989(99)00059-0

[115] Ahissar M, Hochstein S. Task difficulty and the specificity of perceptual learning. Nature. 1997;**387**(6631):401-406. DOI: 10.1038/387401a0

[116] Finnerty GT, Shadlen MN, Jazayeri M, Nobre AC, Buonomano DV. Time in cortical circuits. The Journal of Neuroscience. 2015;**35**(41):13912-13916. DOI: 10.1523/JNEUROSCI.2654-15.2015

[117] Sohn H, Narain D, Meirhaeghe N, Jazayeri M. Bayesian computation through cortical latent dynamics. Neuron. 2019;**103**(5):934-947.e5. DOI: 10.1016/j.neuron.2019.06.012

[118] Bueti D, Buonomano DV. Temporal perceptual learning. Timing and Time Perception. 2014;**2**(3):261-289. DOI: 10.1163/22134468-00002023

[119] Shrager Y, Kirwan CB, Squire LR. Neural basis of the cognitive map: Path integration does not require hippocampus or entorhinal cortex. Proceedings of the National Academy of Sciences. 2008;**105**(33):12034-12038. DOI: 10.1073/pnas.0805414105

Chapter 2

Perspective Chapter: Should the Hippocampus be Considered a Key Part of the Reading Network?

Frédéric Bernard

Abstract

Traditionally associated with memory functions, the hippocampus is now increasingly recognized for its role in language, particularly in reading. This review chapter presents numerous brain imaging and cognitive studies on reading, including studies on healthy participants, people with dyslexia, and neuropsychological patients. These studies demonstrate the necessity of the hippocampus for various aspects of reading, from word decoding to text comprehension. The chapter also explores findings that show how reading practice may contribute to hippocampal development and protection. Given these insights into the deep connections between the hippocampus and reading, it is time to question and potentially redefine the traditional boundaries of the reading network.

Keywords: hippocampus, language, memory, reading, neuropsychology, brain imaging

1. Introduction

The hippocampus is a complex brain structure that remains fascinating even though the frontal cortex partly stole the spotlight from it starting in the 1990s [1]. Its discovery by the Italian anatomist and surgeon Julius Caesar Arantius dates back to the sixteenth century [2]. It was not until the mid-twentieth century that a direct link was established between the hippocampus and memory, particularly through the observation of the effects of bi-hippocampal resection in patient H.M. to treat highly debilitating epileptic seizures [3]. This role was subsequently confirmed in other patients with hippocampal lesions, making this region a key component of the network that underlies declarative memory [4], or even solely episodic memory according to some researchers like Tulving [5].

More recently, since the 1990s, an increasing amount of data has led researchers and clinicians to consider that the hippocampus could also play an important role in language. Thus, for example, a reexamination of data obtained from H.M. suggests that, in addition to memory disorders, he had difficulties understanding language [6, 7]. These language difficulties could also be observed in patients with temporal lobe epilepsy [8, 9]. More recently, Piai et al. have shown, through the recording of electrical activity in the hippocampus, that this structure was involved in language processing [10], leading Covington and Duff to propose extending the 'classic' language network to include the hippocampus [11].

In the rest of this chapter, we will present several results suggesting that the hippocampus may also play a significant role in an even more specific activity, reading. This observation raises the question of whether it would be relevant to include the hippocampus in the reading network, which primarily encompasses the ventral occipito-temporal cortex and the lateral fronto-temporal cortex [12].

In light of the simple model of reading [13], we will first explore the potential role of the hippocampus in the identification of individual words, what is called decoding, before examining the stage of understanding sentences and texts.

2. Decoding or the identification of individual words

2.1 In healthy individuals

Before learning to read and being able to correctly identify written words, children spend their first years expanding their vocabulary by learning thousands of new words that they hear. Each of these words corresponds to an arbitrary association between a combination of elementary sounds called phonemes and at least one meaning. In a functional MRI study, Breitenstein et al. showed that healthy adults who activated the hippocampus the most during exposure to new words were also the most successful in expanding their vocabulary [14]. This finding suggests that the hippocampus is involved in the successful learning of new words that are heard. In another fMRI study, Davis et al. highlighted a significant activation of the left hippocampus in healthy adults when they were hearing entirely unfamiliar novel words compared to consolidated and unconsolidated novel words already heard [15]. Moreover, the magnitude of this activation was positively correlated with the post-scan recognition level of these entirely unfamiliar novel words. These results demonstrate that the hippocampus contributes to the initial acquisition of novel spoken words.

When children learn to read from an alphabetic writing system, they first learn to associate each letter with the corresponding sound or phoneme. This process, called grapheme-phoneme conversion, is part of an indirect or graphophonological pathway and requires the co-activation of the visual word form area (VWFA) located in the occipito-temporal cortex, which processes groups of letters, and a temporo-parietal region, which processes the corresponding sounds. These two regions are connected via the posterior segment of the arcuate fasciculus, which significantly develops during the learning of reading as highlighted by diffusion tensor imaging (DTI) [16]. The graphophonological pathway is particularly useful for reading regular words and pseudowords. Using an artificial orthography in an fMRI study, Quinn et al. showed an increase in hippocampal activity between two consecutive days of training to read words using the grapheme-phoneme conversion process with new artificial and arbitrary association rules [17]. The results of an MEG study, in which Finnish adult participants were trained to associate novel foreign letters with Finnish speech sounds, also suggest that the hippocampal region plays a role in this kind of associative learning enabling grapheme-phoneme conversion [18].

He et al. studied 416 healthy Chinese adults and found that a component called 'form-sound association' was positively associated with gray matter volume in the bilateral hippocampi [19]. This association was measured using a Visual-Auditory Learning test, which involves forming associations between non-language visual stimuli and oral responses, and a Chinese Vocabulary test, which involves reading 40 very low-frequency Chinese characters. This result confirms the role of the hippocampi in the ability to make connections between a new morpheme visually presented and its sound, which mainly relies on the graphophonological pathway.

Another complementary pathway, the direct or orthographical pathway, is increasingly used as children progress in their reading skills. This pathway starts at the VWFA, which processes groups of letters, and leads directly to the lateral temporal cortex, involved in accessing the semantic information associated with a recognized word from its orthographic form. This pathway is particularly useful for reading irregular words and developing spelling ability.

In an fMRI study [20], Abutalebi et al. compared brain activity in 12 healthy participants while they read dialect words for the first time (from a native language in which participants were illiterate) versus German words (from a second language in which participants were literate). This led to the activation of a network that included the left hippocampus. According to the authors, these findings reflect the contribution of the hippocampus in the development of a new orthographic lexicon by creating associations between meanings and orthographic word forms.

In an fMRI study exploring the effects of a 5-week morpheme-based spelling intervention on children with poor spelling and reading abilities, Gebauer et al. highlighted an increase in spelling and reading comprehension, associated with increased activation in the left temporal, parahippocampal, and hippocampal regions during a lexical decision task [21]. This result reflects the role of these regions in the recollection of a newly learned morpheme-based strategy. It aligns with the findings of Krafnick et al., who observed an increase in gray matter volume in the hippocampus of dyslexic children after an 8-week reading intervention [22].

Sterpenich et al. explored the effects of sleep deprivation on the learning and consolidation of visually processed non-words [23]. Compared to a group of participants who had a sleepless night immediately after learning the non-words, another group who had a full night's sleep afterward recognized significantly more non-words, with this better recognition being associated with stronger hippocampal activation. These results confirm the role of the hippocampus in the learning of new lexical representations through the mobilization of the two complementary reading pathways, the graphophonological pathway and the orthographic pathway, and demonstrate the detrimental effects of sleep deprivation on these processes.

In an fMRI study, Tao et al. examined the brain changes associated with orthographic word-form learning in healthy adults [24]. The hippocampus showed a significant increase in activity during learning. Moreover, the level of activity in this region was associated with better post-scan recall scores.

Overall, these results suggest that the hippocampus is involved in the learning and consolidation of new words, non-words, or pseudowords that are read.

2.2 In developmental dyslexia

Paz-Alonso et al. studied the effects of dyslexia on brain activations associated with the reading of single words, pseudowords, and pseudohomophones [25]. They observed that lower accuracy in reading pseudohomophones among individuals with dyslexia was associated with reduced activation in the left angular gyrus and hippocampus. This finding reflects the role these regions play in semantic processing during reading. Moreover, during word reading, although there were no accuracy differences between dyslexic participants and controls, dyslexic participants exhibited stronger functional connectivity between the left hippocampus and the *pars opercularis* of the left inferior frontal gyrus. This may indicate a greater need in dyslexic individuals to integrate and maintain the memory representations required for online reading, facilitated by the hippocampus, in interaction with regions involved in accessing representations for word reading, such as the *pars opercularis*.

2.3 In patients with temporal lobe epilepsy

Lah et al. conducted a systematic review to examine reading in children with temporal lobe epilepsy [26]. The results show that, overall, patients with temporal lobe epilepsy have lower levels of reading accuracy for regular words, irregular words, and non-words compared to normal controls. Although these results support the view that the hippocampus plays a crucial role in decoding, they do not provide details regarding the specific processes associated with decoding that are impaired.

2.4 In patient H.M

MacKay and James found that patient H.M. suffered from deficits in reading low-frequency words and pseudowords aloud [27]. This result has been interpreted as reflecting the crucial role of the hippocampus in creating new connections between nodes or representational units located at the semantic, phonological, or orthographic levels.

2.5 In patients with Alzheimer's disease

Ota et al. evaluated language abilities in 22 patients with Alzheimer's disease [28]. They found significant negative correlations between a score for reading aloud Kanji words and small-world properties (reflecting structural brain networks) in several brain regions, including the bilateral hippocampi. This means that as the reading score decreases, the functions of the highlighted regions become segregated from their surroundings. The authors interpreted this result as reflecting the crucial role of the hippocampi in semantic processes during the reading of Kanji words.

3. Comprehension

3.1 A cognitive model of comprehension

According to one of the most influential models in the cognitive sciences of reading, the Construction-Integration model [29, 30], two forms of representations are activated during reading and text comprehension: (1) the text base and (2) the situation model. The text base includes surface elements (each individual word consisting of an association between a combination of letters and one or several meanings, and the way these words are ordered according to specific syntax) and semantic propositions (associations between a predicate, most often a verb, and one or several arguments, typically nouns). The text base primarily relies on the information contained within the text itself, whereas the situation model involves integrating this information with the reader's memories and knowledge. Therefore, the situation model is likely to differ between readers, while the text base remains relatively consistent across readers. These two forms of representations are activated during the reading of a text, ultimately leading to the construction of a global representation known as the episodic text memory. The representations described here will be referenced in some of the articles presented below.

3.2 At the sentence level

3.2.1 In healthy individuals

In an fMRI study, Cooke et al. measured brain activity while students were reading sentences differing in their grammatical structure [31]. They observed activation of the left hippocampus when contrasting object-relative long antecedent-gap sentences with a pseudofont baseline, and when contrasting object-relative long antecedent-gap sentences with subject-relative long antecedent-gap sentences. At the time, the authors had no precise explanation for this new result. It may have reflected the possible role of this region in single-word processing during lexical encoding and in lexical meaningfulness. However, it seemed unlikely to the authors at the time that this region had a linguistically specific role.

In a Positron Emission Tomography (PET) study, Waters et al. explored the brain regions involved in syntactic processing during the comprehension of written sentences [32]. Participants were divided into two groups based on their sentence processing speed. When contrasting syntactically complex subject-object sentences with syntactically simple object-subject sentences, the authors found that only participants with low processing speed activated several regions, including the right hippocampus. According to the authors, this result was not easily explicable and may reflect the use of visual imagery.

Hoenig and Scheef studied the role of the medial temporal lobe in semantic processing [33]. Twenty-two participants performed a context verification task, making decisions about the semantic fit of congruent and incongruent target words with the overall meaning of preceding sentence contexts. Half of the sentences ended with an ambiguous (homographic) word. The study followed a 2 × 2 factorial design with four experimental conditions: CH (congruent homographic), CN (congruent neutral), IH (incongruent homographic), and IN (incongruent neutral). All these conditions, requiring semantic context verification, resulted in significant activation of a network including the bilateral hippocampi. This region may 'contribute to semantic processing by a mnemonic function that serves to link the target meaning representation with the meaning of a prior sentence context'. A conjunction analysis of the contrasts IH minus IN and CH minus CN yielded significant activation in several left hemisphere regions, including the parahippocampal gyrus. This region may then play a role in the processing of semantic ambiguity.

Using an artificial language, Opitz and Friederici explored the brain regions involved in detecting long-distance and local syntactic violations [34]. Twenty-three participants, previously trained in the new grammar system named BROCANTO, read sentences that were either grammatical or ungrammatical. The authors found that the hippocampus was significantly activated in response to violations of local syntactic dependencies. This result is interpreted as reflecting that a local syntactic violation 'introduces a new relationship between a particular word and its new syntactic role in a sentence', which may require 'increased relational processing demands' mediated by the hippocampus.

Lee and Newman studied the effects of two different sentence presentation paradigms—rapid serial visual presentation (RSVP) and whole sentence presentation—on syntactic processing [35]. Twenty participants read single sentences presented either as a whole on a screen or one word at a time in the middle of the same screen. After reading each sentence, a probe was presented to evaluate comprehension. Comprehension accuracy was significantly higher for sentences presented as a whole. Several regions, including the bilateral hippocampi, were significantly more activated during the reading of sentences presented as a whole compared to those read in RSVP. This result may reflect the role of the hippocampi in a relational binding process, integrating items into a cohesive memory representation, which may be limited during RSVP.

Prat and Just investigated the relationships between interindividual differences in working memory capacity and brain activity during a sentence comprehension task with varying syntactic complexity [36]. They found a positive correlation between working memory capacity and the activation level in several brain regions, including the left hippocampus, when comparing complex sentences to simple ones. In simple terms, participants with higher working memory capacity activated several brain regions more intensely while reading syntactically complex sentences, with the hippocampus specifically associated with memory function in this context.

Citron and Goldberg measured brain activity in 26 participants while they were reading metaphorical sentences [37]. By comparison to literal sentences, metaphorical sentences were associated with the activation of a brain network that included the left hippocampus. Along with the amygdala, which was also activated, the hippocampus may contribute to the memory encoding and/or retrieval of emotional information that occurs while reading metaphorical sentences.

Bonhage et al. explored the brain signature of working memory for sentence structure [38]. Among several contrasts, they compared brain activity measured while 18 participants were reading and encoding sentence fragments to brain activity measured during a baseline condition involving the reading and encoding of ungrammatical word strings. They found that a network of brain regions, including the bilateral hippocampi, was significantly activated. This result may reflect the role of the hippocampi in enriching the information in sentences with semantic information stored in long-term memory. The authors refer to the work of MacKay et al., showing that patient H.M. 'was unable to recognize ambiguities in sentences', a result 'interpreted as reflecting a specific deficit regarding semantic-level binding' [6]. Another complementary explanation is based on results showing an involvement of the hippocampus in syntax processing [39], specifically in detecting syntactic violations after predictive processing, which cannot apply when reading ungrammatical word strings.

A year later, Bonhage et al. used a combination of eye-tracking and fMRI techniques to identify brain regions involved in linguistic predictions via anticipatory eye movements [40]. The correct prediction of the syntactic word category (verb/noun) of a target that would appear after reading a regular sentence or a meaningless jabberwocky sentence was associated with significant activation of several brain regions, including the bilateral hippocampi. This result may reflect the role of the hippocampus in predictive processing at a syntactic level. The finding that the bilateral hippocampi were also significantly more activated for regular sentences than for jabberwocky sentences underscores the role of this region in predictive processing at a lexical-semantic level. These results are considered in light of the predictive coding model [41], which may apply to linguistics. As stated by Ryan and Shen, the use of eye-tracking is highly relevant for studying memory because the oculomotor system is well connected to the hippocampal memory system [42]. By extension, eye-tracking is particularly valuable for studying the role of the hippocampus in reading, as this cognitive ability relies on the complex exploration of sentences and texts through numerous saccades and fixations. These eye movements contribute to the emergence of meaning, in connection with the hippocampus.

In another study combining eye-tracking and fMRI techniques, Schuster et al. explored the effects of word length, frequency, and predictability on brain activity while 56 healthy participants read sentences [43]. Sentence reading was associated with the activation of a large network of brain regions including the hippocampus. There was also a significant negative correlation between the frequency of the words in the sentences and activation in several regions, including the left hippocampus. In simple terms, activity in this region decreased as word frequency increased. However, the authors did not specifically interpret this correlation with the left hippocampus, only considering its well-known role in memory encoding and retrieval. Notably, the predictive coding model [44] was proposed to interpret a negative correlation obtained in the left occipito-temporal cortex, which encompasses the VWFA. Considering the previous study described above, this model could also apply to the left hippocampus.

Pu et al. used a combination of magnetoencephalography (MEG) and eye-tracking techniques to investigate the specific roles of hippocampal theta oscillations in language processing [45]. They found increased theta power in the hippocampus when healthy participants read sentences ending with a semantically incorrect word, which was not the case when sentences ended with a syntactically incorrect word. These results highlight the critical role of the hippocampus in semantic processing during reading. More precisely, the hippocampus could be involved in 'semantic retrieval and prediction based on previous knowledge' (see above) and in an integration process, given that a semantic violation of the last word increases the difficulty of integrating the meaning of the upcoming words into the meaning built up during reading.

In a study combining eye-tracking and fMRI techniques, Schuster et al. investigated the brain regions involved in predictive processing during reading [46]. They presented 39 healthy participants with sentences that ended with a target word that was either congruent or incongruent with the preceding context and had either high- or low-cloze probability. The right hippocampal region was significantly more activated for low-cloze compared to high-cloze sentences in congruent sentence endings. This result was interpreted as reflecting the contribution of this region to language processing and the assembly of semantic meaning by relating incoming words to stored semantic information.

3.2.2 In patients with epilepsy

McCarthy et al. evaluated 64 patients with complex partial epilepsy for resective surgery to relieve intractable seizures [47]. Intracranial electrodes were implanted to localize the seizure foci. Recordings were obtained from these electrodes while the patients were reading sentences. Half of the sentences presented to the patients ended normally, while the other half ended with a semantically anomalous word. The authors found that 'anomalous sentence endings often, but not always, elicited a large negative field potential in the hippocampus'. These results are coherent with those obtained in healthy subjects and described above. They confirm the role of the hippocampus in semantic processing whether it is involved in semantic retrieval, prediction, or integration.

Noppeney et al. explored the compensatory mechanisms associated with good reading skills in patients after left anterior temporal lobe resection for mesial temporal lobe epilepsy [48]. Brain activity was measured using fMRI while 16 patients read nine-word sentences. Reading ability was significantly and positively correlated with activation levels in several regions, including the right hippocampus. Furthermore, in controls and in patients with a reading ability within the normal range, activations were found in the right hippocampus and inferior temporal cortex. The authors interpret this result as indicating that patients with high reading skills might engage more in encoding sentences using the right hippocampus. Additionally, this result suggests that patients without a functional left anterior hippocampus rely on the right hippocampus to maintain proficient reading skills.

3.2.3 In patient H.M.

In a series of four experiments, MacKay and James evaluated patient H.M.'s sentence reading abilities using novel sentences composed of high-frequency words [49]. In all these experiments, patient H.M. produced more misreadings than controls. These misreadings were associated with reduced semantic and syntactic complexity, leading to ungrammaticality. These results were interpreted in light of Node Structure Theory [50] and may reflect the crucial role of the hippocampus in binding or creating new connections between nodes.

3.3 At the text level

3.3.1 Functional brain imaging data obtained in healthy participants

To our knowledge, the first study to observe hippocampal activation during text reading was published in 2005 by Xu et al. [51]. In this fMRI study, 22 right-handed healthy participants with an average age of 34 years were instructed to read Aesop's fables in 46-second blocks. Brain activity measured during this main task was compared to activity measured while the same participants read random consonant letter strings. Among other regions, the left hippocampus was significantly activated during the main task compared to the baseline task. The authors interpreted this result by suggesting that the hippocampus might play a role in either memory encoding or retrieval, which implicitly refers to episodic memory, or in the implicit activation of semantic associations as the story unfolds.

In another fMRI study, Ferstl and von Cramon explored the neural substrates of the temporal, spatial, and emotional dimensions of situation models constructed by 20 healthy subjects while reading short narrative texts comprising two sentences [52]. The comparison of brain activity associated with processing the 'spatial' dimension of the situation model with brain activity associated with processing the 'emotional/temporal' dimensions highlighted the activation of the precuneus/posterior cingulate cortex and the hippocampal region. The activation of this latter region has been interpreted as reflecting its involvement in memory and navigation processes concerning spatial information contained in a situation model.

The same interpretation was proposed by Mano et al. to explain why the hippocampal region was activated in 18 healthy adults while they were reading a narrative text that required processing the emotions of protagonists [53]. This again suggests that this region is involved in the processing of spatial information during narrative comprehension.

In an fMRI study aimed at exploring the neural substrates of analogical reasoning during metaphor comprehension, Prat et al. asked 24 healthy right-handed participants with varying levels of working memory to read three-sentence passages with different processing demands [54]. Unlike several cortical regions, which were activated based on the processing demands of the task, the hippocampus was activated in a similar manner regardless of these demands. This suggests that the hippocampus is recruited as soon as reading and metaphor comprehension are involved, regardless of task difficulty. Furthermore, there was a positive correlation between the participants' working memory capacity and the level of activation in the hippocampus as a function of the supportive context provided. This indicates that participants with higher working memory capacity activate the hippocampus more when the supportive context can be particularly exploited, suggesting a role for the hippocampus in the flexible use of 'working semantic memory' during metaphor comprehension.

Aboud et al. found, in adolescents aged between 9 and 14 years, a positive correlation between activation levels of the left hippocampus (among a larger network) during the reading of documentary texts and the comprehension scores measured thereafter [55]. This result was interpreted as indicating that the best readers, in terms of reading comprehension, have better inferential processing capabilities supported by those regions associated with the default mode network, of which the hippocampus is a part.

Helder et al. showed that in a group of healthy adult participants, the detection of incoherency when reading the sixth and last sentence of a text was accompanied by the activation of a network that includes the hippocampus [56]. The authors suggest that the hippocampal activation could reflect the 'reactivation of episodic memory traces of the text or reactivation of background knowledge' in an attempt to restore coherency, as well as the episodic encoding of this particular situation.

In an fMRI study exploring the brain regions involved in coherence monitoring during the reading of documentary texts, Van Moort et al., asked 31 healthy participants to read 10-sentence-long texts about well-known historical topics [57]. These texts included a target sentence that was either true or false based on the readers' background knowledge. Comparing brain activity measured during the reading of a true target sentence versus a false target sentence highlighted significant activation in several regions, including the left hippocampus. This sensitivity of the left hippocampus to the 'correctness' of information with respect to background knowledge, while a dorso-medial prefrontal region was significantly more sensitive to the 'incorrectness' of information, suggests that a network involving these two regions is engaged in knowledge-based processing. The dorso-medial prefrontal region would 'detect erroneous world-knowledge information and signal to the hippocampus that existing knowledge structure should not be updated', while the hippocampus would be involved in the 'normal' integration processes between what is read and background knowledge.

In a study using eye-tracking, electroencephalography (EEG), and fMRI, Sato et al. explored the mnemonic neural dynamics associated with the natural reading of literature [58]. One of the experiments involved 19 participants reading two essays at a natural pace inside an MRI scanner for 10 minutes. The fMRI results showed negative correlations between brain activity in several regions, including the left hippocampal region, and text correlation scores that reflect the relationship between the content of the read texts and the content reports subsequently written by the participants. This indicates a negative subsequent memory effect for the left hippocampal region, which is unusual since this region is more often associated with a positive subsequent memory effect. The authors suggest that this result may be explained by the long duration of the reading task (10 minutes) and cite a study in which the hippocampus was activated only at the end of an event, while the average activity in this region decreased during the event.

Interestingly, Saito et al. found similar paradoxical results in their study [59]. They compared brain activity between a group of 23 rapid readers and a group of 23 non-rapid readers while reading novels during 60-second blocks (compared to a low-level cross-fixation baseline task). Both reading speed and comprehension scores were higher in rapid readers than in non-rapid readers. During reading, brain activity was significantly lower in rapid readers than in non-rapid readers in several regions, including the hippocampus. Additionally, there was a significant negative correlation between reading speed and activity in these same regions. The authors interpret these results as reflecting the ability of rapid readers to reduce language processes, such as phonological, semantic, and syntactic processes, while maintaining reading comprehension during rapid reading.

In a recent fMRI study aiming to identify the brain regions associated with the level of comprehension of documentary texts, Keller et al. asked 31 healthy participants, with either high or low comprehension skills, to read 65-sentence-long texts three times each [60]. The participants then completed a comprehension test based on multiple-choice questions. Several positive correlations were found between comprehension scores and activity measured during the reading of the texts in various brain regions, including the bilateral hippocampi. This result was interpreted as reflecting the role of the hippocampi in the episodic encoding and consolidation of new declarative knowledge. More precisely, during the reading of texts, this region may enable the encoding and integration of new semantic information from the texts with pre-existing semantic knowledge to construct new knowledge structures.

3.3.2 Brain imaging data obtained in patients

In an fMRI study [61], Malfait et al. investigated the brain regions activated while 19 children (mean age of around 11 years) with benign epilepsy with centro-central spikes (BECTS) read pairs of syntactically complex sentences. They were asked to decide whether the second sentence of each pair was true or false with respect to the first sentence. Performance on this task was comparable between children with BECTS and a control group. During this reading task, in addition to several brain regions commonly activated by both groups, children with BECTS also activated other regions, including the left hippocampus. According to the authors, this additional activation of the left hippocampus was unexpected. They consider its well-known association with memory systems and its more specific role in grapheme decoding, as demonstrated by He et al. (see above) [19].

To our knowledge, the first study to explore the brain structures necessary for text comprehension and memorization was conducted by Hausser et al. using a combined VBM/DTI approach in neuropsychological patients [62]. In this study, comprehension scores (text base and situation model) were obtained after the patients read narrative texts. The results show that the hippocampal region, in connection with the uncinate fasciculus (known to play a role in semantic processing), and the fornix and ventral cingulum (known to play a role in episodic memory), is essential not only for retrieving the text base and the situation model through episodic memory but also for activating the text base during reading and comprehension.

4. The effects of reading practice and literacy on the hippocampus

Sumowsky et al. explored the contribution of various types of cognitive leisure activities to cognitive reserve in patients with multiple sclerosis [63]. The results showed that greater engagement in reading and writing activities was positively correlated with larger hippocampal volume and better memory levels. According to the authors, 'most knowledge acquisition after high school is accomplished through literacy (i.e., reading), which may explain the relationship between reading-writing activity and hippocampal volume reported herein'. These valuable findings thoroughly 'inform the development of targeted evidence-based enrichment programs' aimed at bolstering reserve against memory decline.

In a study published by Sun et al. in *Psychological Medicine* [64], data from over 10,000 American children aged 9–13, as part of the ABCD (Adolescent Brain and Cognitive Development) project, were analyzed. Parents completed a questionnaire about their children's reading for pleasure (RFP), including questions on the duration ('For how many years has your child read for pleasure?') and frequency ('Approximately how many hours per week does your child read for pleasure?'). Children underwent a neurocognitive assessment to measure their cognitive abilities, and parents filled out the Child Behavior Checklist (CBCL) to identify any psychopathological or behavioral symptoms. Additionally, MRI scans were used to measure total brain volume and specific cortical and subcortical regions. Results showed positive correlations between RFP levels and two cognitive scores: a global cognitive score and a verbal memory score. RFP levels also correlated positively with language development and academic success. Negative correlations were found between RFP levels and measures of mental disorders, including dimensional psychopathology, adaptive dysfunction, teacher-reported problems, and impulsivity. Overall, adolescents with higher RFP levels had better cognitive performance and fewer mental disorders. MRI data revealed a significant positive link between RFP levels and total brain volume, particularly in a fronto-temporal network associated with language, including the left hippocampal region. The volumes of these brain regions also correlated positively with cognitive scores and negatively with attention and psychopathological disorders. In summary, this study confirms the positive effects of RFP on cognition, well-being, and brain development in adolescents, highlighting significant relationships with several brain structures, including the hippocampus.

5. Conclusions

This chapter provides a comprehensive exploration of the hippocampus's role in reading, traditionally viewed as a memory-related brain structure. Through an extensive review of brain imaging and cognitive studies in various populations, the hippocampus is established as a crucial component in reading. Key findings highlight its involvement at various stages of reading, from word decoding to text comprehension via sentence comprehension. At the decoding level, the hippocampus is actively engaged in learning grapheme-phoneme associations, orthographic word forms, associations between orthographic word forms and meanings, and forming connections between semantic, phonological, and orthographic units. At the sentence level, the hippocampus plays a significant role in syntactic processing and semantic processing, including semantic prediction and integration. At the text level, the hippocampus is involved in the harmonious use of semantic and episodic memory systems, as well as in inferential processing, enabling readers to create and memorize the text base and situation model that contribute to a coherent episodic text memory. Moreover, this chapter examines how reading practice contributes to hippocampal development and protection. In conclusion, this chapter provides compelling evidence that the hippocampus should be considered an integral part of the reading network. Recognizing its role enhances our understanding of reading's cognitive and neural mechanisms and emphasizes the importance of reading practices in educational, developmental, and therapeutical strategies. This perspective advocates for continued research and practical applications in education and neurocognitive health.

Author details

Frédéric Bernard
University of Strasbourg, Strasbourg, France

*Address all correspondence to: frederic.bernard@unistra.fr

References

[1] Damasio A. Descartes' Error: Emotion, Reason and the Human Brain. New-York: Putman; 1994. 312 p

[2] Bir SC, Ambekar S, Kukreja S, Nanda A. Julius Caesar Arantius (Giulio Cesare Aranzi, 1530-1589) and the hippocampus of the human brain: History behind the discovery. Journal of Neurosurgery. 2015;**122**(4):971-975. DOI: 10.3171/2014.11.JNS132402

[3] Scoville WB, Milner B. Loss of recent memory after bilateral hippocampal lesions. Journal of Neurology, Neurosurgery, and Psychiatry. 1957;**20**(1):11. DOI: 10.1136/jnnp.20.1.11

[4] Zola-Morgan S, Squire LR. Neuroanatomy of memory. Annual Review of Neuroscience. 1993;**16**(1): 547-563

[5] Tulving E, Markowitsch HJ. Episodic and declarative memory: Role of the hippocampus. Hippocampus. 1998;**8**(3):198-204. DOI: 10.1002/(SICI)1098-1063(1998)8:3<198::AID-HIPO2>3.0.CO;2-G

[6] MacKay DG, Stewart R, Burke DM. HM revisited: Relations between language comprehension, memory, and the hippocampal system. Journal of Cognitive Neuroscience. 1998;**10**(3):377-394. DOI: 10.1162/089892998562807

[7] MacKay DG. Beyond memory in H.M., the world's most famous "hippocampal amnesic". In: Burman DD, editor. Hippocampus—More than Just Memory. London, UK: IntechOpen; 2023. DOI: 10.5772/intechopen.111609

[8] Bartha-Doering L, Trinka E. The interictal language profile in adult epilepsy. Epilepsia. 2014;**55**(10):1512-1525. DOI: 10.1111/epi.12743

[9] Yurchenko A, Golovteev A, Dragoy O. Single-word, sentence, and discourse comprehension in individuals with temporal lobe epilepsy. Epilepsy and Behavior. 2020;**110**:107140. DOI: 10.1016/j.yebeh.2020.107140

[10] Piai V, Anderson KL, Lin JJ, Dewar C, Parvizi J, Dronkers NF, et al. Direct brain recordings reveal hippocampal rhythm underpinnings of language processing. Proceedings of the National Academy of Sciences of the United States of America. 2016;**113**(40):11366-11371. DOI: 10.1073/pnas.1603312113

[11] Covington NV, Duff MC. Expanding the language network: Direct contributions from the hippocampus. Trends in Cognitive Sciences. 2016;**20**(12):869-870. DOI: 10.1016/j.tics.2016.10.006

[12] Yeatman JD. The neurobiology of literacy. In: Snowling MJ, Hulme C, Nation K, editors. The Science of Reading. 2nd ed. Hoboken, NJ: Wiley-Blackwell; 2022. pp. 533-555

[13] Gough PB, Tunmer WE. Decoding, reading, and reading disability. Remedial and Special Education. 1986;7:6-10. DOI: 10.1177/074193258600700104

[14] Breitenstein C, Jansen A, Deppe M, Foerster AF, Sommer J, Wolbers T, et al. Hippocampus activity differentiates good from poor learners of a novel lexicon. NeuroImage. 2005;**25**(3):958-968. DOI: 10.1016/j.neuroimage.2004.12.019

[15] Davis MH, Di Betta AM, Macdonald MJ, Gaskell MG. Learning and consolidation of novel spoken words.

Journal of Cognitive Neuroscience. 2009;**21**(4):803-820. DOI: 10.1162/jocn.2009.21059

[16] Thiebaut de Schotten M, Cohen L, Amemiya E, Braga LW, Dehaene S. Learning to read improves the structure of the arcuate fasciculus. Cerebral Cortex. 2014;**24**(4):989-995. DOI: 10.1093/cercor/bhs383

[17] Quinn C, Taylor JSH, Davis MH. Learning and retrieving holistic and componential visual-verbal associations in reading and object naming. Neuropsychologia. 2017;**98**:68-84. DOI: 10.1016/j.neuropsychologia.2016.09.025

[18] Xu W, Kolozsvari OB, Oestenveld R, Hämäläinen JA. Rapid changes in brain activity during learning of grapheme-phoneme associations in adults. NeuroImage. 2020;**220**:117058. DOI: 10.1016/j.neuroimage.2020.117058

[19] He Q, Xue G, Chen C, Chen C, Lu ZL, Dong Q. Decoding the neuroanatomical basis of reading ability: A multivoxel morphometric study. The Journal of Neuroscience. 2013;**33**(31):12835-12843. DOI: 10.1523/JNEUROSCI.0449-13.2013

[20] Abutalebi J, Keim R, Brambati SM, Tettamanti M, Cappa SF, De Bleser R, et al. Late acquisition of literacy in a native language. Human Brain Mapping. 2007;**28**:19-33. DOI: 10.1002/hbm.20240

[21] Gebauer D, Fink A, Kargl R, Reishofer G, Koschutnig K, Purgstaller C, et al. Differences in brain function and changes with intervention in children with poor spelling and reading abilities. PLoS One. 2012;**7**(5):e38201. DOI: 10.1371/journal.pone.0038201

[22] Krafnick AJ, Flowers DL, Napoliello EM, Eden GF. Gray matter volume changes following reading intervention in dyslexic children. NeuroImage. 2011;**57**:733-741. DOI: 10.1016/j.neuroimage.2010.10.062

[23] Sterpenich V, Ceravolo L, Schwartz S. Sleep deprivation disrupts the contribution of the hippocampus to the formation of novel lexical associations. Brain and Language. 2017;**167**:61-71. DOI: 10.1016/j.bandl.2016.12.007

[24] Tao Y, Schubert T, Wiley R, Stark C, Rapp B. Cortical and subcortical mechanisms of orthographic word-form learning. Journal of Cognitive Neuroscience. 2024;**36**(6):1071-1098. DOI: 10.1162/jocn_a_02147

[25] Paz-Alonso PM, Oliver M, Lerma-Usabiaga G, Caballero-Gaudes C, Quiñones I, Suárez-Coalla P, et al. Neural correlates of phonological, orthographic and semantic reading processing in dyslexia. NeuroImage: Clinical. 2018;**20**:433-447. DOI: 10.1016/j.nicl.2018.08.018

[26] Lah S, Castles A, Smith ML. Reading in children with temporal lobe epilepsy: A systematic review. Epilepsy and Behavior. 2017;**68**:84-94. DOI: 10.1016/j.yebeh.2016.12.021

[27] MacKay DG, James LE. Aging, retrograde amnesia, and the binding problem for phonology and orthography: A longitudinal study of "hippocampal amnesic" H.M. Aging Neuropsychology and Cognition. 2002;**9**(4):298-333. DOI: 10.1076/anec.9.4.298.8774

[28] Ota M, Koshibe Y, Higashi S, Nemoto K, Tsukada E, Tamura M, et al. Structural brain network correlated with reading impairment in Alzheimer's disease. Dementia and Geriatric Cognitive Disorders. 2020;**49**:264-269. DOI: 10.1159/000508406

[29] Kintsch W. The role of knowledge in discourse comprehension: A construction-integration model. Psychological Review. 1988;**95**(2):163-182. DOI: 10.1037/0033-295X.95.2.163

[30] Kintsch W. Comprehension: A Paradigm for Cognition. New-York: Cambridge University Press; 1998. 461 p

[31] Cooke A, Zurif EB, DeVita C, Alsop D, Koenig P, Detre J, et al. Neural basis for sentence comprehension: Grammatical and short-term memory components. Human Brain Mapping. 2001;**15**:80-94. DOI: 10.1002/hbm.10006

[32] Waters G, Caplan D, Alpert N, Stanczak L. Individual differences in rCBF correlates of syntactic processing in sentence comprehension: Effects of working memory and speed of processing. NeuroImage. 2003;**19**:101-112. DOI: 10.1016/S1053-8119(03)00007-7

[33] Hoenig K, Scheef L. Mediotemporal contributions to semantic processing: fMRI evidence from ambiguity processing during semantic context verification. Hippocampus. 2005;**15**:597-609. DOI: 10.1002/hipo.20080

[34] Opitz B, Friederici AD. Neural basis of processing sequential and hierarchical syntactic structures. Human Brain Mapping. 2007;**28**:585-592. DOI: 10.1002/hbm.20287

[35] Lee D, Newman SD. The effect of presentation paradigm on syntactic processing: An event-related fMRI study. Human Brain Mapping. 2010;**31**:65-79. DOI: 10.1002/hbm.20845

[36] Prat CS, Just MA. Exploring the neural dynamics underpinning individual differences in sentence comprehension. Cerebral Cortex. 2011;**21**:1747-1760. DOI: 10.1093/cercor/bhq241

[37] Citron FMM, Goldberg AE. Metaphorical sentences are more emotionally engaging than their literal counterparts. Journal of Cognitive Neuroscience. 2014;**26**(11):2585-2595. DOI: 10.1162/jocn_a_00654

[38] Bonhage CE, Fiebach CJ, Bahlmann J, Mueller JL. Brain signature of working memory for sentence structure: Enriched encoding and facilitated maintenance. Journal of Cognitive Neuroscience. 2014;**26**(8):1654-1671. DOI: 10.1162/jocn_a_00566

[39] Meyer P, Mecklinger A, Grunwald T, Fell J, Elger CE, Friederici AD. Language processing within the human medial temporal lobe. Hippocampus. 2005;**15**(4):451-459. DOI: 10.1002/hipo.20070

[40] Bonhage CE, Mueller JL, Friederici AD, Fiebach CJ. Combined eye tracking and fMRI reveals neural basis of linguistic predictions during sentence comprehension. Cortex. 2015;**68**:33-47. DOI: 10.1016/j.cortex.2015.04.011

[41] Friston K, Kiebel S. Predictive coding under the free-energy principle. Philosophical Transactions of the Royal Society B: Biological Sciences. 2009;**364**(1521):1211-1221. DOI: 10.1098/rstb.2008.0300

[42] Ryan JD, Shen K. The eyes are a window into memory. Current Opinion in Behavioral Sciences. 2020;**32**:1-6. DOI: 10.1016/j.cobeha.2019.12.014

[43] Schuster S, Hawelka S, Hutzler F, Kronbichler M, Richlan F. Words in context: The effects of length, frequency, and predictability on brain responses during natural reading. Cerebral Cortex. 2016;**26**:3889-3904. DOI: 10.1093/cercor/bhw184

[44] Friston K. The free-energy principle: A unified brain theory? Nature Reviews

Neuroscience. 2010;**11**(2):127-138. DOI: 10.1038/nrn2787

[45] Pu Y, Cheyne D, Sun Y, Johnson BW. Theta oscillations support the interface between language and memory. NeuroImage. 2020;**215**:116782. DOI: 10.1016/j.neuroimage.2020.116782

[46] Schuster S, Himmelstoss NA, Hutzler F, Richlan F, Kronbichler M, Hawelka S. Cloze enough? Hemodynamic effects of predictive processing during natural reading. NeuroImage. 2021;**228**:117687. DOI: 10.1016/j.neuroimage.2020.117687

[47] McCarthy G, Nobre AC, Bentin S, Spencer DD. Language-related field potentials in the anterior-medial temporal lobe: I. Intracranial distribution and neural generators. The Journal of Neuroscience. 1995;**15**(2):1080-1089. DOI: 10.1523/JNEUROSCI.15-02-01080.1995

[48] Noppeney U, Price CJ, Duncan JS, Koepp MJ. Reading skills after left anterior temporal lobe resection: An fMRI study. Brain. 2005;**128**:1377-1385. DOI: 10.1093/brain/awh414

[49] MacKay DG, James LE. The binding problem for syntax, semantics, and prosody: H.M.'s selective sentence-reading deficits under the theoretical-syndrome approach. Language and Cognitive Processes. 2001;**16**(4):419-460. DOI: 10.1080/01690960042000102

[50] MacKay DG, Burke DM, Stewart R. HM's language production deficits: Implications for relations between memory, semantic binding, and the hippocampal system. Journal of Memory and Language. 1998;**38**(1):28-69. DOI: 10.1006/jmla.1997.2544

[51] Xu J, Kemeny S, Park G, Frattali C, Braun A. Language in context: Emergent features of word, sentence, and narrative comprehension. NeuroImage. 2005;**25**(3):1002-1015. DOI: 10.1016/j.neuroimage.2004.12.013

[52] Ferstl EC, von Cramon DY. Time, space and emotion: fMRI reveals content-specific activation during text comprehension. Neuroscience Letters. 2007;**427**(3):159-164. DOI: 10.1016/j.neulet.2007.09.046

[53] Mano Y, Harada T, Sugiura M, Saito DN, Sadato N. Perspective-taking as part of narrative comprehension: A functional MRI study. Neuropsychologia. 2009;**47**(3):813-824. DOI: 10.1016/j.neuropsychologia.2008.12.011

[54] Prat CS, Mason RA, Just MA. An fMRI investigation of analogical mapping in metaphor comprehension: The influence of context and individual cognitive capacities on processing demands. Journal of Experimental Psychology: Learning, Memory, and Cognition. 2012;**38**(2):282-294. DOI: 10.1037/a0026037

[55] Aboud KS, Bailey SK, Petrill SA, Cutting LE. Comprehending text versus reading words in young readers with varying reading ability: Distinct patterns of functional connectivity from common processing hubs. Developmental Science. 2016;**19**(4):632-656. DOI: 10.1111/desc.12422

[56] Helder A, van den Broek P, Karlsson J, Van Leijenhorst L. Neural correlates of coherence-break detection during reading of narratives. Scientific Studies of Reading. 2017;**21**(6):463-479. DOI: 10.1080/10888438.2017.1332065

[57] van Moort ML, Jolles DD, Koornneef A, van den Broek P. What you read versus what you know: Neural correlates of accessing context information and background knowledge

in constructing a mental representation during reading. Journal of Experimental Psychology: General. 2020;**149**(11):2084-2101. DOI: 10.1037/xge0000764

[58] Sato N, Mizuhara H. Successful encoding during natural reading is associated with fixation-related potentials and large-scale network deactivation. eNeuro. 2018;**5**(5):1-12. DOI: 10.1523/ENEURO.0122-18.2018

[59] Saito Y, Yoshida S, Ueda R, Senoo A. Association of neural activities in language processing and memory with rapid reading. Juntendo Medical Journal. DOI: 10.14789/jmj.JMJ23-0022-OA [Advance Online Publication] Available from: https://www.jstage.jst.go.jp/article/jmj/advpub/0/advpub_JMJ23-0022-OA/_pdf/-char/en

[60] Keller TA, Mason RA, Legg AE, Just MA. The neural and cognitive basis of expository text comprehension. Science of Learning. 2024;**9**(1):21. DOI: 10.1038/s41539-024-00232-y

[61] Malfait D, Tucholka A, Mendizabal S, Tremblay J, Poulin C, Oskoui M, et al. fMRI brain response during sentence reading comprehension in children with benign epilepsy with centro-temporal spikes. Epilepsy Research. 2015;**117**:42-51. DOI: 10.1016/j.eplepsyres.2015.08.009

[62] Hausser LP, Bugaud A, Noblet V, Loureiro de Sousa P, Botzung A, Blanc F, et al. The hippocampal region is necessary for text comprehension and memorization: A combined VBM/DTI study in neuropsychological patients. Brain Imaging and Behavior. 2021;**15**:2367-2376. DOI: 10.1007/s11682-020-00432-1

[63] Sumowski JF, Rocca MA, Leavitt VM, Ricciteli G, Meani A, Comi G, et al. Reading, writing, and reserve: Literacy activities are linked to hippocampal volume and memory in multiple sclerosis. Multiple Sclerosis. 2016;**22**(12):1621-1625. DOI: 10.1177/1352458516630822

[64] Sun Y-J, Sahakian BJ, Langley C, Yang A, Jiang Y, Kang J, et al. Early-initiated childhood reading for pleasure: Associations with better cognitive performance, mental well-being and brain structure in young adolescence. Psychological Medicine. 2024;**54**(2):359-373. DOI: 10.1017/S0033291723001381

Chapter 3

Role of the Hippocampus in Adaptive Forgetting: A Question of Synaptic Depression?

Gaël Malleret

Abstract

This chapter examines the often overlooked but crucial role of the hippocampus in forgetting as a fundamental cognitive process. Challenging the traditional view that forgetting represents a failure of memory, it argues that adaptive forgetting is vital for maintaining cognitive efficiency. In addition to its established functions in learning and memory, the hippocampus is proposed to play a central role in adaptive forgetting by selectively eliminating unnecessary information. This process enhances the storage and retrieval of relevant memories, primarily through synaptic mechanisms such as long-term synaptic depression (LTD). LTD has been shown to facilitate the inhibition or removal of outdated information, thus preventing cognitive overload. The chapter also offers a historical perspective on key discoveries that have shaped this understanding.

Keywords: forgetting, adaptive, synaptic depression, LTD, interference

1. Introduction

The hippocampus is well known for its pivotal roles in memory formation, consolidation, and retrieval [1, 2]. However, its role in forgetting processes is equally significant, though often underappreciated, probably because forgetting itself has long remained obscure, often perceived as a mere lack of memory—a failed process that occurs involuntarily.

Forgetting is a common and often embarrassing experience. "Where did I put my keys? What is his name again?" These are familiar questions and situations we have all encountered. Yet, more frequently than we realize, our objective is actually to forget rather than to remember. For instance, for a waiter taking numerous similar orders throughout a shift, the ability to forget previous orders once they are completed is advantageous and even crucial to his ability to memorize new orders. Despite common complaints about not having a perfect memory, retaining all daily experiences would significantly impair our ability to remember other, more important information.

Studies of hyperthymestic patients—individuals who can recall an abnormally large number of life experiences—reveal that excessive recall of autobiographical

IntechOpen

memories can impair the formation of other types of memory. The case of patients, like Jill Price [3] or Alexander Luria's patient S. [4], shows that too much recall of long-term memory thus comes at the cost of impairment in short-term memory or other important cognitive skills such as reading. These studies suggest that, like memory, forgetting is essential to our cognitive processes and that certain forms of forgetting are adaptive [5, 6]. This chapter explores the mechanisms by which the hippocampus contributes to forgetting, particularly through the process of long-term synaptic depression (LTD). Additionally, it provides historical insights into the development of the concepts surrounding these mechanisms, highlighting key studies and discoveries.

2. What is adaptive forgetting?

2.1 Theories of forgetting

Forgetting is generally defined as the inability to recall information that was once known. However, this loss does not necessarily mean that the information is lost forever. Often, forgotten memories can be retrieved with the right cues, suggesting that forgetting may not be a simple erasure but rather a temporary inability to access information [7]. This coexistence of different forms of forgetting was duly noted by early philosophers and scientists. As early as the seventeenth century, Robert Hooke thus proposed that forgetting could either result from (1) the decay or degradation of memory traces over time or (2) from the interference caused by other competitive memories during the retrieval process of a particular memory [8, 9].

Throughout the twentieth century, traditional theories of forgetting focused on the notion of interference rather than decay. Some thus believed that the classic study by Jenkins and Dallenbach [10] provided evidence against the decay theory. These authors demonstrated that subjects who slept after learning (and therefore who were protected from interference) retained more information than those who stayed awake during the same time (and were potentially submitted to interfering information), supporting the idea that interference, rather than time-based decay, was responsible for forgetting. Because of these findings, decay theory was essentially abandoned and interference theory remained for a long time the main theory to explain *how* (by what means) we forget ([11]; but see [12] and also [13, 14] concerning the particular case of decay in short-term/working memory).

2.2 Forgetting as a competitive advantage

The interference theory not only explains *how* we forget information but also *why* we forget. Adaptive forgetting [6] is thus a concept that challenges the traditional view of forgetting as the negative counterpart of memory. Instead of seeing forgetting as merely the *passive* loss or decay of memory, adaptive forgetting is considered a crucial process that helps maintain cognitive efficiency by *actively* eliminating unnecessary or outdated information. As noted by early psychologists like Théodule Ribot [15], William James [16] or Henri Bergson [17], forgetting would therefore not be a flaw but a necessary condition for the "*health and life*" of memory [15].

Forgetting can be adaptive in various ways. It allows for the modification of behavior in response to new information, prevents cognitive overload by filtering out irrelevant details, and enables the extraction of general rules from specific experiences. Freud, with his concept of repression, argued that people forget stressful episodes in order to gain some immediate psychological advantage [18], even if the long-term consequences of repression can be deleterious. Extinction, the process by which a learned fear is attenuated, was advocated by Freud in the 1920s for the treatment of phobias [19, 20]. Extinction can be tested in the laboratory when studying the extinction of fear conditioning in rats or mice [21]. After conditioning (for instance, by giving an electric foot-shock) an animal to a context or a sound, freezing response (expressing the animal memory for having been shocked) is generally reduced over successive presentation of the context or sound previously associated with the shock. Like repressed memories, however, freezing (the behavioral response associated to the memory for the stressful event) can be reinstated (a process known as "*spontaneous recovery*") after a long period of disuse (of several weeks or months) when confronted again to the context or sound [19, 21]. Extinction is thus generally considered a new learning based on a new link formed by the cues and the absence of the original fearful event(s). It does not consist in the erasure of the original memory but in the temporary inhibition of its retrieval. Extinction nicely exemplifies the adaptive advantage of forgetting, as it seems logical for the animal to withhold (freezing) responses that are no longer associated with expected events. However, the adaptive aspect of spontaneous recovery (the forgetting of extinction) of the freezing response after several weeks is less evident [6]. Extinction involves the existence of two conflicting memories: one for the original conditioning and the other for extinction training. Spontaneous recovery can thus be regarded as a situation in which experience with ambiguous signals renders it adaptive for the animal to express behavioral ambivalence (i.e., an intermediate level of freezing as it is often observed).

2.3 Proactive interference

Fortunately, our daily lives are filled with more neutral events than traumatic or fearful experiences. Proactive interference occurs when older memories interfere with the acquisition and recall of new ones. This type of interference is particularly relevant in situations where environmental conditions or behaviors need to change rapidly. For instance, an animal trained to associate a specific action with a reward might struggle to learn a new association if the old memory persists. In such cases, adaptive forgetting helps by suppressing or inhibiting the retrieval of outdated memories, allowing the individual to focus on the new, more relevant information [22].

Early interference theories suggested that this process involved "*unlearning*" – meaning "the *replacement*" of old memories with new ones [23]. However, later research has shown that old memories are not entirely erased but rather *suppressed* [22, 24]. This suppression mechanism, often referred to as retrieval inhibition, allows for the temporary inaccessibility of certain memories while preserving the potential for their future retrieval [6]. This adaptive process is crucial for navigating a world where both past experiences (that can be useful to retain in certain circumstances) and current demands must be balanced.

2.4 Adaptive forgetting and the construction of memory

Adaptive forgetting plays a critical role in the construction and transformation of memory over time. Memories are not static; they are constantly being updated, reorganized, and integrated with new information. This process is particularly evident in the transition from episodic-to-semantic memory, where specific, context-rich memories are generalized into broader concepts. For example, a child's memory of learning that "*Paris is the capital of France*" may initially include details about the classroom and teacher. Over time, these details fade, leaving only the essential fact that Paris is the capital of France [12, 25]. This transformation is facilitated by adaptive forgetting, which helps strip away the contextual details of episodic memories to create more stable, semantic knowledge. This process is vital for cognitive efficiency, as it allows the brain to maintain a manageable and relevant store of information. However, when adaptive forgetting is disrupted, as in the case of hyperthymesia or extraordinary memory, individuals may struggle to generalize knowledge, leading to difficulties in everyday functioning [4]. This condition underscores the importance of adaptive forgetting in enabling flexible and efficient cognitive processes.

2.5 Short-term/working memory

Forgetting is not only essential for long-term memory but also for the efficient functioning of short-term or working memory. Working memory is responsible for temporarily storing and manipulating information, like remembering a phone number long enough to dial it [26]. However, not all information held in working memory needs to be retained. Adaptive forgetting ensures that only the most relevant information is maintained, preventing cognitive overload [14]. In fact, forgetting is intrinsic to the concept of working memory. Dudchenko [27] wisely noted that "*Working memory is a short-term memory that, once used, should be forgotten or ignored (...) and may not actually be a type of memory, but a type of forgetting*". As information is supposedly only "*temporarily*" stored in working memory, this means that, after a while, such information is not available any longer (i.e., forgotten).

But what if this information sticks in mind? For several authors, forgetting short-term memory in human involves the decay of memory traces [13], whereas others argue it is caused by interference [28]. However, information stored in so-called short-term/working memory can sometimes be stored more permanently, outlasting their purpose and acting as proactive interference on the storage of newer information in working memory [14, 29–31]. Once again, forgetting this interfering information would be essential to our ability to optimally store new information in working memory.

Therefore, whether it is for long-term, semantic, emotional, or working memory, forgetting would be crucial for the optimal use of our cognitive resources. In fact, even if memory and forgetting are certainly two distinct processes, we will see in this chapter that they may be highly interrelated and potentially dependent on one another. Consequently, the major question that needs to be answered is: do they share the same anatomical substrates and cellular mechanisms?

3. Synaptic mechanisms of forgetting: First evidence and discoveries

3.1 Synaptic mechanisms required for optimal memory storage

Memories are stored through plastic changes in the brain known as memory traces or engrams [32, 33]. However, as we have seen, not all memories are maintained equally, and in fact many can subsequently be forgotten. Ryan and Frankland [7] define forgetting as the *reduced retrievability* of information that was once successfully encoded and identify five possible mechanisms able to explain such reduced retrievability: synaptic strength changes, intracellular signaling, inhibitory mechanisms, hippocampal neurogenesis, microglial remodeling, and sleep. However, these authors also acknowledge that some overlap exists among these mechanisms and that any one of these processes, which alters synaptic transmission within a neural network representing the engram of memory, may consequently alter that memory.

The process of memory storage in the brain is indeed complex and tightly regulated, involving a delicate balance of synaptic mechanisms. For memories to be effectively stored and retrieved, synaptic connections within neural circuits must undergo specific structural and functional changes. These changes are particularly significant in hippocampal-neocortical networks, where memory engrams are thought to mature through a reorganization of synaptic connections [32]. This reorganization is driven by the expression of various genes that lead to modifications in synaptic transmission efficacy, which are crucial for encoding and stabilizing memories [1, 2].

One of the most well-studied mechanisms of synaptic plasticity is Long-Term Potentiation (LTP), a process that strengthens synaptic connections. LTP, which has been particularly studied in the hippocampus, is widely considered a cellular model for learning and memory [34]. The induction of LTP involves a rise in intracellular calcium (Ca2+) levels, primarily through the activation of N-methyl-D-aspartate (NMDA) receptors. These receptors, which are ionotropic glutamate receptors, act as coincidence detectors, becoming active only when *presynaptic* glutamate binds to them and the *postsynaptic* membrane is sufficiently depolarized. When this occurs, the magnesium ion (Mg2+) blocking the NMDA receptor is expelled, allowing Ca2+ to enter the cell.

Once inside the cell, the influx of Ca2+ triggers a cascade of biochemical events that are crucial for the maintenance of LTP. These events involve the activation of several protein kinases, including calcium/calmodulin-dependent protein kinase II (CaMKII), which plays a pivotal role in sustaining the increased synaptic efficacy associated with LTP. The activation of CaMKII leads to the phosphorylation of proteins that are responsible for the insertion and clustering of other glutamate receptors at the postsynaptic density (PSD) such as α-amino-3-hydroxy-5-methyl-4-isoxazolepropionic acid (AMPA) receptors. These changes enhance synaptic transmission, making it more likely for the neuron that potentially participates in the memory engram to respond to future stimuli [35].

LTP is generally divided into two phases: early-phase LTP (E-LTP) and late-phase LTP (L-LTP). E-LTP is a transient form of potentiation that lasts for a few hours and does not require new protein synthesis. In contrast, L-LTP is more stable and long-lasting, persisting for days or even longer. The transition from E-LTP to L-LTP requires the synthesis of new proteins and mRNA, which are necessary for the structural changes that support the prolonged increase in synaptic strength [1, 36]. These proteins can be integrated into the synapse, contributing to the formation of new synaptic connections or the strengthening of existing ones. The specificity of these changes is ensured by a process known as synaptic tagging and capture. According to this hypothesis, when a synapse is activated, it is "tagged" in a way that allows it to capture newly synthesized proteins that are distributed throughout the neuron. These proteins are essential for maintaining the changes in synaptic strength that underlie memory storage. Importantly, only the tagged synapses will undergo these long-term changes, ensuring that the memory is encoded in a specific and targeted manner [36].

For memory to be stored effectively, it is crucial that synaptic modifications are highly selective and regulated. This selectivity is maintained through the careful balance of phosphorylation and dephosphorylation events at the synapse, which are mediated by protein kinases and phosphatases. For example, the persistent activity of CaMKII after its initial activation can serve as a synaptic tag, ensuring that the synapse "remembers" the activity that led to its potentiation [37]. Conversely, protein phosphatases like PP1 can dephosphorylate key synaptic proteins, counteracting the effects of kinases and thus providing a mechanism for downregulating synaptic strength when necessary [38].

Research has shown that the activation of protein phosphatases, particularly protein phosphatase 2B (PP2B), also known as calcineurin, can negatively regulate both LTP and memory consolidation. Calcineurin exerts this effect by dephosphorylating key proteins, such as AMPA and NMDA receptors, which are essential for increasing synaptic efficacy (see above). This dephosphorylation decreases the activity of these proteins, thereby reducing their impact on synaptic transmission and memory formation [38]. Given this negative modulation, we and others have explored in the past whether inactivating calcineurin could, conversely, enhance hippocampal-dependent memory and LTP [39]. In studies using the water maze task, it was observed that memory was indeed enhanced in mutant mice expressing a calcineurin inhibitor. This cognitive enhancement was accompanied by an increase in LTP both *in vitro* and *in vivo*. Tonegawa and colleagues also investigated the effects of inhibiting calcineurin using forebrain-specific knockout (KO) mice. In these mice, calcineurin was completely inhibited in selective cell types, particularly in the granule cells of the dentate gyrus (DG) and the pyramidal cells of the CA1 region of the hippocampus [40]. Interestingly, this total inhibition of calcineurin left high-frequency stimulation-induced LTP intact, a finding that contrasts with our previous study, where partial inhibition of calcineurin enhanced LTP [39]. The authors attributed this difference to the substantial endogenous calcineurin activity that remained in the model expressing a calcineurin inhibitor, as opposed to the complete gene deletion in the KO model [40]. However, the deletion of calcineurin in this model also impaired the expression of Long-Term Depression (LTD), another significant and long-lasting form of synaptic plasticity [35].

3.2 Cellular and molecular mechanisms involved in LTD

LTD can either be induced *de novo* or following a pre-induced LTP as a form of depotentiation [41]. In the hippocampus, LTD can be typically induced by prolonged periods of low-frequency stimulation, such as 15 minutes at 1 Hz [42]. One of the most studied forms of LTD is NMDA receptor-dependent LTD, usually induced by low-frequency stimulation, which leads to a slow increase in intracellular calcium (Ca2+) concentration. This contrasts with LTP, which requires a more rapid increase in Ca2+ due to high-frequency stimulation. The slow Ca2+ influx during LTD induction activates calmodulin, which then activates the phosphatase calcineurin [43]. Calcineurin dephosphorylates the inhibitor-1 peptide, leading to the activation of protein phosphatase 1 (PP1). PP1 subsequently dephosphorylates various substrates, including the ser845 site of the GluA1 subunit of AMPA receptors, signaling their internalization and degradation, which results in reduced synaptic transmission and the expression of LTD [44]. Post-synaptically, this reduction in glutamate sensitivity is primarily due to the removal of AMPA receptors from the synapse or a decrease in their conductance properties. Long-term expression of LTD involves more stable modifications, such as the shrinkage and elimination of both pre- and postsynaptic elements, differing from LTP, which generally involves an increase in the volume of small dendritic spines [45].

The mechanisms underlying the induction and expression of LTD thus appear to be similar for some, and opposite for others, to the one associated with LTP. The decay of NMDA receptor-dependent late (but not early) LTP could thus be mediated by active processes such as depotentiation or a reversal of LTP by LTD that also require NMDA receptor activation. While pre-induction and pre-training injection of NMDA antagonist alters both LTP and long- term memory [46], Villareal and colleagues showed that blockade of NMDA receptor-dependent forms of plasticity (including LTD) preserves pre-induced *in vivo* LTP and also increases retention of previously encoded spatial memory [47]. These data suggest that even if memory encoding requires NMDA-dependent synaptic plasticity (LTP) [46], memory persistence can also be altered by activation of NMDA-dependent plasticity, such as NMDA-dependent LTD. They also reveal the existence of active processes contributing to the possible erasing of previously learned, old information. Synaptic depression would thus naturally occur *in vivo* to reverse prior training or pre-induced potentiation. But what would be the "*purpose*" of such a process? One appealing hypothesis is that LTD might be required for the removal of irrelevant information and the flexible use of cognitive resources [48].

In the last decades, a number of studies have thus explored the possible roles of LTD in learning processes. However, LTD deficits were often first reported in the context of a metaplastic shift (i.e., with combined enhancement of LTP) [40, 49]. To explore the role of LTD, it was essential to find precise experimental tools and use, for instance, laboratory animals with genetic manipulations that specifically alter LTD expression while sparing LTP. The characterization of the serum response factor (SRF) KO mice that showed normal hippocampal LTP but impaired LTD thus represented a good system to explore the selective role of LTD in memory processes [50]. Behaviorally, these SRF knockout mice had no issues with non-hippocampal-dependent tasks but displayed significant deficits in spatial learning tasks, including contextual habituation and water maze training. These findings suggested that LTD plays a role in acquiring spatial/contextual information. At the time, they also aligned with *in vivo* studies on synaptic plasticity in the hippocampus during exposure to new spatial environments. Manahan-Vaughan and colleagues thus found that exposure to an empty space reinforced LTP expression in the CA1 region of the hippocampus and impaired LTD. Conversely, introducing new objects into this environment facilitated LTD and weakened LTP [51]. These results suggested that LTD may be crucial for updating hippocampal-dependent information processing, particularly in response to environmental changes.

3.3 LTD, cognitive flexibility, working memory, and proactive interference

In fact, updating information is a key feature of short-term/working memory, a memory form that allows temporary and flexible storage of information [27]. This form of memory was specifically altered in the calcineurin forebrain-specific knockout (KO) mice that displayed a deficit in LTD [40]. Although these calcineurin KO mice displayed no deficits in Ref. memory, which corresponds to the long-term storage of stable information learned across repetitive trials, they struggled with tasks requiring short-term/working memory. In rodents, reference memory corresponds to long-term semantic memory, whereas working memory is the ability to temporarily store and process trial-unique information [52]. This distinction is critical for understanding the specific role of LTD in working memory. Calcineurin KO mice had no difficulties learning the classical water maze task, which was aimed at testing reference memory. In this task, mice must learn the consistent location of an escape platform over several days of training. However, when challenged with a delayed match-to-place task, in which the platform location changed daily, calcineurin KO mice exhibited significant impairments.

Delayed match (or non-match) tasks are the most commonly used procedures to test working memory in numerous subjects including birds, rodents, non-human primates, and humans [30]. The basic match procedure begins by presenting a subject with a stimulus known as the *"sample"* (often a visual pattern/object or a spatially distinct place) that they are required to remember after a short delay. Once this delay elapses, they have then to identify from a subsequent set of stimuli one that *"matches"* the sample. In the water maze delayed match-to-place task used by Tonegawa and colleagues [40], the platform position changed every day and the mice were required to learn this position over 8 daily training sessions. Although this task cannot be considered one of working memory (working memory being trial-unique specific; see above), it still stresses a short-term form of memory for the platform location that is unique for each day but that the mice need to update every day. While control mice readily learned each platform position every day, no such learning was observed in the calcineurin KO mice, suggesting an impairment in episodic-like memory; each platform location learned everyday representing a discreet episode isolated in space and time.

Based on this finding, the authors then explored *"true"* working memory of these mutants in the classical eight-arm radial maze task. During this task, the mice were given one trial per day (respecting the trial-unique contingency associated to working memory) to localize eight food rewards located in each arm of the maze. Each day, during this unique trial, mice were given the opportunity to perform eight visits separated by a short inter-visit delay of 5 seconds. The animals thus had to use a non-match rule to be adequately reinforced; a re-entry (match) in an already visited arm (in which the animal had already retrieved a food pellet) representing a working memory error as no more food was present in this arm. Here again, forebrain-specific calcineurin KO mice showed impaired performance in this working memory task. From these results, the authors concluded that bidirectional synaptic modification (LTP/LTD balance) seems to be critical for one-trial learning-based working/episodic-like memory. In consequence, Tonegawa and colleagues believed that *"LTD does not seem to be a mechanism that constrains memory, but on the contrary and in conjugation with LTP, constitutes the basis for an effective distributed memory system"*. Following this study, Nakao and colleagues [53] tested rats in a spontaneous alternation test aimed to assess spatial working memory and monitored thereafter LTD in response to low-frequency burst stimulation in the dentate gyrus of the same rat under anesthesia. Interestingly, their behavioral parameter of spatial working memory (the degree of spontaneous alternation, a non-match rule) was positively correlated to the magnitude of LTD. Based on their and Tonegawa's findings [40], Nakao's team posited: *"LTD does not merely act to extinguish previous memory or preexisting LTP but does play an active role in memory acquisition, probably by co-working with LTP"*. However, other data described below seem to contradict such hypothesis.

As mentioned earlier, very few models first offered the opportunity to specifically assess the role of LTD (with no metaplastic shift/combined enhancements in LTP). This was the case of transgenic mice expressing an inhibitor of PP2A, a highly abundant serine/threonine protein phosphatase [54]. Indeed, like CaMKII autophosphorylation acts as an important *"switch"* for the maintenance of LTP, PP2A auto-dephosphorylation represents a key event required for LTD. In these mice,

NMDA-induced AMPA receptor internalization as well as NMDA receptor-dependent hippocampal LTD were blocked without affecting the one induced by other glutamate (metabotropic mGluR) receptor activation. These mice thus represented an excellent model to study the function of LTD, and more specifically of NMDA receptor-dependent LTD, as other forms of plasticity (potentiation, depotentiation, and mGluR-dependent LTD) were largely spared. At the behavioral level, PP2A inhibition had no consequence on the mice's ability to learn the standard reference memory water maze task, during which the mice were required to learn the invariable location of an escape platform. However, this PP2A inhibition greatly impaired cognitive flexibility that was required when the mice had to adapt their behavior to a change in the platform location during a transfer test (also called reversal phase; when the platform was relocated to an opposite quadrant of the pool). In this test, transgenic mice displayed a persistent exploratory behavior in the first learned location as compared to control mice that flexibly adapted their spatial search to the new position of the platform (preferring as expected the new location to the old one). This result, in agreement with the work of Duffy and colleagues [55] that links enhanced LTD with an improvement in spatial reversal learning, thus indicated the persistence (impaired forgetting) in the mutant mice memory of information previously learned but that was no longer relevant.

What about working memory? One can wonder if the cognitive inflexibility observed after PP2A inhibition would be sufficient to impair performance in a task requiring constant flexibility such as a working memory task. The Delayed-Non-Match-to-Place task (DNMTP) in a T-maze allows to test if learned information can be erased after each trial in order to reset working memory for subsequent trials – "*Resetting*", defined as the capacity of the subject to erase or reset the contents of working memory at the end of a test session, has been proposed to be a key feature of working memory [29, 52]. In the DNMTP task, food deprived mice have to retrieve a sugar pellet at the end of an arm (pseudo-randomly determined by the experimenter) and memorize this emplacement (left or right). After a short delay, they next have to choose between this emplacement (i.e., right) and the opposite one (i.e., left). The reinforced arm is the one in which food was untouched, and mice are rewarded only if they choose this new arm and avoid the previously visited one (Non-Match). Each trial is unique and different from the previous one; this task requires focused attention on the ongoing trial and forgetting previous trials, as both arms of the maze being presented are always the same. Inhibition of PP2A clearly affected the performance of transgenic mice in this working memory task [54]. After 10 days of training, transgenic mice thus showed a decreased number of correct choices as compared to controls, suggesting that LTD could underlie working memory processing as previously reported by Nakao, Tonegawa, and their colleagues (see above [40, 53]). However, a different conclusion emerged when the performance of mice was analyzed not across days as traditionally done but across trials. The analysis of the results revealed that PP2A inhibition did not impair the transgenic mice in acquiring this task as they clearly performed above chance level and similarly to control mice during the first daily trial. This result suggests that these mice learned the (non-match) rule of the task as well as the control group and displayed normal working memory, unlike what was previously inferred from the role of LTD in working memory [40, 53]. However, this analysis by trials revealed that the performance of transgenic mice was altered by the multiplication of daily trials: although the performance of control and transgenic mice was equal and above chance during the first daily trial, the performance of transgenic mice quickly dropped after the second trial (chance level) and remained low for the remaining trials of the day (as compared to control mice). These results thus showed that inhibition of PP2A decreased both LTD and cognitive flexibility by altering forgetting abilities, leading to impaired performance in a working memory task but not to decreased working memory *per se.* They also suggest that LTD does not play an active role in acquiring information in working memory as previously suggested [40, 53] but does act to extinguish previous irrelevant memories in order to prevent them from interfering with newly learned information.

3.4 Hippocampal LTD and adaptive forgetting

To confirm such role of LTD, we and others proceeded to show that unbalancing the phosphorylation/dephosphorylation equilibrium toward more dephosphorylation, by inhibiting protein kinases, for instance, has the potential to increase LTD, cognitive flexibility, and forgetting. Previous research has provided both pharmacological and genetic evidence for the role of protein kinase A (PKA) in synaptic plasticity and long-term memory formation [56]. In order to specifically study the role of PKA in the hippocampus, we studied a model with a restricted expression of the RIβ regulatory (R(AB)) subunit of PKA to the CA1 area and the dentate gyrus (and superficial cortical layers II and III). This specific inhibition resulted in impaired late-phase LTP in both the dentate gyrus and CA1 regions but spared the CA3 region [57]. Notably, this restricted inhibition also led to an increase in LTD in these areas, with low-frequency stimulation that typically induces short-lasting LTD in control mice initiating a long-lasting form of LTD in the mutant mice. Behaviorally, these mice showed normal performance in the traditional water maze task when trained with four trials per day, a result that can be explained by the fact that repeating trials in a day may provide sufficient training for the mice to alleviate their deficit in PKA-dependent long-term memory [56]. Indeed, when tested with only one trial per day, these mice were not as accurate as controls in locating the exact platform position (although they learned an approximate position). More importantly, when tested 2 weeks later, they were not able to show any remembrance of this position, indicating a deficit in the consolidation of information into long-term memory, a consequence of their impaired LTP [57]. Nevertheless, these transgenic mice also displayed improved performance in other cognitive tasks. They were first shown to be more flexible in a transfer test and thus displayed a net preference as compared to controls for the new platform position after this one had been changed. Strikingly, this enhanced flexibility was accompanied by an increase in performance in various working memory tasks performed in an 8-arms radial maze. As is the case in the water maze or the T-maze, radial maze learning requires the use of spatial orientation and memory (all eight arms being identical, mice have to spatially differentiate them by using distal visual cues). The DNMTP paradigm described before in the T-maze task [54] can also be used in the 8-arms radial maze, permitting alternative use of four different pairs of arms (4 x 2 = 8 arms). This alternative use of four different pairs of arms allowed us to compare mice' performance when these mice were subjected to a low or a high level of interference. When different pairs of arms were used each day for the four daily trials, the level of interference between these four trials was low. This situation thus represented what is called a low level of Interference Working Memory task (or LIWM), each trial being strictly different from one another as they were performed in different pairs of arms. In contrast, when the same pair of arms were used for all trials, the level of interference between these trials was high as the repetitive presentation of the same pair of arms represented conflicting information for the mice. The paradigm thus used was named high level of Interference Working Memory task (or HIWM). Inhibition of PKA in the dentate gyrus and CA1 region increased mutant mice performance compared to the control group, specifically when using the HIWM task [57].

These results suggest that, similarly to its effects on synaptic plasticity, inhibition of PKA alters memory in two opposite ways: first, by decreasing long-term storage/consolidation of information in reference memory, and second, by increasing working memory capacity, specifically when processing a high number of interfering information is required. In agreement with our previous work on PP2A mice [54], the reference memory deficit observed in these R(AB) mice can be attributed to the decrease in LTP and the improved treatment of interference in working memory tasks to LTD persistence. That is to say, LTP and LTD could act as separate and specific mechanisms to support long-term memory and working memory, respectively, as suggested by Tonegawa, Nakao, and their colleagues [40, 53]. Alternatively, LTD and LTP could mechanistically interplay: LTD could function to increase the signal-to-noise ratio between potentiated synapses that participate in a new memory trace (signal) and those that pertain to past – non-relevant – memory information (noise), an idea supported by several studies showing that exposure to new stimuli facilitates stimulus-induced LTD and reverses previously elicited potentiation [51, 58]. If LTD occurs selectively at synapses responsible for encoding information that becomes irrelevant with new learning (such as previous locations of escape platforms in a water maze, or food rewards in a radial maze), then this specificity could explain how information about a location or a task could be modified without affecting unrelated memories. According to this theory, LTD may function to weaken and thus forget previous memory traces, thereby preventing those traces from interfering with newly encoded information when the demands of a task change [25, 54, 57].

4. Molecular mechanisms of forgetting: Later discoveries

4.1 Other synaptic factors involved in the reduced retrievability of memories

Since the demonstration that protein phosphatases can participate in forgetting processes, either passively by opposing the action of protein kinases in memory consolidation [39, 43] or more actively and directly by promoting the removal of previously stored information [54], efforts were made to identify other key synaptic elements contributing to forgetting. Hardt and colleagues thus identified PKM-ζ, another protein kinase synthesized upon LTP induction or memory formation and remaining constitutively active once synthesized and phosphorylated, as a key switch between memory consolidation and forgetting [12]. Transient inhibition of PKM-ζ leads to the extinction of old memories, while its overexpression prolongs weak long-term memories [59]. PKM-ζ would prevent forgetting of these memories by blocking the internalization of GluA2-containing AMPA receptors, especially in the dorsal hippocampus [60]. While early phases of memory formation are characterized by the initial postsynaptic insertion of GluA1-containing AMPA receptors, it is the persistent postsynaptic increase of GluA2 subunits in AMPA receptors that would allow memory to be maintained in the long term [60, 61].

Likewise, learning-induced regulation of NMDA receptor composition has been suggested as a mechanism for preventing further synaptic changes and potential interference, thus contributing to long-term memory stability [62]. NMDA receptors are heteromeric ion channels comprising various subunits (GluN1, GluN2, and GluN3), with GluN2 subunit types (A-D) conferring distinct functional properties to the receptor [63, 64]. GluN2A-containing NMDA receptors have faster kinetics than GluN2B-containing NMDA receptors [63], limiting the time window for detecting presynaptic and postsynaptic coincidence and reducing the likelihood of further synaptic potentiation. If learning increases the ratio of GluN2A/GluN2B-containing NMDA receptors, memory maintenance may result from raising the threshold for additional synaptic strengthening [62]. Eventually, memories could be lost due to a gradual decrease in the GluN2A/GluN2B ratio (as recently shown by [65]) or the inactivation of PKM-ζ, leading to the internalization of GluA2-containing AMPA receptors [60]. Although the role of PKM-ζ in LTP, learning, and memory remains controversial [66], Hardt and colleagues [12] interpret these synaptic changes as evidence of memory loss akin to the idea that synaptic connections weaken over time when memories are not exercised, gradually decaying [67]. A decrease in postsynaptic GluN2A subunit concentration (relative to GluN2B) or the internalization of GluA2-containing AMPA receptors (due to PKM-ζ inactivation) may occur when memory is not reactivated or strengthened over time (suggesting passive forgetting), or when an active signal triggers LTD *via* GluN2B-containing NMDA receptor activation [68]. Hardt and colleagues view this as evidence that forgetting results more from decay than interference, with LTD weakening memory traces.

However, as previously mentioned, interference theory—not mere memory decay—likely explains how memories are forgotten [11]. The theory of memory decay posits that unused information fades over time, whereas interference theory suggests that new information interferes with the recall of past memories. Since interference is unavoidable in daily life, it is difficult to definitively favor one theory over the other. However, our work on mice expressing a PP2A inhibitor suggests that LTD, at least hippocampal NMDA-dependent LTD, plays a specific role in interference-based forgetting rather than simple memory decay [54]. As previously mentioned, these mice exhibit deficits in a reversal task, as they fail to forget irrelevant information about the old platform position in a water maze. These mice persist in revisiting the old position, unlike control animals that adapt by avoiding the old position in favor of the more recent one. However, when trained to learn only one platform position and tested later at different time points (2 and 4 weeks) to assess natural memory decay, PP2A-inhibited mice showed a normal retention curve, performing well at 2 weeks but exhibiting impaired memory after 4 weeks, similar to control mice. These results suggest that (1) the LTD deficit in these animals impairs interference-based forgetting but not time-based memory decay, and (2) these two types of forgetting do not always share the same molecular mechanisms. Moreover, they suggest that phosphatases do not always merely (passively) oppose protein kinases in memory consolidation but may *actively* participate to a dedicated and active/adaptive forgetting system as the one described by Zhong and colleagues in their works on intracellular signals involved in forgetting [69, 70].

These authors identified *Drosophila melanogaster* mutants with enhanced early (short-term) memory, reasoning that this enhancement might result from a defect in forgetting. Upon analyzing these mutants, Rac-signaling genes caught their attention, leading them to investigate Rac's role in forgetting. Rac, a member of the Rho family of small GTPases, regulates cytoskeleton dynamics, potentially facilitating the physiological or morphological changes necessary for erasing memory by influencing activity-dependent structural plasticity [71]. Zhong and colleagues demonstrated that inhibiting Rac activity slows the decay of early memory, extending it from a few hours to over a day. Conversely, increased Rac activity in neurons of the mushroom body (the Drosophila equivalent of the mammalian hippocampus) accelerates memory decay. They also discovered that endogenous Rac activation is more robustly triggered when memory decay is accelerating in normal flies, positioning Rac as a key molecule specifically controlling forgetting. Recent findings in mice further support this hypothesis. Post-training pharmacological inhibition of RAC1 or viral expression of a dominant-negative form of RAC1 in the hippocampus prevents the partial forgetting of contextual memories. Conversely, expressing a constitutively active version of RAC1 accelerates forgetting in these same tasks [72, 73]. These RAC1 changes produce related synaptic effects that can be measured in hippocampal slices, with RAC1 inhibition resulting in prolonged LTP and RAC1 activation leading to synaptic depression/depotentiation [72, 73].

4.2 Neuromodulation, microglia and adult neurogenesis

As mentioned earlier, forgetting can be defined as the reduced retrievability of memories stored in engram cells [7]. So far, we have listed several key intracellular (or membrane-associated) players (phosphatases, AMPA and NMDA receptors, and Rac-signaling genes) able to reduce the strength of excitatory synaptic inputs onto engram cells and the retrieval of their associated memories. We must now consider other/external factors that can have similar roles.

Berry and Davis proposed that dopamine could influence these changes by playing a dual role in memory and forgetting [74]. They observed that while Drosophila's olfactory memory requires dDA1 dopamine receptor activation in the mushroom body, forgetting labile long-term memories was absent in mutant flies lacking another type of dopamine receptor. However, it is GABAergic neuromodulation that has certainly a key role in reducing the accessibility of memories. Numerous studies have demonstrated that GABAergic interneurons shape neuronal activity and play a key role in the formation of neuronal assemblies [75]. In both the hippocampus and neocortex, GABAergic inhibition regulates the induction of LTP [76] and modulates the expression of long-term plasticity [77]. Although their density is significantly lower than that of principal (glutamatergic) neurons, GABAergic interneurons are strategically positioned within cortical networks, allowing them to control neuronal activity effectively [78]. A defining feature of GABAergic interneurons is their division into distinct subgroups, which are located at key points within neuronal assemblies. One subgroup may regulate inputs to principal neurons, while another subgroup of GABAergic interneurons manages their outputs [79].

Parvalbumin-positive basket cells are a prominent type of GABAergic interneuron, delivering strong inhibition to the somas and proximal dendrites of principal neurons. These cells play crucial roles in generating gamma oscillations and coordinating neuronal synchronization. Several studies have identified the role of parvalbumin neurons in the CA1 region in spatial working memory, but not in spatial reference memory [80]. More recently, research has shown that parvalbumin and somatostatin interneurons may have contrasting roles in working memory [81]. Given the involvement of these interneurons in working memory—and the established connection between working memory and forgetting [14]—it can be hypothesized that GABAergic interneurons may also contribute to the inhibition or suppression of hippocampal-dependent long-term memory, thereby playing a role in forgetting. Strengthening inhibitory GABAergic inputs onto excitatory engram cells can silence these cells, rendering them temporarily inaccessible without erasing the plasticity that contributed to the engram formation [7]. This mechanism would allow rapid reversibility under appropriate conditions through targeted disinhibition.

Microglia could also be involved in the reduction of the retrieval of a given memory trace. During brain development, microglia help shape neural circuits by eliminating weaker synaptic connections that have been tagged with complement proteins [82]. Recent research has shown that similar microglia-dependent mechanisms also contribute to natural forgetting in the healthy adult brain [83]. In a series of experiments, mice that were trained in a contextual fear conditioning protocol showed significant forgetting when tested 1 month after training; however, this forgetting was prevented when microglia were pharmacologically or genetically depleted during the retention interval. The observed forgetting was associated with reduced reactivation of tagged hippocampal engram cells, an effect that was also blocked by microglial depletion.

Similarly, the formation of new neurons in the hippocampus (adult neurogenesis) could also reduce the reactivation of tagged hippocampal engram cells. For many years, it was widely believed that the adult mammalian brain could not produce new neurons. However, during the 1990s, this view shifted. The discovery of new neurons in the hippocampus spurred much speculation about the involvement of adult neurogenesis in learning and memory processes [84]. Supporting this notion, studies have shown that suppressing hippocampal neurogenesis typically disrupts memory formation [85], whereas promoting neurogenesis enhances it [86]. Nonetheless, several studies have also explored the role of adult-born hippocampal neurons in forgetting processes. For instance, we first demonstrated that hippocampal neurogenesis could hinder forgetting of proactive interference in working memory [87]. This finding aligns with the recognized role of the dentate gyrus in pattern separation—a process where overlapping or similar representations are transformed into more distinct ones to differentiate between them [88]. However, when processing highly repetitive information in working memory (like it is being done in a HIWM task – [57]), it is unnecessary to differentiate individual trials; rather, past trials must be forgotten to prevent them from interfering with the recall of new ones. By reducing neurogenesis in the dentate gyrus, forgetting proactive interference in working memory could be improved by limiting pattern separation, thereby reducing overlap between neuronal representations of irrelevant past trials [87].

This observation, however, appears to contradict subsequent findings, which indicate that increasing neurogenesis does not impair forgetting or the processing of proactive interference but, in fact, improves it [89, 90]. Consistent with the hypothesis that the addition of new neurons to hippocampal circuits could destabilize existing memories, Frankland and colleagues demonstrated that enhancing neurogenesis after training promoted the forgetting of spatial and contextual remote memories weeks after their formation [90]. They also showed that weakening old memories facilitates the encoding of new, conflicting information, which they described as a reduction in proactive interference [89]. Consequently, these findings seem to contradict our earlier data suggesting that neurogenesis impedes the forgetting of proactive interference in working memory [87]. The key to resolving this contradiction lies in timing. In the short term, neurogenesis confers an advantage in distinguishing highly similar representations in memory (pattern separation) [91], but it counteracts the forgetting required to erase proactive interference (competitive representations) in working memory [87]. Over the long term, however, adult neurogenesis destabilizes older memories [90], thereby enhancing the hippocampus ability to store new memories more effectively [25, 89].

5. Conclusion

In this chapter, we aimed to draw a parallel between forgetting and a process that we believe plays a significant role in the erasure of past memory traces: synaptic depression. Synaptic depression, particularly LTD, would serve two functions: (1) it could facilitate the flexible learning of new information by clearing out previously stored information that is no longer relevant [54, 57], and, paradoxically, (2) it could also enhance memory efficiency by promoting the consolidation of information into semantic memory [12]. For Hardt, Nader, and Nadel, long-term memories gradually shift from being episodic to semantic in nature, as the hippocampal component of these memories fades with time. This episodic-to-semantic transition is similar to context generalization, where behavior initially specific to a particular learning context is eventually expressed in other contexts. Richards and Frankland reviewed evidence suggesting that forgetting may indeed facilitate such generalization by preventing "overfitting" memories to specific past instances that may not accurately predict future outcomes [25]. The concept of overfitting, commonly used in statistics and machine learning, refers to models that are too detailed and complex, fitting the training data so closely that they fail to generalize well to new, unseen data [92]. In other words, overfitting prevents the abstraction of broader rules about the world (semantic memories) by focusing too heavily on the minutiae of specific experiences (episodic memories). Forgetting these details helps to avoid overfitting and promotes the formation of a more adaptable and generalized understanding of the world.

This idea aligns with the trace transformation theory of memory consolidation [93, 94]. According to this theory, episodic memories are initially composed of both central and peripheral details processed by the hippocampus and neocortex. Over time, a more schematic, gist-like version of the memory emerges, retaining only the core elements, which are represented in extra-hippocampal cortical regions. While peripheral details may degrade over time, the detailed episodic memory remains dependent on the hippocampus. Thus, both the detailed episodic memory and the more generalized gist version can coexist, although they exhibit different vulnerabilities to forgetting over time [94]. Although direct evidence linking synaptic depression to the creation of gist-like representations of semantic memory is still limited, Hardt and colleagues showed that preventing forgetting impairs the development of contextual generalization in rats [95]. Under normal conditions, contextual generalization (such as the generalization of fear to environments other than the one originally used for conditioning) can be observed in fear-conditioned rodents tested after a long retention delay [96]. Hardt and colleagues [95] found that inhibiting the endocytosis of hippocampal GluA2-containing AMPA receptors, a molecular mechanism involved in LTD, not only extends the retention of learned tasks over several days but also prevents the gradual development of generalization after conditioning. This result suggests that the same mechanisms responsible for forgetting (LTD) also promote memory generalization. However, although previous studies, including ours, have demonstrated that molecular alterations in LTD-related pathways affect forgetting processes [54, 60, 95], especially in the context of interference processing in working memory [54, 57], direct evidence that forgetting or generalization produces LTD *in vivo* remained elusive.

LTP was discovered 50 years ago and has since drawn substantial interest [97]. Thousands of studies have been conducted on hippocampal LTP, all based on the assumption that LTP reflects a key cerebral mechanism that could potentially explain learning and memory processes. Several studies have thus shown that altering the molecular cascades controlling LTP does also impair learning and memory [98]. However, surprisingly few direct demonstrations have shown that learning actually induces hippocampal LTP [99, 100]. Likewise, until recently, none has shown that forgetting does produce LTD *in vivo*. To palliate this caveat, we conducted a long-term electrophysiological study in freely moving rats to show that cognitive tasks involving forgetting processes do indeed produces LTD in the hippocampus [101]. Rats were trained in a radial maze in either a long-term reference memory task, or one among two different working memory tasks: a low interference (LIWM) or a high interference working memory task (HIWM) involving variable levels of proactive interference (similar to the ones described earlier in this chapter – [30, 57]) that differentially alter their level of performance. Having previously shown that the dentate gyrus of the dorsal hippocampus [31] could play a major role in processing these interferences, we performed long-term recordings of fEPSPs at the perforant path to dentate gyrus synapse during three consecutive days. Our results show that while the efficient processing (forgetting) of proactive interference in WM is correlated to an LTD that is observed immediately after LIWM training, an inefficient processing of these interferences during HIWM training depends on a delayed LTP, probably contributing to the maladaptive consolidation of these interferences in long-term memory, that interferes with the rats' performance in this task the next day. Strikingly, we also found that while reference memory training initially promotes a delayed LTP that is positively correlated with next day performance of the trained rats (confirming the role of hippocampal LTP in Ref. long-term memory), further training in this task replaces this LTP by an LTD once the reference memory rule was fully acquired and semantized, confirming the fact that the hippocampus is not the final resting place of the engram [93] and suggesting that, once consolidated, information about this task could be permanently stored elsewhere (in the neocortex?) [101].

It is possible that this process operates automatically and without conscious awareness [70]. However, it is also conceivable that LTD-dependent forgetting and memory semantization/generalization could be under voluntary control. Motivated forgetting refers to the intentional suppression of memories under cognitive control. This top-down suppression can occur during the retrieval of previously consolidated memories [5]. Research has shown that this suppression is linked to the activity of prefrontal regions involved in resolving retrieval competition during retrieval-induced forgetting. Retrieval-induced forgetting occurs when recalling certain items (e.g., "orange") from a learned category (e.g., "fruit") weakens the recall of other, non-retrieved items (e.g., "apple") from the same category [102]. This type of forgetting suggests that the very act of remembering some memories can be detrimental to others. Anderson and colleagues found that prefrontal areas are engaged in this process, and that activation of these regions predicted later forgetting [5]. These findings highlight a cortical suppression mechanism through which remembering actively shapes which aspects of our past remain accessible. A key question is whether this prefrontal-dependent control can specifically influence our semantic memory by modulating LTD in other brain regions directly involved in memory storage, such as hippocampal-neocortical networks.

Acknowledgements

Our research was supported by grants from *Agence Nationale de la Recherche (ANR-16-CE16-0008-02)*, CNRS (*ATIP* program JP/INSB-2013-211), *Fondation pour la recherche sur le cerveau* (FRC), Rotary Club (*Bourg en Bresse*) and *Région Rhône-Alpes* (ARC2 and *CIBLE* program (RRA Cible #8399265738)).

Conflict of interest

The author declares no conflict of interest.

Author details

Gaël Malleret
Lyon Neuroscience Research Center (CRNL), National Center for Scientific Research (CNRS) Joint Research Unit 5292, National Institute of Health and Medical Research (Inserm) U1028, Claude Bernard University Lyon 1, Bron, France

*Address all correspondence to: gaelmalleret@gmail.com

References

[1] Kandel ER. The molecular biology of memory storage: A dialogue between genes and synapses. Science. 2001;**294**(5544):1030-1038

[2] Miyashita Y. Cognitive memory: Cellular and network machineries and their top-down control. Science. 2004;**306**(5695):435-440

[3] Glannon W. Brain, Body, and Mind. Oxford University Press; 2011

[4] Luria AR. The Mind of a Mnemonist: A Little Book about a Vast Memory. Cambridge, Mass: Harvard University Press; 1987

[5] Wimber M, Alink A, Charest I, Kriegeskorte N, Anderson MC. Retrieval induces adaptive forgetting of competing memories via cortical pattern suppression. Nature Neuroscience. 2015;**18**(4):582-589

[6] Kraemer PJ, Golding JM. Adaptive forgetting in animals. Psychonomic Bulletin & Review. 1997;**4**(4):480-491

[7] Ryan TJ, Frankland PW. Forgetting as a form of adaptive engram cell plasticity. Nature Reviews. Neuroscience. 2022;**23**(3):173-186

[8] Draaisma D. Metaphors of Memory: A History of Ideas about the Mind. Cambridge, U.K.; New York: Cambridge University Press; 2000

[9] Hintzman DL. Robert Hooke's model of memory. Psychonomic Bulletin & Review. 2003;**10**(1):3-14

[10] Jenkins JG, Dallenbach KM. Obliviscence during sleep and waking. The American Journal of Psychology. 1924;**35**:605-612

[11] Wixted JT. The psychology and neuroscience of forgetting. Annual Review of Psychology. 2004;**55**:235-269

[12] Hardt O, Nader K, Nadel L. Decay happens: The role of active forgetting in memory. Trends in Cognitive Sciences. 2013;**17**(3):111-120

[13] Barrouillet P, Portrat S, Camos V. On the law relating processing to storage in working memory. Psychological Review. 2011;**118**(2):175-192

[14] Malleret G, Salin P, Mazza S, Plancher G. Working memory forgetting: Bridging gaps between human and animal studies. Neuroscience and Biobehavioral Reviews. 2024;**163**:105742

[15] Ribot T. Diseases of Memory: An Essay in the Positive Psychology. New York: D. Appleton and company; 1882

[16] James W. The Principles of Psychology. Cambridge (Mass.) London: Harvard University Press; 1981

[17] Bergson H. Rire: Essai Sur la Signification du Comique. Presse Universitaire de France; 1900

[18] Nørby S. Why forget? On the adaptive value of memory loss. Perspectives on Psychological Science : A Journal of the Association for Psychological Science. 2015;**10**(5):551-578

[19] Cammarota M, Bevilaqua LRM, Vianna MRM, Medina JH, Izquierdo I. The extinction of conditioned fear: Structural and molecular basis and therapeutic use. Revista Brasileira de Psiquiatria Sao Paulo Brazil 1999. 2007;**29**(1):80-85

[20] Freud S. In: Freud A, editor. The Standard Edition of the Complete

Psychological Works of Sigmund Freud. London: Hogarth Press; 1953

[21] Myers KM, Davis M. Mechanisms of fear extinction. Molecular Psychiatry. 2007;**12**(2):120-150

[22] Postman L, Underwood BJ. Critical issues in interference theory. Memory & Cognition. 1973;**1**(1):19-40

[23] Melton AW, Irwin JM. The influence of degree of interpolated learning on retroactive inhibition and the overt transfer of specific responses. By Arthur W. Melton, Jean McQueen Irwin, 1940. The American Journal of Psychology. 1987;**100**(3-4):610-641

[24] Underwood BJ. Interference and forgetting. Psychological Review. 1957;**64**(1):49-60

[25] Richards BA, Frankland PW. The persistence and transience of memory. Neuron. 2017;**94**(6):1071-1084

[26] Baddeley A. Working memory: Theories, models, and controversies. Annual Review of Psychology. 2012;**63**:1-29

[27] Dudchenko PA. An overview of the tasks used to test working memory in rodents. Neuroscience and Biobehavioral Reviews. 2004;**28**(7):699-709

[28] Oberauer K, Lewandowsky S. Forgetting in immediate serial recall: Decay, temporal distinctiveness, or interference? Psychological Review. 2008;**115**(3):544-576

[29] Roberts WA, Dale RHI. Remembrance of places lasts: Proactive inhibition and patterns of choice in rat spatial memory. Learning and Motivation. 1981;**12**(3):261-281

[30] Missaire M, Fraize N, Joseph MA, Hamieh AM, Parmentier R, Marighetto A, et al. Long-term effects of interference on short-term memory performance in the rat. PLoS One. 2017;**12**(3):e0173834

[31] Joseph MA, Fraize N, Ansoud-Lerouge J, Sapin E, Peyron C, Arthaud S, et al. Differential involvement of the dentate gyrus in adaptive forgetting in the rat. PLoS One. 2015;**10**(11):e0142065

[32] Tonegawa S, Pignatelli M, Roy DS, Ryan TJ. Memory engram storage and retrieval. Current Opinion in Neurobiology. 2015;**35**:101-109

[33] Semon RW. The Mneme. London, New York: G. Allen & Unwin Ltd.; 1921

[34] Bliss TV, Collingridge GL. A synaptic model of memory: Long-term potentiation in the hippocampus. Nature. 1993;**361**(6407):31-39

[35] Malenka RC, Bear MF. LTP and LTD: An embarrassment of riches. Neuron. 2004;**44**(1):5-21

[36] Frey U, Morris RG. Synaptic tagging and long-term potentiation. Nature. 1997;**385**(6616):533-536

[37] Lisman J, Schulman H, Cline H. The molecular basis of CaMKII function in synaptic and behavioural memory. Nature Reviews. Neuroscience. 2002;**3**(3):175-190

[38] Mansuy IM, Winder DG, Moallem TM, Osman M, Mayford M, Hawkins RD, et al. Inducible and reversible gene expression with the rtTA system for the study of memory. Neuron. 1998;**21**(2):257-265

[39] Malleret G, Haditsch U, Genoux D, Jones MW, Bliss TVP, Vanhoose AM, et al. Inducible and reversible enhancement of learning, memory, and long-term

potentiation by genetic inhibition of Calcineurin. Cell. 2001;**104**(5):675-686

[40] Zeng H, Chattarji S, Barbarosie M, Rondi-Reig L, Philpot BD, Miyakawa T, et al. Forebrain-specific calcineurin knockout selectively impairs bidirectional synaptic plasticity and working/episodic-like memory. Cell. 2001;**107**(5):617-629

[41] Bear MF, Abraham WC. Long-term depression in hippocampus. Annual Review of Neuroscience. 1996;**19**:437-462

[42] Dudek SM, Bear MF. Homosynaptic long-term depression in area CA1 of hippocampus and effects of N-methyl-D-aspartate receptor blockade. Proceedings of the National Academy of Sciences of the United States of America. 1992;**89**(10):4363-4367

[43] Mansuy IM. Calcineurin in memory and bidirectional plasticity. Biochemical and Biophysical Research Communications. 2003;**311**(4):1195-1208

[44] Collingridge GL, Isaac JTR, Wang YT. Receptor trafficking and synaptic plasticity. Nature Reviews. Neuroscience. 2004;**5**(12):952-962

[45] Becker N, Wierenga CJ, Fonseca R, Bonhoeffer T, Nägerl UV. LTD induction causes morphological changes of presynaptic boutons and reduces their contacts with spines. Neuron. 2008;**60**(4):590-597

[46] Morris RG, Anderson E, Lynch GS, Baudry M. Selective impairment of learning and blockade of long-term potentiation by an N-methyl-D-aspartate receptor antagonist, AP5. Nature. 1986;**319**(6056):774-776

[47] Villarreal DM, Do V, Haddad E, Derrick BE. NMDA receptor antagonists sustain LTP and spatial memory: Active processes mediate LTP decay. Nature Neuroscience. 2002;**5**(1):48-52

[48] Tsumoto T. Long-term depression in cerebral cortex: A possible substrate of "forgetting" that should not be forgotten. Neuroscience Research. 1993;**16**(4):263-270

[49] Chen A, Muzzio IA, Malleret G, Bartsch D, Verbitsky M, Pavlidis P, et al. Inducible enhancement of memory storage and synaptic plasticity in transgenic mice expressing an inhibitor of ATF4 (CREB-2) and C/EBP proteins. Neuron. 2003;**39**(4):655-669

[50] Etkin A, Alarcón JM, Weisberg SP, Touzani K, Huang YY, Nordheim A, et al. A role in learning for SRF: Deletion in the adult forebrain disrupts LTD and the formation of an immediate memory of a novel context. Neuron. 2006;**50**(1):127-143

[51] Kemp A, Manahan-Vaughan D. Hippocampal long-term depression and long-term potentiation encode different aspects of novelty acquisition. Proceedings of the National Academy of Sciences of the United States of America. 2004;**101**(21):8192-8197

[52] Olton DS, Papas BC. Spatial memory and hippocampal function. Neuropsychologia. 1979;**17**(6):669-682

[53] Nakao K, Ikegaya Y, Yamada MK, Nishiyama N, Matsuki N. Hippocampal long-term depression as an index of spatial working memory. The European Journal of Neuroscience. 2002;**16**(5):970-974

[54] Nicholls RE, Alarcon JM, Malleret G, Carroll RC, Grody M, Vronskaya S, et al. Transgenic mice lacking NMDAR-dependent LTD exhibit deficits in behavioral flexibility. Neuron. 2008;**58**(1):104-117

[55] Duffy S, Labrie V, Roder JC. D-serine augments NMDA-NR2B receptor-dependent hippocampal long-term depression and spatial reversal learning. Neuropsychopharmacology : Official Publication of the American College of Neuropsychopharmacology. 2008;**33**(5):1004-1018

[56] Abel T, Nguyen PV, Barad M, Deuel TA, Kandel ER, Bourtchouladze R. Genetic demonstration of a role for PKA in the late phase of LTP and in hippocampus-based long-term memory. Cell. 1997;**88**(5):615-626

[57] Malleret G, Alarcon JM, Martel G, Takizawa S, Vronskaya S, Yin D, et al. Bidirectional regulation of hippocampal long-term synaptic plasticity and its influence on opposing forms of memory. Journal of Neuroscience: The Official Journal of the Society for Neuroscience. 2010;**30**(10):3813-3825

[58] Manahan-Vaughan D, Braunewell KH. Novelty acquisition is associated with induction of hippocampal long-term depression. Proceedings of the National Academy of Sciences of the United States of America. 1999;**96**(15):8739-8744

[59] Shema R, Haramati S, Ron S, Hazvi S, Chen A, Sacktor TC, et al. Enhancement of consolidated long-term memory by overexpression of protein kinase Mzeta in the neocortex. Science. 2011;**331**(6021):1207-1210

[60] Migues PV, Hardt O, Wu DC, Gamache K, Sacktor TC, Wang YT, et al. PKMzeta maintains memories by regulating GluR2-dependent AMPA receptor trafficking. Nature Neuroscience. 2010;**13**(5):630-634

[61] Kessels HW, Malinow R. Synaptic AMPA receptor plasticity and behavior. Neuron. 2009;**61**(3):340-350

[62] Quinlan EM, Lebel D, Brosh I, Barkai E. A molecular mechanism for stabilization of learning-induced synaptic modifications. Neuron. 2004;**41**(2):185-192

[63] Monyer H, Sprengel R, Schoepfer R, Herb A, Higuchi M, Lomeli H, et al. Heteromeric NMDA receptors: Molecular and functional distinction of subtypes. Science. 1992;**256**(5060):1217-1221

[64] Vicini S, Wang JF, Li JH, Zhu WJ, Wang YH, Luo JH, et al. Functional and pharmacological differences between recombinant N-methyl-D-aspartate receptors. Journal of Neurophysiology. 1998;**79**(2):555-566

[65] Bessières B, Dupuis J, Groc L, Bontempi B, Nicole O. Synaptic rearrangement of NMDA receptors controls memory engram formation and malleability in the cortex. Science Advances. 2024;**10**(35):eado1148

[66] Tsokas P, Hsieh C, Yao Y, Lesburguères E, Wallace EJC, Tcherepanov A, et al. Compensation for PKMζ in long-term potentiation and spatial long-term memory in mutant mice. eLife. 2016;**5**:e14846

[67] Thorndike EL. Educational Psychology: The Psychology of Learning. Teachers College: Columbia University; 1913

[68] Dalton GL, Wu DC, Wang YT, Floresco SB, Phillips AG. NMDA GluN2A and GluN2B receptors play separate roles in the induction of LTP and LTD in the amygdala and in the acquisition and extinction of conditioned fear. Neuropharmacology. 2012;**62**(2):797-806

[69] Shuai Y, Zhong Y. Forgetting and small G protein Rac. Protein & Cell. 2010;**1**(6):503-506

[70] Davis RL, Zhong Y. The biology of forgetting-a perspective. Neuron. 2017;**95**(3):490-503

[71] Etienne-Manneville S, Hall A. Rho GTPases in cell biology. Nature. 2002;**420**(6916):629-635

[72] Liu Y, Du S, Lv L, Lei B, Shi W, Tang Y, et al. Hippocampal activation of Rac1 regulates the forgetting of object recognition memory. Current Biology : CB. 2016;**26**(17):2351-2357

[73] Hayashi-Takagi A, Yagishita S, Nakamura M, Shirai F, Wu YI, Loshbaugh AL, et al. Labelling and optical erasure of synaptic memory traces in the motor cortex. Nature. 2015;**525**(7569):333-338

[74] Berry JA, Cervantes-Sandoval I, Nicholas EP, Davis RL. Dopamine is required for learning and forgetting in drosophila. Neuron. 2012;**74**(3):530-542

[75] Isaacson JS, Scanziani M. How inhibition shapes cortical activity. Neuron. 2011;**72**(2):231-243

[76] Davies CH, Starkey SJ, Pozza MF, Collingridge GL. GABA autoreceptors regulate the induction of LTP. Nature. 1991;**349**(6310):609-611

[77] Hensch TK. Critical period plasticity in local cortical circuits. Nature Reviews. Neuroscience. 2005;**6**(11):877-888

[78] Klausberger T, Somogyi P. Neuronal diversity and temporal dynamics: The unity of hippocampal circuit operations. Science. 2008;**321**(5885):53-57

[79] Kvitsiani D, Ranade S, Hangya B, Taniguchi H, Huang JZ, Kepecs A. Distinct behavioural and network correlates of two interneuron types in prefrontal cortex. Nature. 2013;**498**(7454):363-366

[80] Murray AJ, Sauer JF, Riedel G, McClure C, Ansel L, Cheyne L, et al. Parvalbumin-positive CA1 interneurons are required for spatial working but not for reference memory. Nature Neuroscience. 2011;**14**(3):297-299

[81] Kim D, Jeong H, Lee J, Ghim JW, Her ES, Lee SH, et al. Distinct roles of Parvalbumin- and somatostatin-expressing interneurons in working memory. Neuron. 2016;**92**(4):902-915

[82] Schafer DP, Lehrman EK, Kautzman AG, Koyama R, Mardinly AR, Yamasaki R, et al. Microglia sculpt postnatal neural circuits in an activity and complement-dependent manner. Neuron. 2012;**74**(4):691-705

[83] Wang C, Yue H, Hu Z, Shen Y, Ma J, Li J, et al. Microglia mediate forgetting via complement-dependent synaptic elimination. Science. 2020;**367**(6478):688-694

[84] Drew LJ, Fusi S, Hen R. Adult neurogenesis in the mammalian hippocampus: Why the dentate gyrus? Learning & Memory (Cold Spring Harbor, N.Y.). 2013;**20**(12):710-729

[85] Saxe MD, Battaglia F, Wang JW, Malleret G, David DJ, Monckton JE, et al. Ablation of hippocampal neurogenesis impairs contextual fear conditioning and synaptic plasticity in the dentate gyrus. Proceedings of the National Academy of Sciences of the United States of America. 2006;**103**(46):17501-17506

[86] Sahay A, Scobie KN, Hill AS, O'Carroll CM, Kheirbek MA, Burghardt NS, et al. Increasing adult hippocampal neurogenesis is sufficient to improve pattern separation. Nature. 2011;**472**(7344):466-470

[87] Saxe MD, Malleret G, Vronskaya S, Mendez I, Garcia AD, Sofroniew MV, et al.

Paradoxical influence of hippocampal neurogenesis on working memory. Proceedings of the National Academy of Sciences of the United States of America. 2007;**104**(11):4642-4646

[88] Colgin LL, Moser EI, Moser MB. Understanding memory through hippocampal remapping. Trends in Neurosciences. 2008;**31**(9):469-477

[89] Epp JR, Silva Mera R, Köhler S, Josselyn SA, Frankland PW. Neurogenesis-mediated forgetting minimizes proactive interference. Nature Communications. 2016;**7**:10838

[90] Akers KG, Martinez-Canabal A, Restivo L, Yiu AP, De Cristofaro A, Hsiang HLL, et al. Hippocampal neurogenesis regulates forgetting during adulthood and infancy. Science. 2014;**344**(6184):598-602

[91] Sahay A, Wilson DA, Hen R. Pattern separation: A common function for new neurons in hippocampus and olfactory bulb. Neuron. 2011;**70**(4):582-588

[92] Hawkins DM. The problem of overfitting. Journal of Chemical Information and Computer Sciences. 2004;**44**(1):1-12

[93] Winocur G, Moscovitch M, Bontempi B. Memory formation and long-term retention in humans and animals: Convergence towards a transformation account of hippocampal-neocortical interactions. Neuropsychologia. 2010;**48**(8):2339-2356

[94] Sekeres MJ, Bonasia K, St-Laurent M, Pishdadian S, Winocur G, Grady C, et al. Recovering and preventing loss of detailed memory: Differential rates of forgetting for detail types in episodic memory. Learning & Memory (Cold Spring Harbor, N.Y.). 2016;**23**(2):72-82

[95] Migues PV, Liu L, Archbold GEB, Einarsson EÖ, Wong J, Bonasia K, et al. Blocking synaptic removal of GluA2-containing AMPA receptors prevents the natural forgetting of long-term memories. Journal of Neuroscience: The Official Journal of the Society for Neuroscience. 2016;**36**(12):3481-3494

[96] Desmedt A, Marighetto A, Piazza PV. Abnormal fear memory as a model for posttraumatic stress disorder. Biological Psychiatry. 2015;**78**(5):290-297

[97] Bliss TV, Lomo T. Long-lasting potentiation of synaptic transmission in the dentate area of the anaesthetized rabbit following stimulation of the perforant path. The Journal of Physiology. 1973;**232**(2):331-356

[98] Kandel ER, Dudai Y, Mayford MR. The molecular and systems biology of memory. Cell. 2014;**157**(1):163-186

[99] Gruart A, Muñoz MD, Delgado-García JM. Involvement of the CA3-CA1 synapse in the acquisition of associative learning in behaving mice. Journal of Neuroscience: The Official Journal of the Society for Neuroscience. 2006;**26**(4):1077-1087

[100] Whitlock JR, Heynen AJ, Shuler MG, Bear MF. Learning induces long-term potentiation in the hippocampus. Science. 2006;**313**(5790):1093-1097

[101] Missaire M, Fraize N, Comte JC, Truchet B, Parmentier R, Salin PA, et al. Working and reference memory tasks trigger opposed long-term synaptic changes in the rat dentate gyrus. Cerebral Cortex (New York, N.Y. : 1991). 2021;**31**(6):2980-2992

[102] Anderson MC, Neely JH. Interference and inhibition in memory retrieval. In: Memory. Elsevier; 1996. pp. 237-313

Chapter 4

Hippocampal Plasticity and Navigational Skills in Blindness

Maxime Bleau, Daniel-Robert Chebat, Fabien C. Schneider and Maurice Ptito

Abstract

Navigation is a fundamental cognitive ability that relies on the hippocampus, a brain region that is known for its role in spatial representation and memory. In individuals with congenital blindness, the absence of visual input leads to significant neuroplastic adaptations that support alternative navigation strategies. This review examines the structural and functional modifications of the hippocampus in individuals who are blind and explores the broader neural mechanisms underlying their spatial abilities. We discuss how cross-modal plasticity repurposes the visual cortex for navigation, the role of sensory substitution devices in facilitating spatial learning, and behavioral performance in navigation tasks. Additionally, we highlight the implications of these findings for assistive technologies and brain-machine interfaces designed to enhance mobility in blind individuals. By synthesizing recent research, this review provides insights into the remarkable adaptability of the brain in response to sensory loss and underscores the importance of understanding neural plasticity for developing effective navigation aids.

Keywords: congenital blindness, navigation, hippocampus, sensory substitution, brain plasticity

1. Introduction

The brain is not a static entity but a dynamic, evolving structure shaped by experience and necessity throughout development [1]. This ability of the brain to adapt, known as *plasticity*, is particularly evident in congenital blindness (CB) and early-onset blindness (EB), in which the absence of visual input triggers extensive neural reorganization to compensate for the missing sense [2]. For clarity in this review, CB and EB are defined as the absence or loss of vision around birth (CB) or before 3 years of age (EB). By this definition, both conditions are often used interchangeably, as CB and EB samples are frequently combined in the reviewed literature. Nonetheless, EB and CB mark a profound change in the subsequent postnatal development of physical and cognitive abilities, with significant repercussions for the brain. This phenomenon is especially prominent in the visual system, particularly in the visual pathways and structures from the retina to the primary visual cortex (V1), which

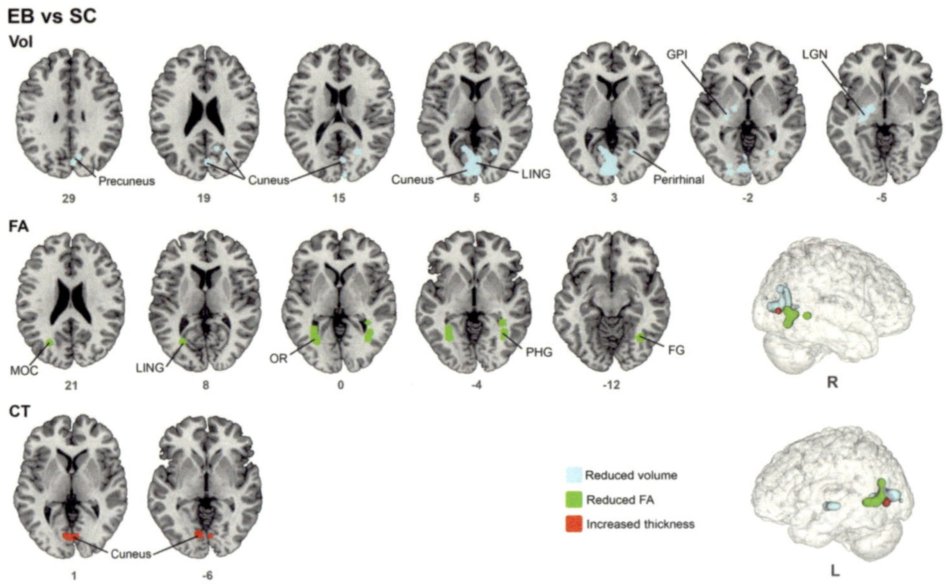

Figure 1.
Structural alterations in the brains of EB (including CB) individuals. Changes in volume (vol), connectivity as measured with fractional anisotropy (FA), and cortical thickness (CT) are consistently recorded in the occipital (visual) cortex and in the retinofugal pathway (optic radiations, lateral geniculate nucleus). FG, fusiform gyrus; GPI, globus pallidus internus; LING, lingual gyrus; MOC, middle occipital cortex; OR, optic radiations; PHG, parahippocampal gyrus.

undergo anatomical and functional modifications to support or enhance nonvisual processing, such as touch, sound, smell, and proprioception. This process is known as cross-modal plasticity [2–4], and it has been vastly studied in numerous samples of CB/EB individuals in the past three decades. The consensus from the literature investigating anatomical and neural connectivity changes in the brains of CB and EB individuals has been reported in a recent meta-analysis study [5]. These differences in terms of volume, fractional anisotropy, and cortical thickness between EB and sighted controls (SC) are illustrated in **Figure 1** and are discussed.

The ability of the brain for cross-modal plasticity is facilitated by a vast array of compensatory strategies and abilities that CB and EB individuals must develop, train, and rely on for everyday tasks. Indeed, by reallocating brain regions typically dedicated to vision, they can accomplish and even reach expertise in many nonvisual tasks, including reading through Braille and spatial navigation using nonvisual aids such as the white cane or other technological devices [for review, see Ref. [6]]. They can also perform spatial tasks and gain knowledge about their environment to orient themselves. This raises an important question: How do parts of the brain, particularly those outside the visual system responsible for spatial cognition and navigation, adapt to the complete loss of visual input? This chapter will explore these areas, notably the hippocampus and its associated navigation network, in both blind and sighted humans and animals.

2. The hippocampus and navigation

In humans, the hippocampus is deeply embedded within the medial temporal lobe and consists of an elongated structure with a club-shaped head resembling a seahorse

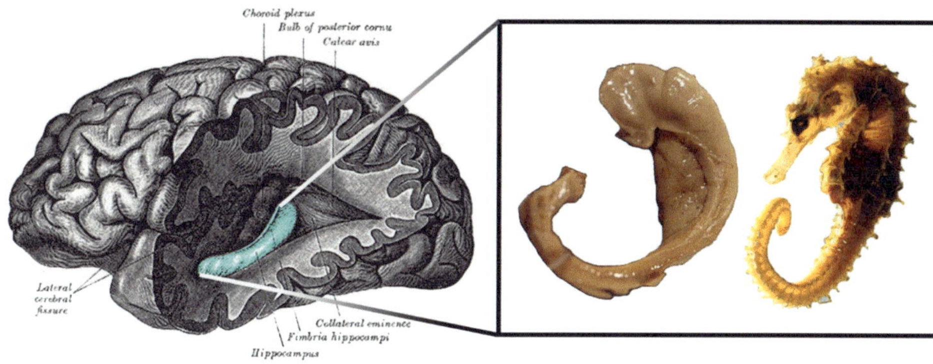

Figure 2.
The human hippocampus in situ. On the left, a drawing by Henry Vandyke Carter from Henry Gray's book, Anatomy of the Human Body *[9]. This illustration depicts the human brain, from which the temporal lobe has been removed, exposing the hippocampus (highlighted in blue). On the right is an ex vivo hippocampus preparation by Laszlo Seress alongside a seahorse (from URL: https://commons.wikimedia.org/wiki/File:Hippocampus_and_seahorse.JPG; under a CC-BY-SA license).*

that begins posterior to the amygdala and arches around the mesencephalon [7, 8]. The hippocampus has two primary gray matter folds: the Cornu Ammonis (CA) fields (hippocampus proper) and the dentate gyrus. Past research has often divided it into three parts: an anterior segment, the head; an intermediate segment, the body; and a posterior segment, the tail (see **Figure 2**).

Functionally, it is highly involved in memory formation, object classification, and motivating complex behaviors such as navigation [10]. Along with its network of other cortical regions, the hippocampus enables humans and other animals to form, through experience-based learning, associations between sensory inputs, objects, and specific locations or events. In that process, they build what is called a "cognitive map" of their environment [11, 12] or a cognitive representation of locations (i.e., a shelter or a food source) and the spatial relationships linking them (i.e., directions, distances, and paths). By using cognitive map-based strategies, humans and animals can adapt to both familiar and new environments and, while in locomotion, keep track of their position in space [13]. This behavior occurs through the continuous comparison of perceived features with prior knowledge embedded in the cognitive map, which is the information ingrained in the neuronal responses of the hippocampus and its network.

2.1 Place cells in the hippocampus

Animal studies have largely demonstrated the critical role played by the hippocampus in spatial navigation. On the one hand, lesion studies in rats have shown that the hippocampus is necessary for solving spatial tasks such as radial mazes [14] and Morris's water maze [15]. On the other hand, most of the knowledge on the functional aspects of the *Hippocampus comes* from electrophysiological recordings, including the pioneering work of O'Keefe and Dostrovsky [16], who first described the presence of "place cells" in this structure. Place cells are widely believed to form the foundation of spatial memory and navigation, as they fire when the animal is in specific "preferred" locations within an environment [12, 17, 18]. Thus, populations of place cells can represent the whole surface of an environment and allow the representation of distances between locations [19, 20]. These internal representations can remain stable for significant periods [21–23], and the hippocampus has been shown to store multiple maps of either different environments or various states of the same environment, with the remapping of the representation of place cells [24]. Furthermore, place cell activity is independent of head direction and visual input [25]. In the absence of visual information, rodents' place cells are modulated by other cues, such as olfaction, path integration, and environmental borders [26–30]. Furthermore, place cell activity is not confined to 2D spaces, as they can encode volumetric space, such as cubic environments [31], which is particularly apparent in flying animals such as bats [32].

Therefore, place cells generate an internal map-like neuronal representation of space, allowing for precise localization and supporting movement planning. The hippocampus has thus been proposed to function as a *memory compression system*, where place cell activity emerges as a byproduct of encoding sensory experiences [33]. This suggests that place cells are influenced by both spatial and nonspatial variables, reflecting recent sensory experiences rather than solely representing static locations. Notably, place cell activity is highly variable and is not only determined by excitatory synaptic inputs. This variability, termed "excess firing variance," suggests that place cells encode additional signals beyond the animal's current head location, contributing to the complexity of spatial representations [34].

2.2 Spatial view cells in primates

In addition to place cells, "spatial view cells" were identified in primates and humans, for whom vision plays a dominant role in spatial processing [35]. Indeed, unlike rodents, which primarily rely on olfactory and/or tactile cues and direct exploration for path integration [36], humans and primates primarily use visual landmarks to navigate from one location to another [37]. Therefore, spatial view cells are known to respond to specific parts of the environment being viewed, regardless of the observer's own location or gaze direction [35]. In other words, spatial cells encode spatial information in a "world-centered" or "allocentric" (independent of the individual's position and point of view) reference frame. This characteristic is fundamental to supporting landmark-based navigation, a key strategy in primates, as it allows for stable object location encoding and, thus, visual landmark recognition [38]. These cells also participate in episodic memory formation, as they provide spatial context for remembering where events occurred and how to move through an environment [35, 39]. This suggests that spatial view cells play a more dominant role in primates than in other mammals [38], but their function may vary across species due to differences in sensory reliance.

Spatial view cells receive input from the ventral visual stream and parietal cortex, which provide detailed information about the visual scene [38]. Through these cells, the hippocampus can integrate sensory information from the visual and parietal cortices to construct a spatial framework for efficient navigation and memory organization [38]. However, even without direct visual input, spatial view cells help maintain an accurate sense of location by updating spatial representations through self-motion cues [38]. This property is beneficial when environmental details are obscured and allows individuals to orient themselves effectively [40].

2.3 Navigation-relevant cells beyond the hippocampus: An interconnected network

The hippocampus, while important, does not function alone but is part of a network of interconnected cortical and subcortical structures. As such, hippocampal

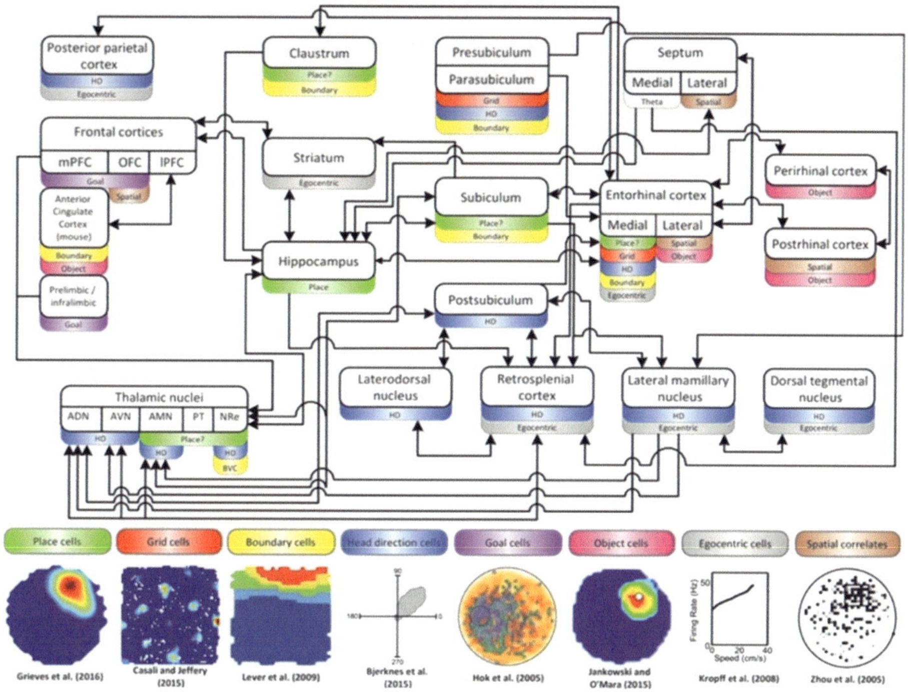

Figure 3.
The different types of neurons engaged in navigation and their location and connectivity in the rodent brain. This schematic illustrates the navigation network in rodents and depicts all the interconnected regions involved in processing navigation-relevant information. The types of cells found in each of these regions are also depicted, including those mentioned in this chapter (place cells, grid cells, head direction cells, and boundary cells). Figure from Ref. [25], reprinted with permission (license no. 6015990335147, Elsevier).

place cells interact closely with grid cells, primarily situated in the entorhinal cortex [41]. This special type of cell provides spatial metrics for place cells in the hippocampus, as they encode specific locations in an environment according to a hexagonal grid system [25]. The combined function of grid and place cells is essential for precise navigation, particularly in complex or cluttered environments [42]. Moreover, to facilitate complex spatial behaviors, these cells also interact with other specialized neurons, such as whole-body motion cells and head direction cells, which, as their name suggests, are sensitive to the facing direction [43]. While most come from animal studies, recent work on human neuronal recordings has confirmed the existence of place cells [44] and grid cells in humans [45]. **Figure 3** illustrates the various types of navigation-relevant cells in the hippocampus and other structures.

2.4 The hippocampus in humans: Neuroimaging and lesion studies

In humans, the role of the hippocampus became explicitly clear following original reports and studies investigating patients with temporal lesions, including the famous patient HM [46]. Following the removal of the medial temporal lobe (including the hippocampus), HM experienced profound memory loss and severe impairment in spatial cognition. Particularly, HM's spatial navigation and spatial memory abilities, strategies now known to be dependent on the hippocampus, were severely affected [47]. Subsequently, exhaustive work using neuroimaging techniques such as PET, fMRI, and

MEG has also demonstrated the critical involvement of the hippocampus in spatial navigation, particularly in the encoding, processing, and retrieval of spatial information, supporting cognitive map formation and wayfinding [for a review, see 48]. Hippocampal activity, mostly in its posterior part, has been found to correlate with Euclidean distances between locations [48, 49] and to be engaged during directional responses in early learning phases [50], mental navigation [51], virtual navigation [52], and other spatial tasks such as path integration and distance judgments [49, 53, 54]. Furthermore, lesion studies validate its role in encoding spatial locations within an allocentric framework: damage to this structure impairs spatial memory, thus preventing individuals from forming or retrieving cognitive maps [55–57]. More recently, studies involving intracranial recordings [58] further demonstrate how the human hippocampus encodes one's location in an environment [59–62] and constructs internal models of space, reflected in its oscillatory patterns, which bear striking similarities to those found in rodents [59, 63, 64].

Therefore, research supports the idea that the hippocampus is essential for allocentric, cognitive map-based navigational strategies rather than egocentric strategies. There is a clear distinction between these two forms of navigation. "Response-based" navigation (mostly reliant on the egocentric reference frame) is governed by the caudate nucleus and not the hippocampus. In contrast to the hippocampus, the caudate nucleus plays a role in procedural learning, enabling navigation through learned sequences of actions [65, 66].

2.5 The broader human navigation network (HNN)

The role of the hippocampus in cognitive map formation and navigation is possible through its interactions with other brain regions, which are also known for their space-related activity. Navigation research constantly shows the involvement of multiple structures in the medial temporal lobe, the (pre)frontal cortex, and the parietal cortex, including parts of the dorsal and ventral visual streams [67]. This network of spatially involved areas is now commonly referred to as the human navigation network (HNN). Most importantly, a meta-analysis of the navigation literature has highlighted that most navigation tasks consistently activate three key regions of this network [68]: the parahippocampal place area (PPA) situated in the parahippocampal gyrus (PHG), the retrosplenial complex (RSC)—or "medial place area" (MPA)—and the occipital place area (OPA). These regions are scene-selective areas that, as the name suggests, are primarily sensitive to the viewing of scenes containing context for spatial navigation, such as landmarks, edges, and paths [54, 68–70]. The PPA specializes in analyzing spatial properties of the immediate environment and responds strongly to navigationally relevant landmarks [71, 72]. In contrast, the RSC plays a key role in situating local scenes within a broader spatial context, translating egocentric information (from the parietal cortex) into an allocentric reference frame [72, 73]. The RSC is also sensitive to directional cues at decision points [50] and encodes information about an individual's position and heading, functioning similarly to head direction cells in rodents [74, 75]. As for the OPA, its role may be more perceptive, as it is sensitive to scene information that forms key aspects to guide navigation, such as edges and materials [69, 76]. Furthermore, the hippocampus collaborates with the entorhinal cortex to encode spatial features and environmental cues, thereby forming cognitive maps [41, 68]. Indeed, as part of the HNN, the entorhinal cortex retains its grid-like coding in humans, as proved by many studies, which demonstrated a "hexadirectional" coding that corresponds to the hexagonal grid built by grid cells [77, 78].

Finally, the HNN also includes parts of the parietal, frontal, and prefrontal cortices, forming a separate system to dictate how individuals can interact with the local environment [79]. Contrary to the scene-selective regions that contribute to the "allocentric" representations of space for more long-distance navigation, the posterior parietal cortex is involved in perceiving space according to an egocentric point of view, in other words, the individual's point of view [80, 81]. The parietal cortex, therefore, mediates interactions with the local environment and enables humans (and other animal species) to select and perform actions (i.e., walking, leaping, climbing, reaching, grasping, and bringing objects to the mouth) that are relevant to the contextual environment. The parietal cortex also closely interacts with the prefrontal cortex, including the frontal eye fields, to direct attention and make decisions. In short, this frontoparietal system is central in spatial navigation as it is sensitive to all kinds of affordances (i.e., objects/landmarks to reach, objects to grasp, obstacles to avoid, salient visual targets to look at) present in the local environment, and it specifies all potential actions (grasping position, direction of locomotion, obstacle avoidance strategy) that are available to the individual [79]. Furthermore, the prefrontal cortex, as part of the HNN, is also crucial for route planning, memory retrieval, maintaining goals in working memory, and integrating input from the PHG [82–84]. These characteristics allow the brain to compare sensory inputs to learned rules and, thus, to predict upcoming landmarks and guide decisions and route selection by dynamically retrieving relevant spatial memories [80, 82].

2.6 The stream of visual information from V1 to the hippocampus

In summary, although they are not visual processing areas *per se*, the hippocampus and HNN play a crucial role in processing sensory information relevant to space, memory, and scene recognition to support spatial navigation, including locomotion and, on a larger scale, spatial orientation. Indeed, navigation-relevant visual information from V1 is distributed to higher-order areas through many interconnected paths, or visual streams. Traditionally, there are two visual streams: the dorsal stream ("where" pathway), which sends visual information for integration in the posterior parietal cortex, involved in spatial awareness and motion, and the ventral stream ("what" pathway), which sends information to the inferotemporal cortex for object recognition. However, regions in the HNN make a second, more medial "where" visual stream that funnels scene- and navigation-relevant information from the visual cortex to the hippocampus, passing through the RSC, PHG, and entorhinal cortex [85–87].

Indeed, scene information is passed from the RSC to the medial temporal lobe, where it is integrated by the PPA and the perirhinal cortex, which plays a key role in object memory [88]. Visual information is then transmitted from these regions to the entorhinal cortex, the primary interface between the neocortex and the hippocampus. This structure conveys contextual spatial (medial entorhinal) and object-related (lateral entorhinal) information to the hippocampus through the tri-synaptic circuit [89]: from the entorhinal cortex to the dentate gyrus (DG), to CA3 via mossy fibers, from CA3 to CA1 via Schaffer collaterals, and to the subiculum, which sends projections back to the entorhinal and other brain regions. Through this circuitry, the hippocampus and HNN support the encoding, consolidation, and retrieval of spatial memory via the visual sensory channel. Additionally, feedback loops from the hippocampus to the entorhinal, prefrontal, and posterior parietal cortices allow it to modulate ongoing visual processing, attention, and decision-making.

2.7 Multisensory integration and plasticity in the hippocampus

To conclude this part of the chapter, it is important to recognize two key aspects of the hippocampus and its capacity to form cognitive maps. First, the hippocampus does not construct cognitive maps by solely relying on visual cues but rather through multisensory integration, in other words, by synthesizing external visual, auditory, and tactile cues and internal proprioceptive and vestibular inputs [67, 90, 91]. All animals, including humans, navigate in multisensory environments and are thus guided by ever-changing spatial information from these sensory inputs. To achieve this, the hippocampus creates a map of space that combines different sensory and abstract reference frames, and this mapping is influenced by behavioral goals and the sensory modalities used [92, 93].

Second, the hippocampus can be considered a hub for neuronal plasticity, i.e., the ability of neurons and, consequently, the brain to change their connections and functions over time and in response to contextual needs. Not only has the hippocampus been shown to be one of the rare regions with neurogenesis, or the generation of new neuronal cells [94], but it is also prone to significant morphological changes dependent on the environment and the individual's experiences [95]. Indeed, in one of the most influential works in human navigation, Maguire and Gadian [96] have shown volumetric variations in the posterior hippocampus linked to navigation expertise, as seen in London taxi drivers and students undergoing spatial inference training [96, 97]. This morphological adaptation highlights that functional plasticity in the hippocampus follows environmental demands and navigational experience, or in more technical terms, plasticity is "experience-dependent."

3. The hippocampus in individuals with congenital blindness

Due to the reliance of humans and other primates on visual cues for navigation, many questions remain unanswered. What occurs in the hippocampus following complete vision loss? How does it adapt to the loss of the most essential input for navigation and orientation? As we know, congenital blindness leads to some of the most significant behavioral adaptations observed in humans. Individuals who are congenitally blind develop compensatory strategies for spatial navigation, relying on alternative sensory inputs and increasing their dependence on memory capacities, which suggests certain hippocampal adaptations. While research has consistently shown that the absence of visual input leads to structural alterations in the visual parts of the brain [2], only a handful of studies have paid closer attention to the hippocampus [5, 98].

3.1 Anatomical and functional changes in the hippocampus

Most notably, structural neuroimaging studies focusing on hippocampal differences between blind and sighted individuals have revealed that CB individuals exhibit a smaller right posterior hippocampus [99, 100] and/or a larger right anterior hippocampus compared to sighted individuals (see **Figure 4**) [100–102]. Furthermore, hippocampal size in CB correlated with wayfinding performance in a maze task [101] and with their learning rate in an obstacle course using a sensory substitution device [103]. Finally, a comprehensive meta-analysis of brain structural changes associated with blindness highlighted a few alterations in the hippocampal formation [5], but no

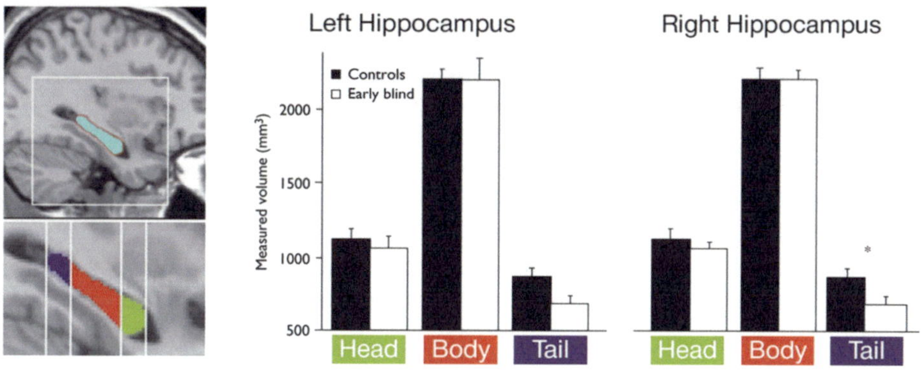

Figure 4.
Example of volumetric changes in the hippocampus of early blind individuals. The posterior (tail) part of the right hippocampus is reduced in volume. Modified, with permission, from Chebat et al., [99].

clear consensus in the literature, which suggests a high interindividual variability in the hippocampal morphometry that is not solely a byproduct of visual deprivation.

As with anatomical studies, a limited body of research has examined the functional reorganization of the hippocampus in blindness [98]. However, those who attempted this endeavor have found that it is still involved in spatial processing and navigation tasks. For example, the hippocampus in CB individuals is involved when they solve tactile mazes and improve their performance over time [104] and when they estimate Euclidean distances using auditory cues [105]. Furthermore, more recent work has investigated the neural patterns associated with cognitive map formation and found no hippocampal adaptation differences between blind and sighted participants while learning a tactile map [106]. These results strongly suggest that the function of the hippocampus is preserved and flexible enough to support spatial cognition, cognitive map formation, and navigation strictly through alternative sensory channels [107]. This flexibility is highlighted in the functional connectivity of the hippocampus in CB, which is increased with many parts of the brain [108, 109]. These include cortical areas such as the primary visual cortex, parts of the ventral and dorsal visual streams, and, most importantly, other areas of the HNN [108, 109], an aspect that may facilitate the processing and integration of nonvisual cues for navigation.

In the animal literature, however, a little more is known about neuronal and molecular changes at the level of the hippocampus following sensory loss [110]. Most notably, blindness is associated with a decreased GABA receptor expression and altered metabotropic glutamate receptor expression, including a reduced expression of the GluN1 subunit and an altered GluN2A:GluN2B ratio [110–113]. This shows that, on a molecular level, the hippocampus seems to revert to a state similar to a critical period, typically recorded between birth and 3 months of age, and is maintained this way throughout adulthood, showing no evidence of full functional recovery [112, 114]. These molecular changes have also been recorded along with a chronic impairment in hippocampal synaptic plasticity, specifically long-term potentiation, throughout adulthood, which only exhibits partial recovery as animals get older [111–113]. Interestingly, at the level of the place cells' response, EB rats exhibit hippocampal place cells that display location-specific firing patterns, similarly to those found in sighted rats [26]. This preservation indicates that vision is not essential for the establishment of the place cells network and that motion-related information and nonvisual stimuli are sufficient to support place cell activity in the absence of visual cues [26].

3.2 The HNN in blindness

While results on the hippocampus are scarce, most research has investigated how areas in the HNN respond to nonvisual spatial cues, including auditory, tactile, and proprioceptive information. These studies highlight the activation of scene-selective PPA and RSC during haptic exploration of scenes [115], when differentiating large nonmanipulable objects (i.e., landmarks) from small objects and non-objects [116], and in a mental navigation task [117]. These activations in CB were either similar to those in sighted individuals [117] or stronger [115, 116]. Furthermore, the parahippocampal gyrus, likely including the PPA, is also involved in tactile maze navigation

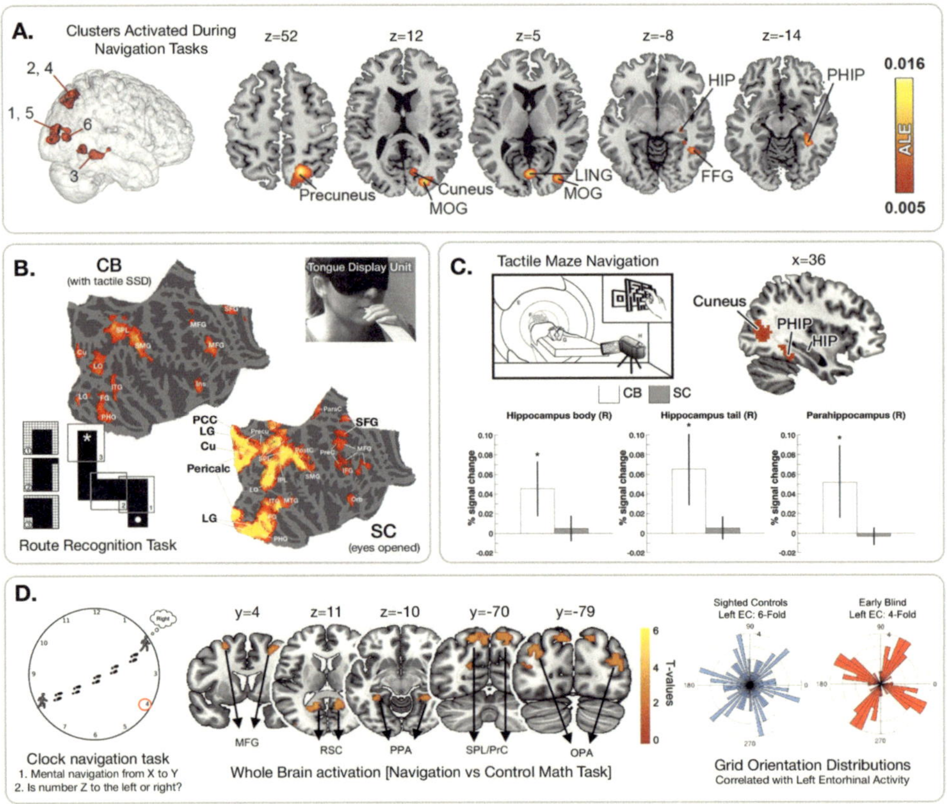

Figure 5.
The hippocampus and Human Navigation Network (HNN) are involved in spatial navigation tasks in CB/EB individuals. A. A meta-analysis of the neuroimaging literature revealed consistent clusters of activation, including parietal and medial temporal cortices, in blind individuals. Clusters include the visual cortex (clusters 1, 5, and 6; cuneus, MOG, and LING), the parietal cortex [clusters 2 and 4; precuneus and superior parietal lobule (SPL)], and the (medial) temporal cortex (cluster 3; FFG, PHIP, and HIP). Adapted from Bleau et al., [98], under a CC BY 4.0 license. B. The HNN is involved in virtual route recognition using a sensory substitution device (SSD). Modified, with permission, from Kupers et al., [118]. C. The hippocampus (HIP) and para-hippocampus (PHIP) are recruited during tactile maze navigation in CB. Adapted, with permission, from Gagnon et al., 2012 [104]. D. The HNN is consistently activated during a clock navigation task, but the entorhinal cortex shows an altered grid-like coding pattern, four-fold instead of six-fold (in sighted individuals). Adapted from Sigismondi et al., 2024 [117], under a CC BY 4.0 license. CB, congenitally blind; Cu, cuneus; FFG, fusiform gyrus; HIP, hippocampus; LING, lingual gyrus; MFG, middle frontal gyrus; MOG, middle occipital gyrus; OPA, occipital place area; PCC, posterior parietal cortex; Pericalc, pericalcarine; PHIP, parahippocampal gyrus; PPA, parahippocampal place area; PrC, precuneus; RSC, retrosplenial complex; SC, sighted controls; SPL, superior parietal lobule.

[104], route recognition using a visual-to-tactile sensory substitution device [118], and material discrimination (an essential aspect of nonvisual navigation) with the use of echolocation in the case of CB expert echolocators [119]. Furthermore, the OPA in CB is activated in mental [117] and echolocation-guided navigation [120]. These scene-selective regions in CB, along with the ventral and dorsal visual streams, also benefit from increased functional connectivity with each other [108, 116] and, as previously said, with the hippocampus [108].

Beyond these scene-processing areas, other areas of the HNN in the parietal, temporal, and frontal cortices are still activated in navigation and spatial processing tasks in CB [98, 117, 118]. The parietal cortex is associated with Euclidean distance estimation via auditory cues [105] and nonvisual route recognition [118], while the temporal-parietal junction is active during virtual navigation using tactile and auditory feedback [121, 122] in a way that reflects the general navigation skills of CB individuals [122]. In the temporal cortex, the superior temporal gyrus is activated in imagined locomotion [123], while the entorhinal cortex remains involved in mental navigation [117]. However, the hexadirectional grid-like coding in the entorhinal cortex is altered in CB individuals, exhibiting a four-fold rather than a six-fold symmetry [117]. This functional change may be linked to the adoption of different navigational strategies, such as relying on 90-degree turns to avoid disorientation [117]. Finally, prefrontal areas and parts of the ventral and dorsal streams, such as the precuneus, fusiform gyrus, and lateral occipital cortex, still emerge as involved in spatial processing and navigation tasks [98, 117–119, 124]. **Figure 5** illustrates the neural network involved in nonvisual spatial navigation in CB.

The recruitment of these multiple cortical regions across different sensory modalities in both CB and sighted individuals suggests that the HNN is, on the one hand, commonly solicited for the processing of multisensory spatial information to support navigation in humans and, on the other hand, resilient to the complete loss of visual input [117]. These findings align with the hypothesis of amodal spatial representations, which stipulates that those representations, including cognitive maps, are constructed with inputs from multiple senses but stored in a modality-independent manner [98, 125]. These functional aspects of the hippocampus and HNN are essential for blind individuals to maintain efficient levels of spatial competence despite the absence of visual input.

4. Navigation abilities in the blind

4.1 Behavioral performance in navigation tasks and enhanced nonvisual abilities

As previously mentioned, CB individuals can learn various compensatory strategies to retain spatial awareness, navigate safely, and learn the layout of their environment for orientation, thereby preserving function throughout the HNN in the process. However, the volume alterations in CB may reflect high variability in those compensatory strategies and their travel habits, as it has been evidenced that hippocampal size is a reliable predictor of navigation abilities in humans [126].

Navigating the environment requires the ability to perceive and respond to external cues [127], and evidence suggests that blindness leads to the enhancement of nonvisual abilities, as they often outperform sighted controls in auditory and tactile tasks of spatial and nonspatial nature. Indeed, CB individuals often exhibit superior auditory localization skills [128–130], which also correlates with activation in the visual cortex [129]. Furthermore, they can, with the use of sensory substitution devices (SSDs), locate and avoid obstacles as efficiently or better than blindfolded sighted individuals using tactile or auditory information [131–137], sometimes even performing as well as non-blindfolded sighted individuals using vision [138]. However, other studies suggest that EB exhibits impairments in other auditory and proprioceptive spatial tasks [139–143]. As for spatial navigation itself, the literature provides no clear consensus. Some studies find that CB can navigate their surroundings as effectively as sighted individuals using assistive technologies or can even outperform them in simple obstacle avoidance [133, 135, 138, 144] or in nonvisual path integration [145]. However, when it comes to "allocentric" navigation, studies show that blind individuals are either equivalent to their sighted counterparts or that they fail to achieve the same level of proficiency [104, 106, 146–153]. **Figure 6ABC** illustrates performances of CB in spatial navigation tasks involving the allocentric reference frame such as maze learning and mental navigation in a clock task.

Hence, there is no denying that CB leads to complex behavioral changes that vary according to the types of paradigms, contextual cues, and different factors, including age, gender, blindness onset, travel habits, expertise with assistive technology, and specialized mobility training [154–156]. Nevertheless, the cognitive mapping abilities associated with the hippocampus exhibit significant variability in CB, likely resulting from the diverse adaptive strategies and compensatory skills developed in response to the complete loss of visual input. Indeed, CB individuals increase their reliance on egocentric strategies, such as route following, instead of allocentric ones, an adaptation from which may stem the recorded structural alterations in the hippocampus. Additional research is necessary to explore ways to enhance CB individuals' access to spatial information and improve their cognitive mapping abilities [154, 156]. As an example, Bleau and van Acker [152] have shown that increasing the amount of available information in accessible tactile maps can eliminate the differences in cognitive mapping performances between CB individuals, sighted individuals, and those who have late-onset blindness (individuals who had prior visual experience).

4.2 Impact of sensory substitution devices

Sensory substitution devices (SSDs) convert visual information into auditory or tactile feedback to support blind individuals in navigating their environment or accomplishing other tasks such as reading or recognizing objects [6]. The incorporation of SSDs into the daily lives of blind individuals not only offers insights into how perceptual learning and cross-modal plasticity occur [155] but also how it is possible to augment perception and spatial awareness in this population to better support nonvisual navigation. Some SSDs, such as the EyeCane [137], have been developed specifically to support efficient navigation by providing spatial information in a form that the brain can easily interpret [121]. By converting spatial information (e.g., the presence and distance of obstacles and walls) directly into auditory or tactile cues, they can provide real-time feedback about the environment, its content, and its layout, and help blind individuals avoid obstacles and make navigation decisions [134, 144].

Indeed, CB participants navigating with the tongue display unit (TDU), a visual-to-tactile SSD, can detect and avoid obstacles and achieve a significantly faster pace than blindfolded sighted individuals performing the same tasks in the same conditions [138]. **Figure 6DEF** illustrates spatial navigation abilities of CB using SSDs. In their utilization, these devices engage, through cross-modal

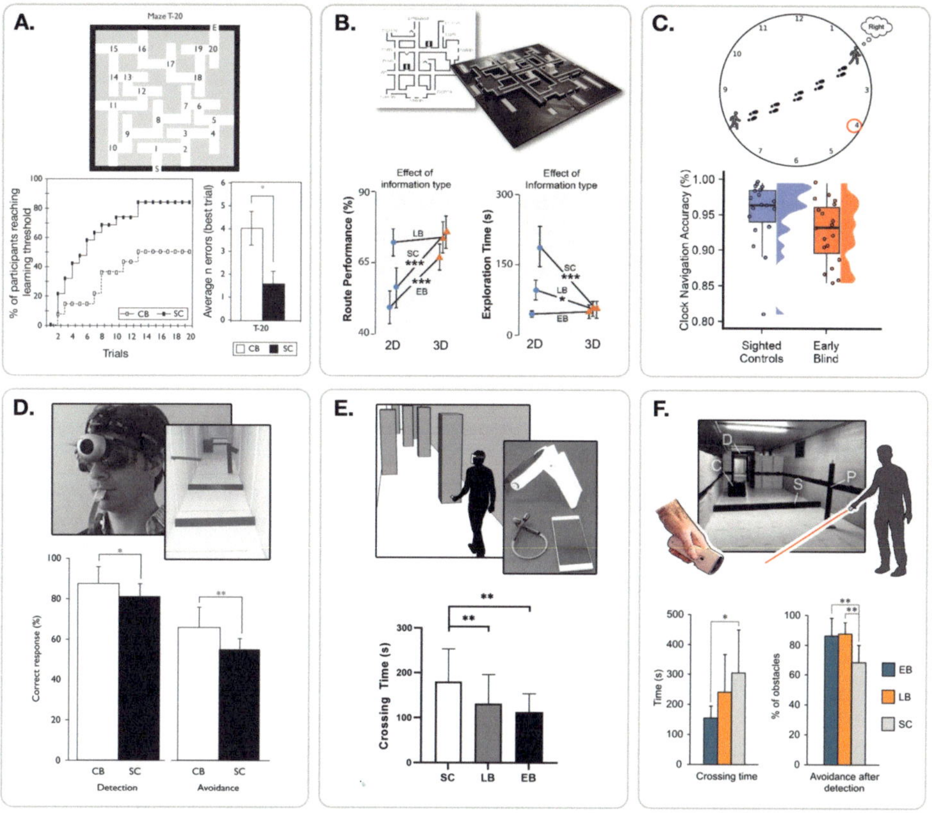

Figure 6.
Behavioral performances of CB and sighted individuals in navigation tasks involving sensory substitution. A. CB makes more errors in tactile maze solving and learns the task at a lower rate than their sighted counterparts. Adapted, with permission, from Gagnon et al., 2010 [153]. B. When using a 3D tactile maze instead of a 2D embossed tactile maze, CB, LB, and sighted individuals form equivalent cognitive maps, enabling them to improvise routes between points of interest. Adapted from Bleau et al., [152], under a CC BY 4.0 license. C. CB performs worse than sighted individuals in a clock navigation task involving allocentric spatial coding. Adapted from Sigismondi et al., 2023 [117], under a CC BY 4.0 license. D-E-F. CB outperform sighted individuals in navigation tasks involving detecting and avoiding obstacles using tactile and auditory sensory substitution devices, such as the tongue display unit (D; adapted, with permission, from Chebat et al., [133], the auditory GSSD (E; adapted from Paré et al., [135], under a CC BY 4.0 license), and the EyeCane (F; adapted from Bleau et al., [134], under a CC BY 4.0 license). CB, congenitally blind; EB, early blind; LB, late blind; SC, sighted controls; T-20, maze with 20 T-shaped intersections.

plasticity, brain areas typically associated with vision, including the primary visual cortex, and other higher-order areas involved in motion, shape, and spatial perception, including the area HMT+, lateral occipital cortex, and area V6 [118, 121, 157]. These devices and how the CB brain adapts to use them suggest that blind individuals utilize the same brain regions typically involved in vision to process spatial information from other senses [158, 159].

SSDs thus have the potential to increase spatial awareness when combined with—not without—more traditional navigational aids (i.e., white cane or guide dog) to make navigation safer and more effective [134]. These insights from SSDs have other practical implications. They suggest that training programs and assistive technologies designed for blind individuals can and should capitalize on the brain's capacity for cross-modal plasticity [160]. By enhancing the use of nonvisual cues for navigation, it may be possible to further augment the adaptive changes in the brain and provide additional spatial information to the hippocampus and its network, thus better supporting the development of spatial abilities in the process.

4.3 Future research directions and potential applications

As technology advances, new and improved SSDs and brain-machine interfaces (BMIs) will likely play an even greater role in enhancing navigation capabilities and promoting independence for individuals living with blindness. Indeed, our growing understanding of the brain's capacity to reconfigure itself in response to changes in sensory input has implications for both theoretical neuroscience and practical applications, such as the development of neuroscience-based training programs and refined SSDs. Indeed, currently available or tested SSDs still require significant training and time for users to process environmental data efficiently. Studies have shown that training for relatively simple tasks or environments with optimal contrast and minimal complexity takes long hours [6, 155]. Further research is needed to optimize these devices for greater accuracy and ease of use. Improving SSDs with AI to provide intelligible and customized feedback, tailored to the task and user's needs, will become crucial in making SSDs more widely adopted as augmented reality tools.

BMIs, on the other hand, hold great potential for the more seamless integration of assistive feedback into the brain's navigation networks and even directly into the hippocampus to trigger spatial learning. However, challenges remain in making these devices widely accessible, as they require complex hardware and software, as well as a deep understanding of the brain's neural pathways related to spatial cognition. Continued advancements in neurotechnology, signal processing, and cross-modal plasticity will be crucial in making BMIs a more viable and practical tool for aiding navigation in individuals who are blind. Moreover, integrating SSDs and BMIs could hold the key to further enhancing navigational independence.

Further studies are needed to refine their usability and efficacy in real-world settings. Research should also explore how training with these technologies can further enhance brain plasticity and improve cognitive mapping abilities. In that same goal, virtual reality and virtual environments could be beneficial when combined with more sensory substitution capacities. Additionally, longitudinal studies on the long-term effects of sensory substitution and BMIs on brain plasticity are essential. These studies could provide valuable insights into the sustained benefits of assistive technologies for blind individuals and their impact on cognitive functions such as memory, attention, and spatial reasoning.

5. Conclusion

Blindness is associated with significant structural and functional alterations induced by brain plasticity, particularly in regions traditionally associated with vision. Studies highlight how the visual cortex, through cross-modal plasticity, is repurposed for non-visual processing to improve compensatory skills and support spatial navigation in blind individuals. Beyond the visual system, areas associated with navigation and spatial awareness, including the hippocampus, maintain their function by processing and integrating information from multiple senses. However, structural changes in the hippocampus are linked to behavioral changes and high variability in compensatory strategies used for daily orientation, a sphere where blind individuals often develop deficits that limit their independence. To aid in improving navigational and cognitive mapping skills, new technology such as sensory substitution devices, AI, augmented reality, and even brain-machine interfaces can play a pivotal role by providing real-time, refined, and contextualized sensory feedback and feeding it to neural networks mediating these abilities.

Acknowledgements

This work was supported by the Canadian Institutes of Health Research (CIHR; 163014-2019: MP) and scholarships from the CIHR (MB) and the Centre Interdisciplinaire de Recherche sur le Cerveau et l'Apprentissage (CIRCA), University of Montreal (MB).

Conflict of interest

The authors declare no conflict of interest.

Author details

Maxime Bleau[1*], Daniel-Robert Chebat[2], Fabien C. Schneider[3] and Maurice Ptito[2,4,5]

1 École d'optométrie, Université de Montréal, Québec, Canada

2 Visual and Cognitive Neuroscience Laboratory (VCN Lab), The Department of Psychology, Ariel University, Ariel, Israel

3 Université Jean Monnet Saint-Etienne, CHU Saint-Etienne, Unité de recherche TAPE, Saint-Etienne, France

4 Department of Applied Mathematics and Computer Science, Visual Computing, Danish Technical University, Lyngby, Denmark

5 Faculté de Médecine, Institute of Neuroscience (IoNS), Université Catholique de Louvain (UCL), Brussels, Belgium

*Address all correspondence to: maxime.bleau.1@umontreal.ca

References

[1] Torres RF et al. Environmental enrichment and epigenetic changes in the brain: From the outside to the deep inside. In: van Zundert B, Montecino M, editors. Neuroepigenetics Mechanisms in Health and Disease. Cham: Springer Nature Switzerland; 2025. pp. 217-230

[2] Kupers R, Ptito M. Compensatory plasticity and cross-modal reorganization following early visual deprivation. Neuroscience & Biobehavioral Reviews. 2014;**41**:36-52

[3] Sadato N et al. Activation of the primary visual cortex by braille reading in blind subjects. Nature. 1996;**380**(6574):526-528

[4] Zhang C et al. Properties of cross-modal occipital responses in early blindness: An ALE meta-analysis. NeuroImage: Clinical. 2019;**24**:102041

[5] Paré S et al. Brain structural changes in blindness: A systematic review and an anatomical likelihood estimation (ALE) meta-analysis. Neuroscience & Biobehavioral Reviews. 2023;**150**:105165

[6] Ptito M et al. Brain-machine interfaces to assist the blind. Frontiers in Human Neuroscience. 2021;**15**:46

[7] Anand KS, Dhikav V. Hippocampus in health and disease: An overview. Annals of Indian Academy of Neurology. 2012;**15**(4):239-246

[8] Dekeyzer S et al. "Unforgettable" – A pictorial essay on anatomy and pathology of the hippocampus. Insights Into Imaging. 2017;**8**(2):199-212

[9] Gray H. Anatomy of the human body. Annals of Surgery. 1918;**68**(5):564-566

[10] Stella F et al. Self-organization of multiple spatial and context memories in the hippocampus. Neuroscience & Biobehavioral Reviews. 2012;**36**(7):1609-1625

[11] Tolman EC. Cognitive maps in rats and men. Psychological Review. 1948;**55**(4):189

[12] O'Keefe J, Nadel L. The Hippocampus as a Cognitive Map. Oxford, England: Clarendon Press; 1978

[13] Golledge RG. Wayfinding Behavior: Cognitive Mapping and Other Spatial Processes. Baltimore, US: JHU Press; 1999

[14] Olton DS, Walker JA, Gage FH. Hippocampal connections and spatial discrimination. Brain Research. 1978;**139**(2):295-308

[15] Morris RGM et al. Place navigation impaired in rats with hippocampal lesions. Nature. 1982;**297**(5868):681-683

[16] O'Keefe J, Dostrovsky J. The hippocampus as a spatial map: Preliminary evidence from unit activity in the freely-moving rat. Brain Research. 1971;**34**:171-175

[17] O'Keefe J. A review of the hippocampal place cells. Progress in Neurobiology. 1979;**13**(4):419-439

[18] O'Keefe J, Conway DH. Hippocampal place units in the freely moving rat: Why they fire where they fire. Experimental Brain Research. 1978;**31**(4):573-590

[19] O'Keefe J. Place units in the hippocampus of the freely moving rat. Experimental Neurology. 1976;**51**(1):78-109

[20] Wilson MA, McNaughton BL. Reactivation of hippocampal ensemble memories during sleep. Science. 1994;**265**(5172):676-679

[21] Hill AJ. First occurrence of hippocampal spatial firing in a new environment. Experimental Neurology. 1978;**62**(2):282-297

[22] Muller RU, Kubie JL, Ranck JB. Spatial firing patterns of hippocampal complex-spike cells in a fixed environment. Journal of Neuroscience. 1987;7(7):1935-1950

[23] Thompson LT, Best PJ. Long-term stability of the place-field activity of single units recorded from the dorsal hippocampus of freely behaving rats. Brain Research. 1990;**509**(2):299-308

[24] Colgin LL, Moser EI, Moser M-B. Understanding memory through hippocampal remapping. Trends in Neurosciences. 2008;**31**(9):469-477

[25] Grieves RM, Jeffery KJ. The representation of space in the brain. Behavioural Processes. 2017;**135**:113-131

[26] Save E et al. Spatial firing of hippocampal place cells in blind rats. Journal of Neuroscience. 1998;**18**(5):1818-1826

[27] Save E, Nerad L, Poucet B. Contribution of multiple sensory information to place field stability in hippocampal place cells. Hippocampus. 2000;**10**(1):64-76

[28] Quirk GJ, Muller RU, Kubie JL. The firing of hippocampal place cells in the dark depends on the rat's recent experience. Journal of Neuroscience. 1990;**10**(6):2008-2017

[29] Zhang S et al. Spatial representations of place cells in darkness are supported by path integration and border information. Frontiers in Behavioral Neuroscience. 2014;**8**:222

[30] Markus EJ et al. Spatial information content and reliability of hippocampal CA1 neurons: Effects of visual input. Hippocampus. 1994;**4**(4):410-421

[31] Grieves RM et al. The place-cell representation of volumetric space in rats. Nature Communications. 2020;**11**(1):789

[32] Ulanovsky N, Moss CF. Hippocampal cellular and network activity in freely moving echolocating bats. Nature Neuroscience. 2007;**10**(2):224-233

[33] Benna MK, Fusi S. Place cells may simply be memory cells: Memory compression leads to spatial tuning and history dependence. Proceedings of the National Academy of Sciences. 2021;**118**(51):e2018422118

[34] Fenton AA, Muller RU. Place cell discharge is extremely variable during individual passes of the rat through the firing field. Proceedings of the National Academy of Sciences. 1998;**95**(6):3182-3187

[35] Rolls ET. Spatial view cells and the representation of place in the primate hippocampus. Hippocampus. 1999;**9**(4):467-480

[36] Rowland DC, Yanovich Y, Kentros CG. A stable hippocampal representation of a space requires its direct experience. Proceedings of the National Academy of Sciences. 2011;**108**(35):14654-14658

[37] Ekstrom AD. Why vision is important to how we navigate. Hippocampus. 2015;**25**(6):731-735

[38] Rolls ET. Hippocampal spatial view cells for memory and navigation, and

their underlying connectivity in humans. Hippocampus. 2023;**33**(5):533-572

[39] Georges-François P, Rolls ET, Robertson RG. Spatial view cells in the primate hippocampus: Allocentric view not head direction or eye position or place. Cerebral Cortex. 1999;**9**(3):197-212

[40] Robertson RG, Rolls ET, Georges-François P. Spatial view cells in the primate hippocampus: Effects of removal of view details. Journal of Neurophysiology. 1998;**79**(3):1145-1156

[41] Neupane S, Fiete I, Jazayeri M. Mental navigation in the primate entorhinal cortex. Nature. 2024;**630**(8017):704-711

[42] Moser EI, Kropff E, Moser M-B. Place cells, grid cells, and the brain's spatial representation system. Annual Review of Neuroscience. 2008;**31**:69-89

[43] Taube JS. Head direction cells and the neurophysiological basis for a sense of direction. Progress in Neurobiology. 1998;**55**(3):225-256

[44] Ekstrom AD et al. Cellular networks underlying human spatial navigation. Nature. 2003;**425**(6954):184-188

[45] Jacobs J et al. Direct recordings of grid-like neuronal activity in human spatial navigation. Nature Neuroscience. 2013;**16**(9):1188-1190

[46] Scoville WB, Milner B. Loss of recent memory after bilateral hippocampal lesions. Journal of Neurology, Neurosurgery, and Psychiatry. 1957;**20**(1):11

[47] Bohbot V, Iaria G, Petrides M. Hippocampal function and spatial memory: Evidence from functional neuroimaging in healthy participants and performance of patients with medial temporal lobe resections. Neuropsychology. 2004;**18**(3):418-425

[48] Morgan LK et al. Distances between real-world locations are represented in the human hippocampus. Journal of Neuroscience. 2011;**31**(4):1238-1245

[49] Howard LR et al. The hippocampus and entorhinal cortex encode the path and Euclidean distances to goals during navigation. Current Biology. 2014;**24**(12):1331-1340

[50] Wolbers T, Büchel C. Dissociable retrosplenial and hippocampal contributions to successful formation of survey representations. Journal of Neuroscience. 2005;**25**(13):3333-3340

[51] Ghaem O et al. Mental navigation along memorized routes activates the hippocampus, precuneus, and insula. Neuroreport. 1997;**8**(3):739-744

[52] Maguire EA et al. Knowing where and getting there: A human navigation network. Science. 1998;**280**(5365):921-924

[53] Wolbers T et al. Differential recruitment of the hippocampus, medial prefrontal cortex, and the human motion complex during path integration in humans. Journal of Neuroscience. 2007;**27**(35):9408-9416

[54] Ziegler MG et al. Differential involvement of the anterior and posterior hippocampus, parahippocampus, and retrosplenial cortex in making precise judgments of spatial distance and object size for remotely acquired memories of environments and objects. Cerebral Cortex. 2023;**33**(18):10139-10154

[55] Bohbot VD et al. Spatial memory deficits in patients with lesions to the right hippocampus

and to the right parahippocampal cortex. Neuropsychologia. 1998;**36**(11):1217-1238

[56] Abrahams S et al. Spatial memory deficits in patients with unilateral damage to the right hippocampal formation. Neuropsychologia. 1997;**35**(1):11-24

[57] Feigenbaum JD, Morris RG. Allocentric versus egocentric spatial memory after unilateral temporal lobectomy in humans. Neuropsychology. 2004;**18**(3):462

[58] Axmacher N. Intracranial EEG: A Guide for Cognitive Neuroscientists. Berlin, Germany: Springer Nature; 2023

[59] Seeber M et al. Human neural dynamics of real-world and imagined navigation. Nature Human Behaviour. 2025;**9**(4):781-793

[60] Stangl M et al. Boundary-anchored neural mechanisms of location-encoding for self and others. Nature. 2021;**589**(7842):420-425

[61] Liu J et al. Multi-scale goal distance representations in human hippocampus during virtual spatial navigation. Current Biology. 2023;**33**(10):2024-2033

[62] Huang Z et al. Human hippocampal theta oscillations organise distance to goal coding. bioRxiv. 2024:2024.12.12.628182

[63] Bohbot VD et al. Low-frequency theta oscillations in the human hippocampus during real-world and virtual navigation. Nature Communications. 2017;**8**(1):14415

[64] Seger SE et al. Memory-related processing is the primary driver of human hippocampal theta oscillations. Neuron. 2023;**111**(19):3119-3130

[65] Iaria G et al. Cognitive strategies dependent on the hippocampus and caudate nucleus in human navigation: Variability and change with practice. Journal of Neuroscience. 2003;**23**(13):5945-5952

[66] Bohbot VD et al. Caudate nucleus-dependent response strategies in a virtual navigation task are associated with lower basal cortisol and impaired episodic memory. Neurobiology of Learning and Memory. 2011;**96**(2):173-180

[67] Ekstrom AD, Arnold AEGF, Iaria G. A critical review of the allocentric spatial representation and its neural underpinnings: Toward a network-based perspective. Frontiers in Human Neuroscience. 2014;**8**:803

[68] Epstein RA et al. The cognitive map in humans: Spatial navigation and beyond. Nature Neuroscience. 2017;**20**(11):1504-1513

[69] Epstein RA, Baker CI. Scene perception in the human brain. Annual Review of Vision Science. 2019;**5**(1):373-397

[70] Marchette SA et al. Outside looking in: Landmark generalization in the human navigational system. The Journal of Neuroscience. 2015;**35**(44):14896

[71] Epstein R, Kanwisher N. A cortical representation of the local visual environment. Nature. 1998;**392**(6676):598-601

[72] Epstein RA. Parahippocampal and retrosplenial contributions to human spatial navigation. Trends in Cognitive Sciences. 2008;**12**(10):388-396

[73] Alexander AS et al. Rethinking retrosplenial cortex: Perspectives and predictions. Neuron. 2023;**111**(2): 150-175

[74] Shine JP et al. The human retrosplenial cortex and thalamus code head direction in a global reference frame. Journal of Neuroscience. 2016;**36**(24):6371-6381

[75] Lu Z et al. A neural compass in the human brain during naturalistic virtual navigation. bioRxiv. 2024:2024.04.18.590112

[76] Julian JB et al. The occipital place area is causally involved in representing environmental boundaries during navigation. Current Biology. 2016;**26**(8):1104-1109

[77] Nau M et al. Hexadirectional coding of visual space in human entorhinal cortex. Nature Neuroscience. 2018;**21**(2):188-190

[78] Wagner IC et al. Entorhinal grid-like codes and time-locked network dynamics track others navigating through space. Nature Communications. 2023;**14**(1):231

[79] Cisek P. Evolution of behavioural control from chordates to primates. Philosophical Transactions of the Royal Society B: Biological Sciences. 2021;**377**(1844):20200522

[80] Moghadam M, Towhidkhah F, Gharibzadeh S. A fuzzy-oscillatory model of medial prefrontal cortex control function in spatial memory retrieval in human navigation function. Frontiers in Systems Neuroscience. 2022;**16**:972985

[81] Galati G et al. The neural basis of egocentric and allocentric coding of space in humans: A functional magnetic resonance study. Experimental Brain Research. 2000;**133**:156-164

[82] Spiers HJ. Keeping the goal in mind: Prefrontal contributions to spatial navigation. Neuropsychologia. 2008;**46**(7):2106-2108

[83] Patai EZ, Spiers HJ. The versatile Wayfinder: Prefrontal contributions to spatial navigation. Trends in Cognitive Sciences. 2021;**25**(6):520-533

[84] Das A, Menon V. Replicable patterns of causal information flow between hippocampus and prefrontal cortex during spatial navigation and spatial–verbal memory formation. Cerebral Cortex. 2022;**32**(23):5343-5361

[85] Rolls ET et al. A ventromedial visual cortical 'where' stream to the human hippocampus for spatial scenes revealed with magnetoencephalography. Communications Biology. 2024;**7**(1):1047

[86] Read M-L et al. Multimodal MEG and Microstructure–MRI investigations of the human hippocampal scene network. The Journal of Neuroscience. 2025;**45**(22):e1700242025

[87] Rah YJ, Shin JH, Lee SA. The visual scene network and hippocampus represent spatial boundary structures for temporal episodic memory organization. Journal of Cognitive Neuroscience. 2025:1-16. Available from: https://direct.mit.edu/jocn/article-abstract/doi/10.1162/jocn_a_02229/123925/The-Visual-Scene-Network-and-Hippocampus-Represent?redirectedFrom=fulltext

[88] Burke SN et al. Shared functions of Perirhinal and Parahippocampal cortices: Implications for cognitive aging. Trends in Neurosciences. 2018;**41**(6):349-359

[89] Ben-Simon Y et al. A direct excitatory projection from entorhinal layer 6b neurons to the hippocampus contributes to spatial coding and memory. Nature Communications. 2022;**13**(1):4826

[90] Taube JS, Valerio S, Yoder RM. Is navigation in virtual reality with fMRI really navigation? Journal of Cognitive Neuroscience. 2013;**25**(7):1008-1019

[91] Jeffery KJ. Integration of the sensory inputs to place cells: What, where, why, and how? Hippocampus. 2007;**17**(9):775-785

[92] Radvansky BA et al. Behavior determines the hippocampal spatial mapping of a multisensory environment. Cell Reports. 2021;**36**(5):109444

[93] Park SA et al. Map making: Constructing, combining, and inferring on abstract cognitive maps. Neuron. 2020;**107**(6):1226-1238.e8

[94] Kempermann G et al. Human adult neurogenesis: Evidence and remaining questions. Cell Stem Cell. 2018;**23**(1):25-30

[95] Boecker H et al. Hippocampal subfield plasticity is associated with improved spatial memory. Communications Biology. 2024;**7**(1):271

[96] Maguire EA et al. Navigation-related structural change in the hippocampi of taxi drivers. Proceedings of the National Academy of Sciences. 2000;**97**(8):4398-4403

[97] Woollett K, Maguire EA. Acquiring "the knowledge" of London's layout drives structural brain changes. Current Biology. 2011;**21**(24):2109-2114

[98] Bleau M et al. Neural substrates of spatial processing and navigation in blindness: An activation likelihood estimation meta-analysis. Frontiers in Neuroscience. 2022;**16**:1010354

[99] Chebat DR et al. Alterations in right posterior hippocampus in early blind individuals. Neuroreport. 2007;**18**(4):329-333

[100] Lepore N et al. Pattern of hippocampal shape and volume differences in blind subjects. NeuroImage. 2009;**46**(4):949-957

[101] Fortin M et al. Wayfinding in the blind: Larger hippocampal volume and supranormal spatial navigation. Brain. 2008;**131**(11):2995-3005

[102] Pan N et al. Morphometry difference of the hippocampal formation between blind and sighted individuals. Frontiers in Neuroscience. 2021;**15**:715749

[103] Chebat DR, Schneider FC, Ptito M. Neural networks mediating perceptual learning in congenital blindness. Scientific Reports. 2020;**10**:495. DOI: 10.1038/s41598-019-57217-w

[104] Gagnon L et al. Activation of the hippocampal complex during tactile maze solving in congenitally blind subjects. Neuropsychologia. 2012;**50**(7):1663-1671

[105] Chan CC et al. Cross auditory-spatial learning in early-blind individuals. Human Brain Mapping. 2012;**33**(11):2714-2727

[106] Ottink L et al. Mental maps without vision: Neural signatures of cognitive maps based on haptic input in the hippocampal formation. bioRxiv. 2023:2023.10.20.563338

[107] Ottink L et al. Cognitive map formation supported by auditory, haptic, and multimodal information in persons with blindness. Neuroscience & Biobehavioral Reviews. 2022;**140**:104797

[108] Qin W et al. Functional connectivity density in congenitally and late

blind subjects. Cerebral Cortex. 2015;**25**(9):2507-2516

[109] Ma G, Yang D, Qin W, Liu Y, Jiang T, Yu C. Enhanced functional coupling of hippocampal sub-regions in congenitally and late blind subjects. Frontiers in Neuroscience. 2017;**10**:612

[110] Desgent S, Ptito M. Cortical GABAergic interneurons in cross-modal plasticity following early blindness. Neural Plasticity. 2012;**2012**(1):590725

[111] Hagena H, Feldmann M, Manahan-Vaughan D. Lifelong changes of neurotransmitter receptor expression and debilitation of hippocampal synaptic plasticity following early postnatal blindness. Scientific Reports. 2022;**12**(1):9142

[112] Feldmann M et al. Early loss of vision results in extensive reorganization of plasticity-related receptors and alterations in hippocampal function that extend through adulthood. Cerebral Cortex. 2019;**29**(2):892-905

[113] Beckmann D et al. Hippocampal synaptic plasticity, spatial memory, and neurotransmitter receptor expression are profoundly altered by gradual loss of hearing ability. Cerebral Cortex. 2020;**30**(8):4581-4596

[114] Quinlan EM, Olstein DH, Bear MF. Bidirectional, experience-dependent regulation of N-methyl-D-aspartate receptor subunit composition in the rat visual cortex during postnatal development. Proceedings of the National Academy of Sciences. 1999;**96**(22):12876-12880

[115] Wolbers T et al. Modality-independent coding of spatial layout in the human brain. Current Biology. 2011;**21**(11):984-989

[116] He C et al. Selectivity for large nonmanipulable objects in scene-selective visual cortex does not require visual experience. NeuroImage. 2013;**79**:1-9

[117] Sigismondi F et al. Altered grid-like coding in early blind people. Nature Communications. 2024;**15**(1):3476

[118] Kupers R et al. Neural correlates of virtual route recognition in congenital blindness. Proceedings of the National Academy of Sciences. 2010;**107**(28):12716

[119] Milne JL et al. Parahippocampal cortex is involved in material processing via echoes in blind echolocation experts. Vision Research. 2015;**109**:139-148

[120] Norman LJ, Thaler L. The occipital place area is recruited for echo-acoustically guided navigation in blind human echolocators. The Journal of Neuroscience. 2023;**43**(24):4470

[121] Aggius-Vella E et al. Activation of human visual area V6 during egocentric navigation with and without visual experience. Current Biology. 2023;**33**(7):1211-1219.e5

[122] Halko MA et al. Real world navigation Independence in the early blind correlates with differential brain activity associated with virtual navigation. Human Brain Mapping. 2014;**35**(6):2768-2778

[123] Deutschlander A et al. Imagined locomotion in the blind: An fMRI study. NeuroImage. 2009;**45**(1):122-128

[124] Struiksma ME et al. Spatial language processing in the blind: Evidence for a supramodal representation and cortical reorganization. PLoS One. 2011;**6**(9):e24253

[125] Loomis JM et al. Spatial working memory for locations specified by vision and audition: Testing the amodality hypothesis. Attention, Perception, & Psychophysics. 2012;**74**(6):1260-1267

[126] Schinazi VR et al. Hippocampal size predicts rapid learning of a cognitive map in humans. Hippocampus. 2013;**23**(6):515-528

[127] Wolbers T, Hegarty M. What determines our navigational abilities? Trends in Cognitive Sciences. 2010;**14**(3):138-146

[128] Voss P et al. Early- and late-onset blind individuals show supra-normal auditory abilities in far-space. Current Biology. 2004;**14**(19):1734-1738

[129] Gougoux F et al. A functional neuroimaging study of sound localization: Visual cortex activity predicts performance in early-blind individuals. PLoS Biology. 2005;**3**(2):e27

[130] Doucet ME et al. Blind subjects process auditory spectral cues more efficiently than sighted individuals. Experimental Brain Research. 2005;**160**(2):194-202

[131] Segond H, Weiss D, Sampaio E. Human spatial navigation via a visuo-tactile sensory substitution system. Perception. 2005;**34**(10):1231-1249

[132] Auvray M, Myin E. Perception with compensatory devices: From sensory substitution to sensorimotor extension. Cognitive Science. 2009;**33**(6):1036-1058

[133] Chebat D-R et al. Navigation with a sensory substitution device in congenitally blind individuals. Neuroreport. 2011;**22**(7):342-347

[134] Bleau M et al. Blindness and the reliability of downwards sensors to avoid obstacles: A study with the EyeCane. Sensors (Basel). 2021;**21**(8):2700

[135] Paré S et al. Spatial navigation with horizontally spatialized sounds in early and late blind individuals. PLoS One. 2021;**16**(2):e0247448

[136] Stoll C et al. Navigating from a depth image converted into sound. Applied Bionics and Biomechanics. 2015;**2015**:543492

[137] Maidenbaum S et al. The "EyeCane", a new electronic travel aid for the blind: Technology, behavior & swift learning. Restorative Neurology and Neuroscience. 2014;**32**(6):813-824

[138] Chebat D-R, Maidenbaum S, Amedi A. Navigation using sensory substitution in real and virtual mazes. PLoS One. 2015;**10**(6):e0126307

[139] Cappagli G, Gori M. Auditory spatial localization: Developmental delay in children with visual impairments. Research in Developmental Disabilities. 2016;**53-54**:391-398

[140] Gori M, Amadeo MB, Campus C. Spatial metric in blindness: Behavioural and cortical processing. Neuroscience and Biobehavioral Reviews. 2020;**109**:54-62

[141] Gori M et al. Impairment of auditory spatial localization in congenitally blind human subjects. Brain. 2014;**137**(Pt. 1):288-293

[142] Zwiers MP, Van Opstal AJ, Cruysberg JR. A spatial hearing deficit in early-blind humans. The Journal of Neuroscience : The Official Journal of the Society for Neuroscience. 2001;**21**(9):RC142: 1-RC142: 5

[143] Lewald J. Opposing effects of head position on sound localization

in blind and sighted human subjects. European Journal of Neuroscience. 2002;**15**(7):1219-1224

[144] Buchs G et al. Waist-up protection for blind individuals using the EyeCane as a primary and secondary mobility aid. Restorative Neurology and Neuroscience. 2017;**35**(2):225-235

[145] Loomis JM et al. Nonvisual navigation by blind and sighted: Assessment of path integration ability. Journal of Experimental Psychology: General. 1993;**122**(1):73

[146] Fortin M et al. Impact of vision on the development of topographical orientation abilities. Neuroreport. 2006;**17**(4):443-446

[147] Pasqualotto A et al. Visual experience facilitates allocentric spatial representation. Behavioural Brain Research. 2013;**236**:175-179

[148] Iachini T, Ruggiero G, Ruotolo F. Does blindness affect egocentric and allocentric frames of reference in small and large scale spaces? Behavioural Brain Research. 2014;**273**:73-81

[149] Ruggiero G, Ruotolo F, Iachini T. How ageing and blindness affect egocentric and allocentric spatial memory. Quarterly Journal of Experimental Psychology. 2021;**75**(9):1628-1642. 17470218211056772

[150] Ruggiero G, Ruotolo F, Iachini T. Congenital blindness limits allocentric to egocentric switching ability. Experimental Brain Research. 2018;**236**(3):813-820

[151] Ottink L et al. Cognitive map formation through tactile map navigation in visually impaired and sighted persons. Scientific Reports. 2022;**12**(1):11567

[152] Bleau M et al. Cognitive map formation in the blind is enhanced by three-dimensional tactile information. Scientific Reports. 2023;**13**(1):9736

[153] Gagnon L et al. Tactile maze solving in congenitally blind individuals. Neuroreport. 2010;**21**(15):989-992

[154] Schinazi VR, Thrash T, Chebat DR. Spatial navigation by congenitally blind individuals. Wiley Interdisciplinary Reviews: Cognitive Science. 2016;**7**(1):37-58

[155] Chebat D-R et al. Sensory substitution and the neural correlates of navigation in blindness. In: Pissaloux E, Velazquez R, editors. Mobility of Visually Impaired People: Fundamentals and ICT Assistive Technologies. Berlin, GE: Springer International Publishing; 2018. pp. 167-200

[156] Giudice NA. Navigating without vision: Principles of blind spatial cognition. In: Handbook of Behavioral and Cognitive Geography. Cheltenham, UK: Edward Elgar Publishing; 2018

[157] Ptito M et al. Recruitment of the middle temporal area by tactile motion in congenital blindness. Neuroreport. 2009;**20**(6):543-547

[158] Proulx MJ et al. Multisensory perceptual learning and sensory substitution. Neuroscience & Biobehavioral Reviews. 2014;**41**:16-25

[159] Saccone EJ, Tian M, Bedny M. Developing cortex is functionally pluripotent: Evidence from blindness. Developmental Cognitive Neuroscience. 2024;**66**:101360

[160] Chebat D-R, Schneider FC, Ptito M. Spatial competence and brain plasticity in congenital blindness via sensory substitution devices. Frontiers in Neuroscience. 2020;**14**:815

Chapter 5

Perspective Chapter: Hippocampus and Limbocortical Networks in Emotional Regulation and Functional Neurological Disorders

Nick Tsarouchas, Nicholas Tsarouchas and Constantin Tsarouchas

Abstract

The hippocampus constitutes a core component of the most extensive integrated network of the human brain, the limbocortical network, involved in memory, learning processes, and emotional and behavioral regulation. In this essay, we model the limbocortical network and demonstrate by means of dynamic modular neuronal networks the role of the hippocampus in emotional regulation. The hippocampus is a hub integrated within small-to-large scale neuronal networks through reciprocal excitatory and inhibitory connections, and positive and negative feedback loops, driving oscillatory behaviour in neuronal assemblies. The hippocampal formation, the circuit of Papez and the limbocortical network, are the integral components of large-scale brain networks (default-mode, salience, attention, executive) that underpin higher-order cognitive, emotional, and behavioral functions. Emotions or 'e-motions' are more than just cognitive and affective appraisals, they represent dynamic drives that set human behavior into motion. From an evolutionary perspective, emotions act as homeostatic mechanisms to balance and regulate the internal and external environments of organisms, crucial for the survival and reproduction of the individual and the species. Emotions have evolved in the social mammalian brain, reaching incredible richness and complexity that drives communication, learning, imagination and social interaction—all aspects of human life, behavior and culture. The superposition and competition of emotional states, multimodal sensory integration with episodic memories and motor behaviors, defines a unique abstract perception of psychosocial space, flow of time and sense of self for every human individual. Emotional dysregulation is associated with misperceptions or distortions, biases and prediction errors of the self and the world, resulting in psychological or psychiatric and functional neurological disorders.

Keywords: hippocampus, limbic system, limbocortical networks, memory, emotion, emotional regulation, oscillopathies, movement disorders, functional neurological disorders, post-traumatic stress disorders, behavioral disorders, emotional dysregulation, default mode network, salience network, central executive network, learning, cognition, oscillations, neurology, neurophysiology

 IntechOpen

1. Introduction

The limbocortical network, the brain's most extensive and integrated network, is at the core of memory and learning processes and the regulation of emotions and behavior. It serves as a framework for large-scale neuronal communication by intertwining diverse inputs from various cortical areas within limbic circuits. This integration enables the network-level storage, processing, and representation of information, which, in turn, allows for the emergence of higher-order systemic properties underpinning complex cognitive and emotional processes that ultimately govern motor and behavioral output [1]. The limbic system (integral part of the limbocortical network) is composed of cortical and subcortical components.

Cortical components of the limbic system include the hippocampus, which is essential for memory formation, spatial navigation, and time perception; the amygdala, which is pivotal in processing emotions, particularly fear and pleasure; and the cingulate gyrus, which plays a critical role in emotional regulation, linking behavioral outcomes to motivation. The parahippocampal gyrus contributes to memory encoding and retrieval, while the subcallosal gyrus and the orbitofrontal cortex are involved in mood regulation, decision-making, and processing of rewards. The insular cortex connects our bodily states to emotional experiences and consciousness. The *medial prefrontal cortex* plays a key role in evaluating and integrating emotional and social information, modulating the activity of other limbic regions, and contributing to decision-making processes and social behavior [1–3].

Subcortical components include the thalamus, which relays sensory and motor signals and is integral to consciousness; the hypothalamus, which governs autonomic functions and the endocrine system; and the mammillary bodies, which assist in memory recollection. The fornix serves as a major output pathway of the hippocampus, linking it to the septal nuclei, which are associated with reward and reinforcement. The nucleus accumbens is a critical hub in the brain's reward circuitry, influencing pleasure and motivation. The olfactory bulb, while primarily involved in the sense of smell, also triggers emotional and memory responses. Finally, the anterior commissure plays a role in interhemispheric communication and the perception of pain and emotion [1–3].

The hippocampal formation is a complex primordial structure within the deep temporal lobe built from phylogenetically ancient Allocortex. This is composed of the 3-layered archiocortex consisting of polymorphic, pyramidal, and molecular layers (strata alveole/oriens, pyramidale, radiatum/lacunosum-moleculare). The limbic system is further composed of Paleocortex, which contains 3–5 layers of cells located in the parahippocampal gyrus (entorhinal, perirhinal, and parahippocampal cortex), uncus (piriform cortex), and lateral olfactory gyrus. The mesocortex, a transitional form between the allocortex and isocortex (neocortex), contains 3–6 layers and is found in the insula and cingulate gyrus. Embryologically the hippocampus initially forms a crescent ridge along the floor of the temporal horn of the lateral ventricle. As it expands and rotates, the limbic system develops and grows in tandem with the brain vesicles to create a highly integrated system that connects to all lobes (cerebral cortex) and subcortical structures (diencephalon, basal ganglia, brainstem) (**Figure 1a** and **b**) [2–4].

The hippocampus, parahippocampal gyrus (entorhinal, perirhinal and parahippocampal cortex), the uncus (piriform cortex), lateral olfactory gyrus, the insula and cingulate gyrus, and the orbitofrontal cortex are thus phylogenetically associated structures, implying deeper reciprocal connectivity between the hippocampus and these limbic system areas [3, 4]. The hippocampus and the limbic system function as a

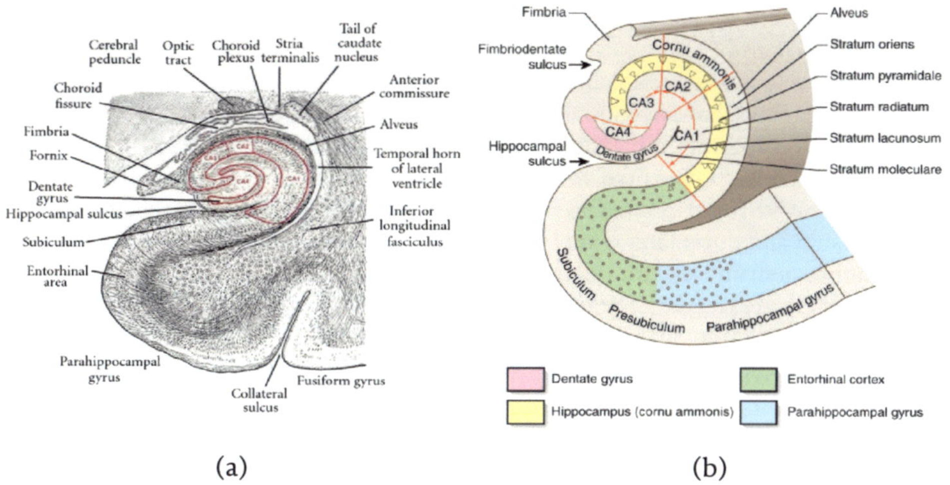

Figure 1.
(a) https://en.wikipedia.org/wiki/Hippocampus (Creative Commons 4.0 International (CC BY-SA 4.0)) J. A. Kiernan modified from Edinger, 1899 (Ref.) Epilepsy Research and Treatment Vol 2012, Article ID 176157, 12pages.doi:10.1155/2012/176157 - https://www.hindawi.com/journals/ert/2012/176157.fig. 004.jpg - Hippocampus and Cornu Ammonis regions (CA1, CA2, CA3, CA4). (b) https://medicine.en-academic.com/3923. Schematic diagram of the hippocampal formation showing the disposition of the various cell fields. CA1-4 denotes a classification scheme for subdividing the cornu ammonis region into a series of radially disposed fields. Credit: Medical dictionary: medicine.academic.ru/3923y.

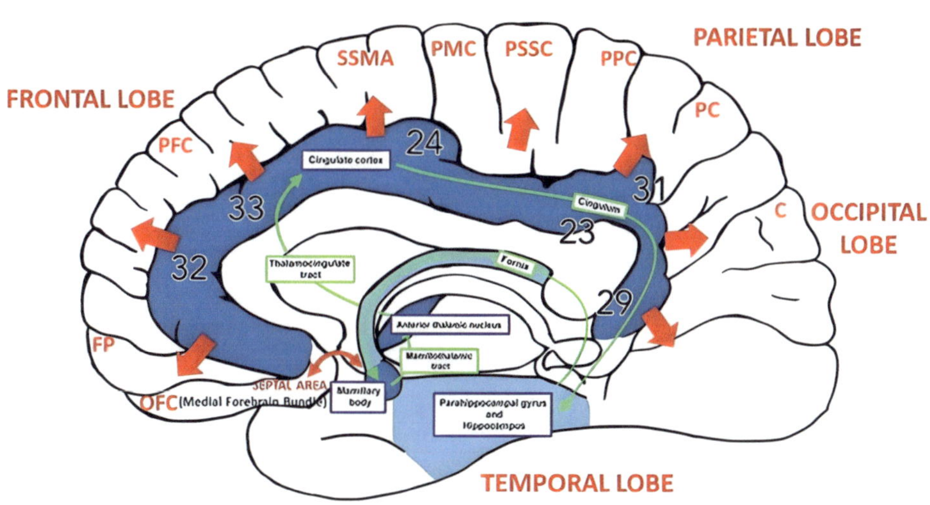

Figure 2.
Limbic system or circuit of Papez. Modified with permission from Weininger et al. [5]. OFC: orbitofrontal cortex, FP: frontopolar, PFC: prefrontal cortex, SSMA: supplementary sensorimotor area, PMC: primary motor cortex, PSSC: primary somatosensory cortex, PPC: posterior parietal cortex, PC: precuneus, C: cuneus. (Creative Commons 4.0 International (CC BY 4.0)) Reproduced from [6].

central hub (local area network) within larger scale limbocortical networks interconnected through reciprocal excitatory and inhibitory connections forming positive and negative feedback loops (**Figure 2**) [1, 7–10].

The hierarchical organization and flexible operation of the human brain via functional modular neural networks gives rise to three macro-scale canonical networks: (1) the default mode network (DMN), which the hippocampus is an integral part of; (2) the frontoparietal network (FPN), also known as central executive network (CEN); and (3) the salience network (SN) [11]. Their interaction seems to play a crucial role in almost all cognitive, emotional, and behavioral dysfunctions–the triple-network model of psychopathology (**Table 1** and **Figure 3**) [13, 14].

The DMN is involved in internally focused thought (self-referential thought, introspection), and FPN is involved in goal-directed behavior (task-related attention and executive functions). The salience network, primarily composed of the anterior insula and dorsolateral anterior cingulate cortex (AI-dACC), contains the von Economo neurons [15] and is cardinal for detecting and integrating emotionally and physiologically relevant stimuli. This network helps in dynamically switching between the other large-scale brain networks, such as the default mode network (DMN) and the central executive network (FPN). The co-activation of the amygdala-hippocampus complex and other SN subcortical nodes in response to various experimental tasks indicates a general role in identifying homeostatically relevant competing internal and external stimuli [16, 17]. Its function is thus essential for processing reward, motivation, emotion, and pain [18].

Limbocortical and thalamocortical networks are intertwined via hierarchical modular organization and reciprocal connectivity across different levels of neural organization, giving rise to large-scale oscillatory activity. Their derangements will be referred to as oscillopathies in our second chapter. This network architecture enables

Large-scale network	Subnetwork components	Function
Default Mode Network (DMN)	Medial Prefrontal Cortex (mPFC)	Self-referential processing and decision-making
	Posterior Cingulate Cortex (PCC)/ Precuneus	Episodic memory retrieval and awareness
	Inferior Parietal Lobule (IPL)	Integrating sensory information and attention
	Hippocampus/Parahippocampal Cortex	Memory consolidation and retrieval
	Lateral Temporal Cortex	Processing semantic memory and language
Frontoparietal Network (FPN) or Central Executive Network (CEN)	Dorsolateral Prefrontal Cortex (DLPFC)	Working memory, planning, and decision-making
	Anterior Cingulate Cortex (ACC)	Error detection, attention regulation, and emotional processing
	Posterior Parietal Cortex (PPC)	Spatial attention, working memory, and sensory information integration
	Inferior Frontal Junction (IFJ)	Task switching and inhibitory control
Salience Network (SN)	Anterior Insula (AI)	Interoception, emotional awareness, and sensor>'information integration
	Anterior Cingulate Cortex (ACC)	Evaluating salience of emotional and cognitive information
	Dorsal Anterior Cingulate Cortex (dACC)	Cognitive control and conflict monitoring
	Amygdala	Emotion processing and detection of salient stimuli
	Ventral Striatum	Reward processing and decision-making

Table 1.
Large-scale brain networks: Default mode network (DMN), frontoparietal or central executive network (FPN/ CEN) and salience network (SN) with their key modular components, along with their respective functions. The highlighted modular (subnetwork) components are highly integrated with the Hippocampus via reciprocal connections forming larger scale limbo-cortical networks, crucial for cognitive, emotional and behavioral regulation.

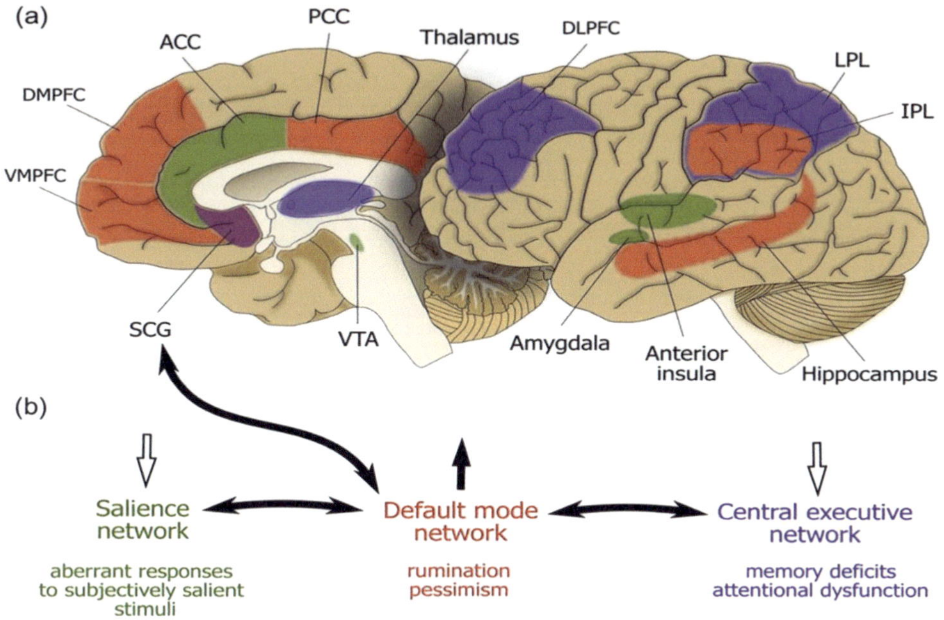

Figure 3.
Large-scale brain networks integrating limbocortical and thalamocortical networks – Default mode network (HPC, PHC/LTC, mPFC, PCC/Precuneus), salience network (AMG, AI, ACC, VStr, VTA) and central executive network (TH, DLPFC, PPC). Reproduced with permission from Ref. [12].

parallel processing across multiple levels, including the brainstem, diencephalon, basal ganglia, limbic system, and various cortical regions. Simultaneous direct and indirect short-cuts through the circuitry optimize complex cognitive and emotional processing and enable rapid and eloquent behavioral responses [1, 3, 11, 17].

2. From the hippocampal formation (trisynaptic circuit) to the limbic system

The primary input to the hippocampus comes from the entorhinal cortex (EC), which is strongly and reciprocally connected with numerous cortical and subcortical structures—including different thalamic nuclei (anterior and midline groups), the medial septum (medial septal nucleus and diagonal band of Broca), the supramammillary nucleus of the hypothalamus, the raphe nuclei, ventral tegmental area, and locus coeruleus of the brainstem. The EC thus serves as a critical interface between neocortical regions (e.g., parahippocampal gyrus, perirhinal cortex) and subcortical structures, coupling them to the hippocampus (**Figure 4**) [18].

The local hippocampal network consists of several interconnected regions, each with distinct excitatory and inhibitory components. The EC sends excitatory projections directly to the distal apical dendrites of CA1 pyramidal neurons (direct perforant pathway) and to the dentate gyrus (DG) and CA3 regions via the indirect perforant pathway. The DG, receiving input from the EC, transmits excitatory signals to CA3 through mossy fibers, while local interneurons provide inhibitory feedback to regulate granule cells within the DG. Mossy fibers play a crucial role in transmitting these excitatory signals from DG granule cells to CA3 pyramidal cells (**Figure 4**) [19].

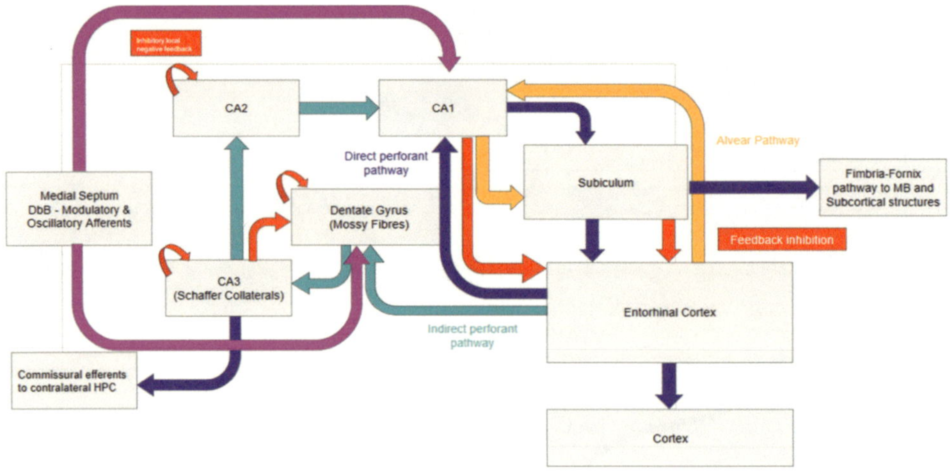

Figure 4.
Hippocampal Formation. The trisynaptic circuit and its internal organization with subregions, pathways and connections.

The alvear pathway originates from EC layer III, travels through the alveus, and targets basal and proximal apical dendrites (closer to the soma) of CA1 neurons (takes a more ventral route compared to the perforant path). The direct perforant pathway (axons also originating from EC layer III) forms synapses on the distal apical dendrites of CA1 neurons (monosynaptic circuit). The indirect perforant pathway (axons from EC layer II) reaches CA1 via the trisynaptic circuit: granule cells in the DG (first synapse) transmit signals via mossy fibers to pyramidal neurons in CA3 (second synapse), which then project via the Schaffer collaterals to pyramidal neurons in CA1 (third synapse) (**Figure 2**) [19].

Within CA3, excitatory connections include inputs from the DG via mossy fibers and projections to CA1 through the Schaffer collateral pathway. CA3 also contains recurrent excitatory connections that facilitate autoassociative memory processes. Local interneurons in CA3 provide inhibitory feedback to control excitatory activity. The CA2 region receives excitatory input from CA3 and projects excitatory signals to CA1 and the EC, with local interneurons regulating these signals. In the CA1 region, excitatory inputs from CA3 are received via the Schaffer collateral pathway, and outputs are sent to the subiculum and EC, with inhibitory interneurons modulating both excitatory inputs and outputs. The subiculum receives excitatory inputs from CA1 and projects to the EC and other brain regions, with local interneurons regulating the excitatory output for proper signaling (**Figure 4**) [19].

This intricate network of excitatory and inhibitory components within the hippocampal formation generates from low to high frequency dynamic oscillatory activity. Based on rhythmic volleys of inhibitory inputs to principal cell populations, inhibition-disinhibition patterns are generated, providing alternating temporal windows of relatively reduced and enhanced excitability in neuronal networks. These serve as temporal frames to bind or group neuronal activity into cell assemblies and sequences of assemblies on a large scale, effectively exchanging information among cortical networks that play a crucial role in memory processing and spatiotemporal navigation. For example, the trisynaptic pathway allows to rapidly form memories for specific experiences, while the monosynaptic pathway slowly learns generalities [20].

The major output of the hippocampus consists of axons from CA1, which project back to the EC both directly and via the subiculum, completing the trisynaptic circuit (**Figure 4**). The trisynaptic circuit is organized transversely along the hippocampus, while association and commissural fibers are organized along the anteroposterior axis. Hilar mossy cells and CA3 pyramidal cells contribute to ipsilateral hippocampal association fibers, which connect to the dendrites of granule cells and GABAergic interneurons of the inner molecular layer of the DG, as well as contralateral commissural fibers [19, 20].

Hippocampal commissural connections, which are primarily excitatory, are less abundant and have evolutionary declined in monkey and humans [21]. Schaffer collaterals, axon collaterals from CA3 pyramidal cells of the ipsilateral and contralateral hippocampi, project information to the pyramidal neurons of the CA1 hippocampal area. These Schaffer collateral synapses make excitatory glutamatergic synapses (provide positive feedback) that support activity-dependent plasticity and development of memory processing and formation [22]. In CA3, basket cells receive excitatory input from pyramidal cells and provide inhibitory feedback, forming a powerful recurrent inhibition circuit that dampens excitatory responses and shapes the hippocampus's oscillatory activity (**Figure 4**) [23].

The hippocampal trisynaptic loop, with its extensive feedforward and feedback projections, is a fundamental mechanism of controlled recurrent excitation that underpins memory, learning, and emotion within the limbocortical networks (Papez circuit) (**Figures 2**, **3** and **5**). Numerous brain structures transmit information to and from the trisynaptic circuit, and their activity can be directly or indirectly modulated by the activity of the whole trisynaptic loop. Major outputs are via the fornix to the lateral septal area and the mammillary body of the hypothalamus, while additional outputs are to other cortical areas, including the anterior cingulate and prefrontal cortex (**Figures 3** and **4**).

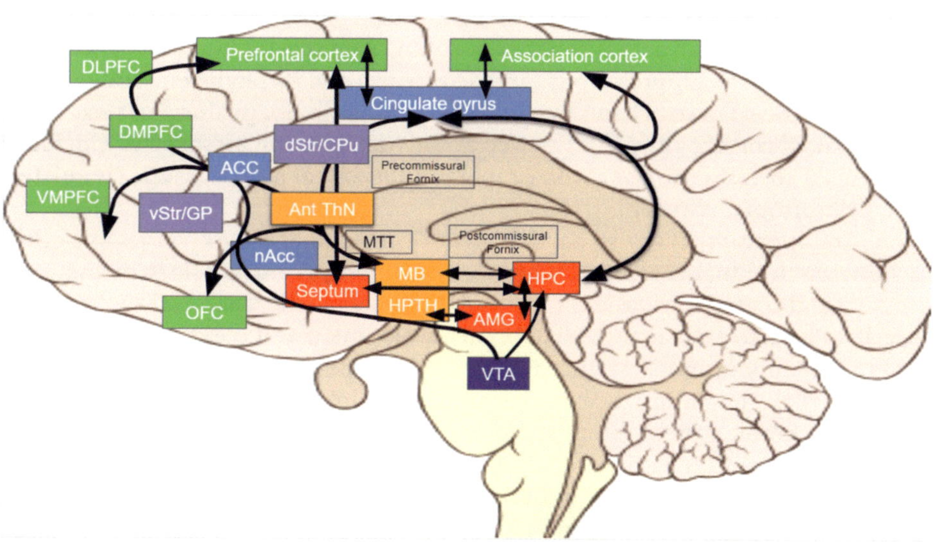

Figure 5.
The complexity of the limbocortical network - integration of the hippocampus and the limbic system with large-scale brain networks that essentially interconnect the Hippocampus-Amygdala Complex (Archicortex-Paleocortex) with the Prefrontal Cortex (Neocortex).

The crura of the fornix connect through the corpus callosum and hippocampal commissures with bilateral hippocampal formations. CA3 connects to the lateral and medial septum via the alveus and fimbria fornix. CA1 and the subiculum are connected to the parahippocampal regions, the entorhinal cortex, and nucleus accumbens, projecting to the septal nuclei, preoptic nuclei, ventral striatum, orbital cortex, and anterior cingulate cortex (via the precommissural fornix), as well as to the anterior and lateral dorsal nuclei of the thalamus, the mammillary bodies, and ventromedial hypothalamus (via the postcommissural fornix) (**Figure 2**) [24, 25]. The information from the hippocampal formation received by the mammillary bodies via the fornix is relayed to the anterior nuclei of the thalamus and the anterior cingulate cortex (Brodmann areas 24, 32, 33) via the mammillothalamic tract [5], while the subiculum relays information to the posterior cingulate cortex (Brodmann 23) [25].

Through the cingulate gyrus and thalamic nuclei, primary sensory and association cortical areas are reached, integrating information at a higher level to process complex stimuli from external and internal environments (**Figure 3**). The temporal association cortex identifies the nature of stimuli (perception), while the frontal association cortex plans responses to the stimuli (behavior). These association cortices project to other cortical association areas and subcortical structures, including the hippocampus, thalamus, basal ganglia, cerebellum, and brainstem [25].

The hippocampus also receives modulatory inputs from the cholinergic, serotoninergic, noradrenergic, and dopaminergic systems; the amygdala; the nucleus reuniens of thalamus; and the medial septum. The supramammillary nucleus of the hypothalamus is strongly connected via the medial forebrain bundle to the medial septum, diencephalon, and brainstem (**Figures 2** and 5) [25].

3. From the limbic system (multi-loop circuit) to large-scale limbocortical networks

The limbic system is a complex network comprising several interconnected regions, including the hippocampus (archaeocortex) and its phylogenetically associated paleocortex structures (such as the olfactory bulb, piriform cortex, periamygdaloid cortex, amygdala) as well as the transitioning mesocortex (including the perirhinal cortex, entorhinal cortex, parahippocampal gyrus, insula, cingulate cortex, orbitofrontal cortex) [5].

The parahippocampal gyrus, particularly the entorhinal cortex, serves as a critical relay between the hippocampus and neocortex, playing a central role in memory processing and spatial navigation. As one of the oldest cortical areas, the entorhinal cortex dates back to early mammalian brain development and is extensively connected to the hippocampus, particularly through the perforant pathway [25].

The amygdala, including the broader periamygdaloid complex, is a crucial component of the limbic system, deeply involved in processing emotional responses, particularly fear and aggression. Situated adjacent to the hippocampus, it forms a complex network that integrates emotional significance with memory and decision-making. The amygdala receives sensory inputs from various cortical and subcortical regions, including the olfactory bulb and the thalamus, enabling it to assess and react to emotionally salient stimuli. Its reciprocal connections with the hippocampus and other limbic structures facilitate the modulation of emotional experiences and memories, influencing behavioral responses and learning (**Figure 6**) [25].

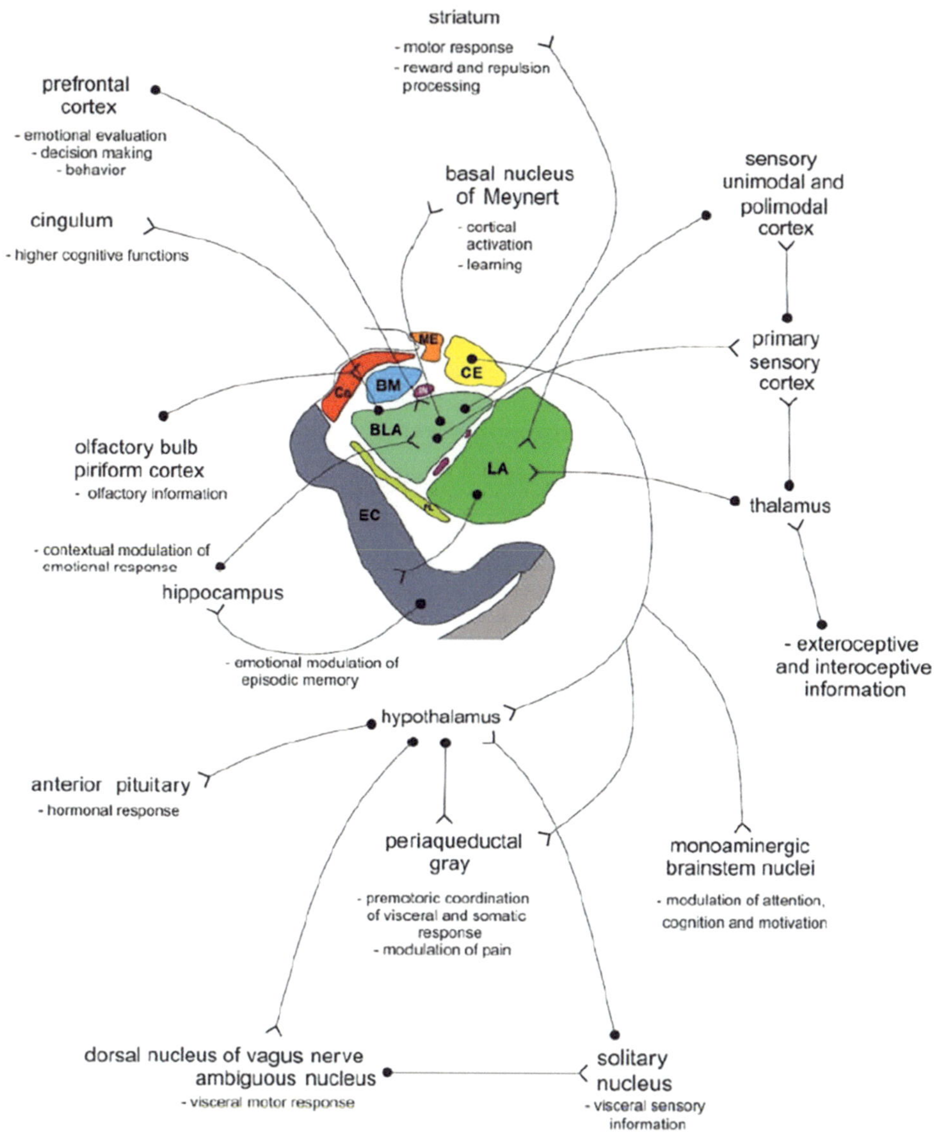

Figure 6.
Schematic of the connections of the amygdaloid complex nuclei with cortical and subcortical structures (reproduced with permission from [26] – under Creative Commons Attribution CC BY 4.0). BLA—basolateral (basal) nucleus; BM—basomedial (accessory basal) nucleus; CE—central nucleus; Co—cortical nucleus; EC—entorhinal cortex; IN—intercalated neurons; ME—medial nucleus; LA—lateral nucleus; PL—paralaminar nucleus.

The uncus, which includes the piriform cortex, represents an ancient olfactory processing area reflecting the primordial significance of the sense of smell in early vertebrates. Its connection with the hippocampus highlights the role of olfactory cues in memory and spatial navigation, underscoring the evolutionary link between olfaction and hippocampal function. Similarly, the lateral olfactory gyrus, involved in processing olfactory information crucial for early mammalian survival, interacts with the hippocampus, preserving the pathway from olfaction to memory systems [25].

The insula integrates sensory, emotional, and cognitive information, playing a role in homeostasis and self-awareness, with connections to the hippocampus that reflect the integration of visceral and emotional states with memory processes, rooted in the brain's evolutionary history [27].

The cingulate gyrus, a key component of the ancient limbic system, is involved in emotion formation, processing, learning, and memory. Its robust reciprocal connections with the hippocampus facilitate the integration of emotional and cognitive aspects of memory [25].

Finally, the orbitofrontal cortex, evolved to handle complex social and environmental interactions, is involved in decision-making and reward processing. Its connections with the hippocampus enable the integration of complex sensory information and past experiences to guide behavior and decision-making [27].

These interconnected regions highlight the evolutionary significance, and the deep reciprocal connectivity with the hippocampus reveals their functional integration in collectively supporting memory, spatial navigation, emotional regulation, and decision-making [25].

The two major pathways into and out of the hippocampus are the fornix and entorhinal cortex (via the cingulate cortex). The pre-commissural branch of the fornix connects to the septal nuclei, preoptic nuclei, ventral striatum, orbitofrontal cortex, and anterior cingulate cortex. The post-commissural branch of the fornix links to the anterior nucleus of the thalamus and the mammillary bodies of the hypothalamus. Damage to the mammillary bodies, as seen in Korsakoff's syndrome due to alcohol exposure and thiamine deficiency, leads to profound difficulty in forming new memories. Additionally, since the mammillo-thalamic tract also extends to the anterior thalamic nucleus, the hippocampus can influence the thalamus indirectly as well as directly [28].

The hippocampus has direct connections (outputs) to the entorhinal cortex (via the subiculum) and the amygdala. The entorhinal cortex projects to the cingulate cortex. The anterior thalamic nuclei also connect to the cingulate cortex. Therefore, the hippocampus can affect the cingulate cortex through either the anterior thalamic nucleus or the entorhinal cortex. The input paths to the hippocampus mirror the aforementioned outputs: the pre-commissural branch of the fornix brings inputs from the septal nuclei, part of the median medial forebrain bundle (including also the nucleus basalis of Meynert and substantia innominata), and the post-commissural branch of the fornix receives inputs from the mammillary bodies (hypothalamus) (**Figures 2** and 5) [27].

The cingulate cortex, temporal lobe cortex, amygdala, orbital cortex, and olfactory bulb are all intricately interconnected and project via the entorhinal cortex of parahippocampal gyrus back to the hippocampus, forming a major loop called the Papez circuit. The Papez circuit like many other components of the limbocortical network is involved in learning, memory, emotion, and social behavior. It was originally proposed by James Papez to be the anatomical substrate for emotional experience. The hippocampus and amygdala complex (allocortex-palleocortex), along with the prefrontal cortex (neocortex), are integral to processing and experiencing emotions (**Figure 6**) [28].

The prefrontal cortex (neocortex) is formed from isocortex. It represents the most recent and largest part of the human cortex, comprising up to 90% of its surface. It forms the cortical regions of all brain lobes except for the limbic system. The isocortex is organized into six layers, each with distinct functions: the four most superficial layers (I-IV) serve as input stations, receiving corticopetal fibers from other cortical areas and the thalamus, whereas the two deeper layers (V-VI) are output stations that send corticofugal projections to subcortical structures. However, the development of these layers varies across different regions of the neocortex, resulting in anatomical architectural and functional connectivity differences. For example, the motor cortex, which is involved in movement, features a high density of pyramidal cells, particularly in layers II-V, while having few granular cells (agranular cortex). In contrast, the primary sensory cortex (somatosensory, visual, auditory) is heavily filled with stellate (granular) cells (especially in layer IV) that receive, process, and relay sensory information from the thalamus to other cortical layers, hence containing a relatively small population of pyramidal cells (granular cortex) (**Figure 5**) [27, 28].

Additionally, widespread neurotransmitter systems modulate these processes. Noradrenaline from the locus coeruleus (LC) regulates mood/arousal, anxiety, pain, sleep/wake cycles, and motor activity. Serotonin from the raphe nuclei (RN) regulates mood, emotions, sleep/wake cycles, dominance/aggression, and anxiety. Dopamine from the ventral tegmental area (VTA) and substantia nigra (SN) in the midbrain is essential for emotional reward and drive. Acetylcholine from the basal nucleus of Meynert and septal nuclei affects cognitive processing, arousal, and attention. Glutamate has an excitatory effect (from neuronal activation to stress excitotoxicity), and GABA has a major inhibitory effect in the adult brain. These neurotransmitter systems project throughout the cortex, modulating in particular the prefrontal cortex (**Figure 7**) [27].

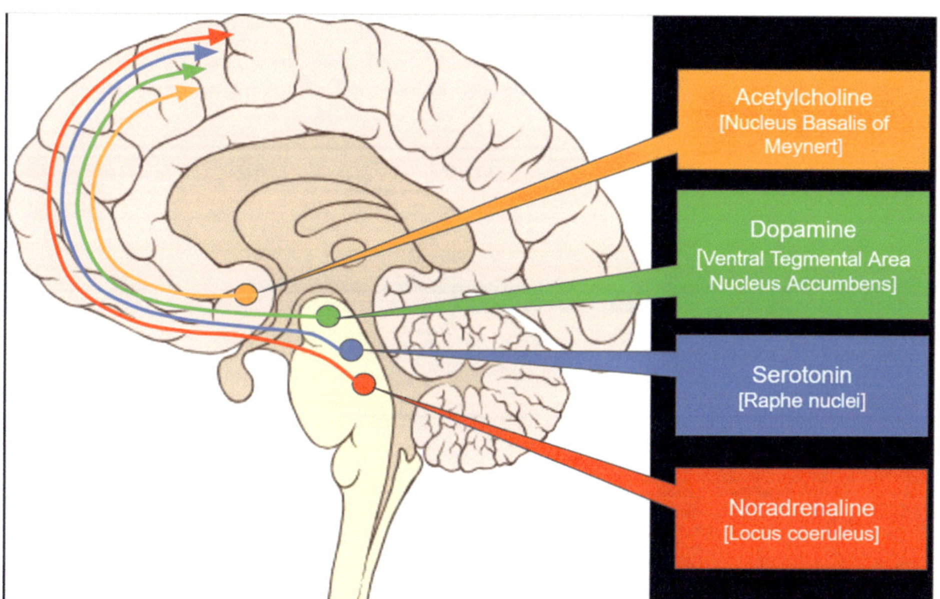

Figure 7.
Projections of brainstem structures of cholinergic (NBM), noradrenergic neurons (LC), dopaminergic Neurons (SNc, VTA, nAcc), serotoninergic (RN), directly and indirectly through allocortical (HPC), mesocortical (parahippocampal gyrus, entorhinal cortex, uncus, lateral olfactory gyrus, insula, cingulate gyrus, orbitofrontal cortex), diencephalic (thalamus, hypothalamus, subthalamus) and basal ganglia (caudate nucleus, putamen, globus pallidus, subthalamic nucleus, and substantia nigra) to the prefrontal cortex the end-target.

4. Neurophysiology of emotions

Emotions, as the name implies ("e-motions"), are fundamental drives that set our behavior (mind and personality) into motion. Emotions have evolved as survival mechanisms across all organisms, facilitating interaction and communication with our environment and providing feedback responses to internal and external stimuli. Emotions are essentially 'homeostatic' behavioral drives that help maintain the balance of the organism with its internal and external environments [29].

Even simple organisms like insects (Drosophila) have elementary emotional responses: they move toward hedonic stimuli such as food and mating opportunities and away from stressors, indicating a rudimentary form of pleasure and aversion. This suggests that emotions have contextual cues that guide purposeful behavior [29].

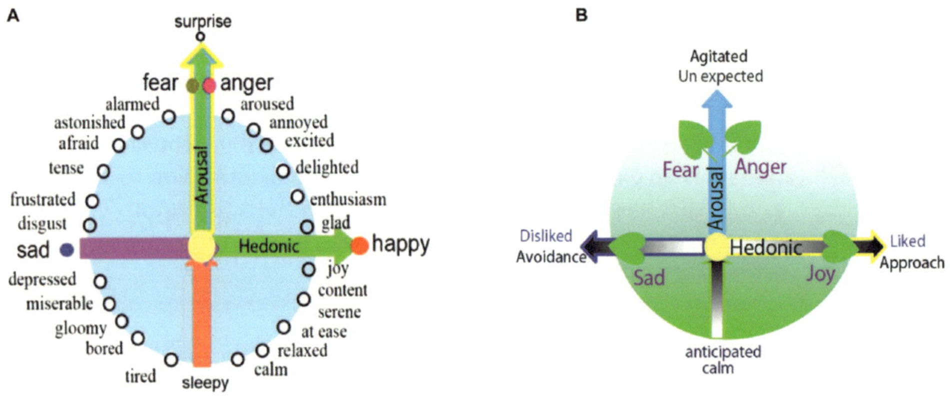

(a)

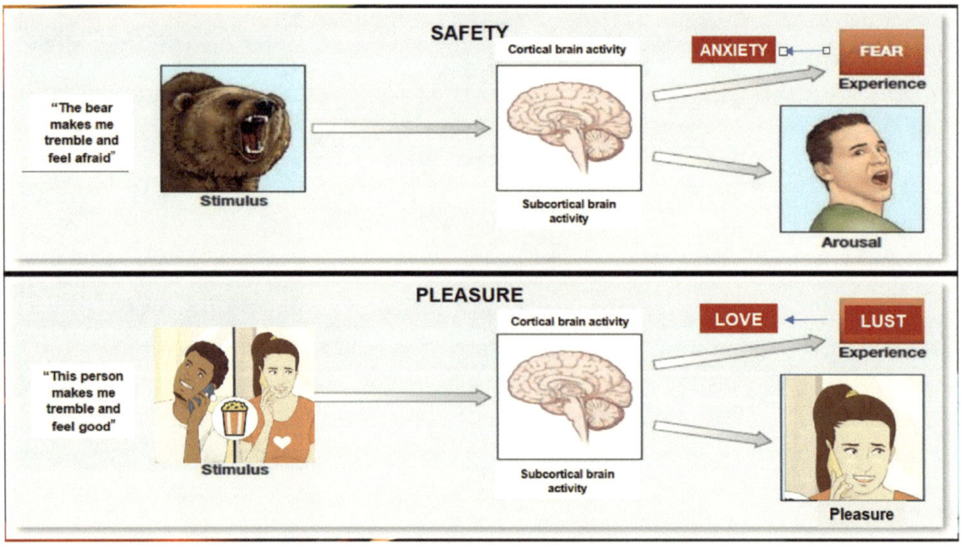

(b)

Figure 8.
(a) Ref. [29]. (b) Modified from https://www.brainkart.com/article/The-Many-Facets-of-Emotion_29432/to illustrate the Cannon-Bard theory of emotion (W. B. Cannon, 1927).

In more complex organisms such as humans, avoidance of pain and stress responses are processed in primordial brain structures like the periaqueductal gray matter (a collection of neurons) that acts as a 'gatekeeper' and filters incoming stimuli to assess their threat level and trigger physiological stress responses (**Figure 8a** and **b**) [30, 31].

According to Aristotle (384–322 BC), emotions (*pathos*) are drives of human life that cannot be ignored; ethics cultivates them in developing character; rhetoric manages them to produce belief [32]. Descartes (1649) identified six passions (wonder, love, hate, desire, joy, and sadness), while William James (1890) reduced them to four basic emotions: fear, grief, love, and rage, based on bodily involvement [22]. Wilhelm Max Wundt (1897), the father of modern psychology, distinguished three dimensions based on pleasure/unpleasure, arousal/subdue, and strain/relaxation [22]. In more recent years, James Russell (1980) proposed the Circumplex model of Emotion (based on two dimensions of Arousal and Valence) (**Figure 9a** and **b**) [33].

Emotions are network-level phenomena arising from complex interactions across the limbocortical network, including multiple cortical areas and deeper subcortical structures, such as the amygdala, hippocampus, basal ganglia, and brainstem structures. These interactions trigger rapid (instinctual) responses for survival and influence higher-order cognitive and affective functions. Conversely, top-down attentional pathways influence lower-level sensory processing, and emotional regulation impacts decision-making, affecting experiences and social behavior. Thus, even seemingly rational decisions are often influenced by underlying emotional drives. Emotional dysregulation can lead to a range of cognitive, affective, behavioral, and even seizure disorders, highlighting the profound impact of emotions on human behavior (**Figures 3**, **5** and **6**) [26, 34].

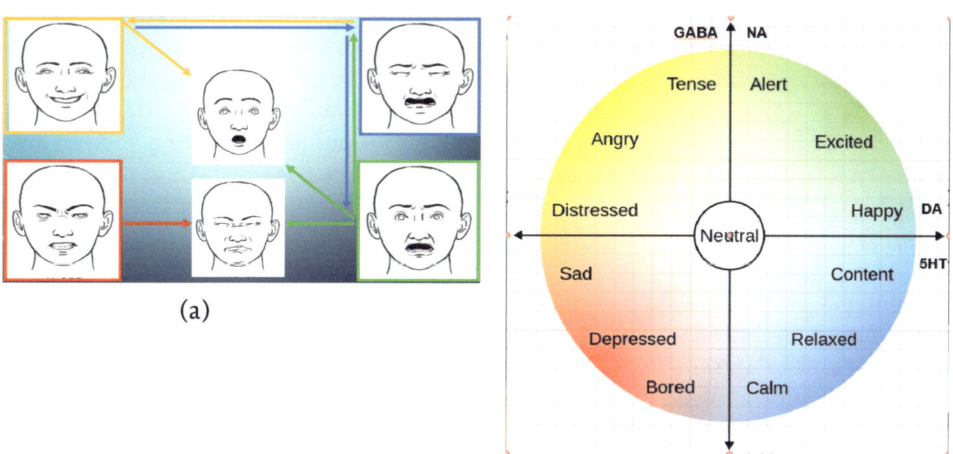

(a)

(b)

Figure 9.
(a) Circumplex theory of emotions with 4 primary emotions (joy, sadness, fear, anger) and combinations in-between, like surprise/startle (a mixture of joy and fear) and disgust (a mixture of anger and fear). (*b*) *Circumplex model of emotion has two axes: Valence (driven and regulated by dopaminergic and serotoninergic transmission pathways respectively) and Arousal (driven and regulated by noradrenergic and GABAergic transmission pathways respectively). File: Circumplex model of emotion. Svg. (2024, March 17). Wikimedia Commons. Retrieved 18:20, 03.08.2024 from https://commons.wikimedia.org/w/index.php?title=File:Circumplex_model_of_emotion.svg&oldid=861227692.*

5. Evolution of emotion circuits from the reptilian to the mammalian brain

Ontogenesis (the development of an organism) often mirrors the broader evolution of life on earth. According to the triune brain theory by neuroscientist Paul MacLean, the human brain has evolved from primordial structures including the hindbrain (myelencephalon, metencephalon and cerebellum), midbrain, and forebrain (diencephalon and telencephalon or cerebrum) [35].

The most primitive of them, known as the 'Reptilian' brain, encompasses the basal ganglia and thalamic structures (derived from the floor of the forebrain during development). This part of the brain governs basic survival functions, like aggression, dominance, and territoriality, operating largely on instinct with minimal emotional processing [35].

Following this, the paleomammalian complex, which includes interconnected limbic system structures such as the medial septum, hypothalamus, hippocampal-amygdala complex, anterior cingulate cortex, and orbitofrontal cortex, evolved early in mammalian history. This complex is responsible for driving motivations and emotions related to feeding, reproduction, and parental care, as well as more complex social behaviors.

Neuroscientist Jaak Panksepp further identified seven primary affective systems within the limbic structure; SEEKING (expectancy), FEAR (anxiety), RAGE (anger), LUST (sexual excitement), CARE (nurturance), PANIC/GRIEF (sadness), and PLAY (social joy) [36].

The most recent evolutionary development is the neomammalian complex (cerebral neocortex), a structure that is more developed in higher mammals, especially humans. This structure enables advanced cognitive functions such as language, abstraction, planning, and perception, supporting a complex circuitry of cognitive, affective, and behavioral processes.

Within this framework, the hippocampus-amygdala complex connects to the thalamic nuclei and cingulate gyrus, enabling the brain to integrate sensory information at a higher level. These pathways extend to primary sensory and association cortical areas, which process and perceive complex stimuli from both external and internal environments. The temporal, parietal, and occipital association cortical areas are involved in sensory processing and perception, while the frontal and prefrontal association areas are responsible for planning and executing responses to these stimuli. These cortical association areas project to other association cortical areas and loop back to subcortical structures, including the hippocampus-amygdala, thalamus, basal ganglia, cerebellum, and brainstem [25].

The brain's overarching function is to integrate sensory inputs and translate them into motor and behavioral outputs, with large-scale networks of sensory–motor integration having evolved through different levels of neural organization. The hippocampus plays a key role in this integration by raising reward expectations in the ventromedial prefrontal cortex (limbic input) [1] through its connections with the anterior thalamus/cingulate cortex and the ventral striatum (including globus palludis, nucleus accumbens and sub-thalamic nucleus) (**Figure 10**) [25, 26].

Decision-making, particularly regarding cost/benefit assessment of specific reward value, occurs in the orbitofrontal cortex, which is intimately connected to the hippocampal-amygdala complex via the uncinate fasciculus.

The dorsolateral prefrontal cortex projects back with cortical input for decision making and action selection through the dorsal striatum (globus pallidus internus

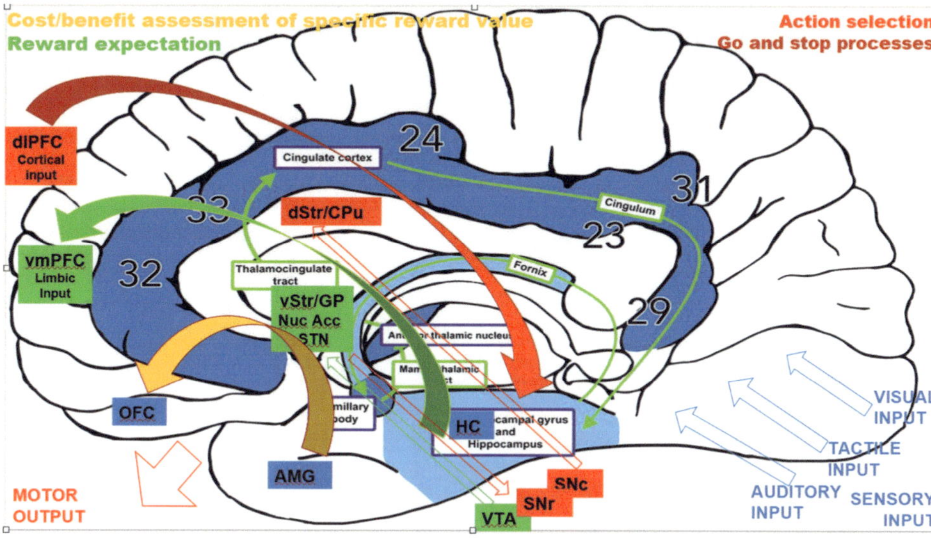

Figure 10.
Limbocortical Network - Large scale integrated behavioral (emotion) networks – crucial interactions of Hippocampus-Amygdala Complex with Prefrontal Cortex (PFC) in cost/benefit assessment of specific reward value (Orbitofrontal Cortex: OFC), reward expectation (Ventral Striatum: vStr, Globus Pallidus: GP, Nucleus Accumbens: Nuc Acc, Subthalamic Nucleus: STN, limbic input into the Ventromedial Prefrontal Cortex: vmPFC), Action Selection via Go-and-Stop processes (Dorsolateral Prefrontal Cortex: dlPFC, via the dorsal Striatum: dStr, Caudate nucleus: C and Putamen: Pu). In addition the upstream hippocampal-prefrontal network receives input from the Ventral Tegmental Area (VTA), while behavioral/motor output is controlled downstream by the dlPFC, and regulated by the basal ganglia network with modulatory inputs from the Substantia Nigra Compacta (SNc) and Substantia Nigra Reticulata (SNr).

GPi) down to the substantia nigra (pars reticulata SNr), the ventral anterior nucleus (VA) and ventral lateral nucleus of the thalamus (VL), and brainstem [37–39]. Through this direct pathway, the basal ganglia initiate voluntary movements by disinhibiting thalamic neurons that drive upper motor neurons [40, 41] (regulated by dopamine secreted by the striatum onto the D1 dopamine receptor on the substantia nigra compacta SNc).

An indirect pathway from the cortex, through the putamen, to the thalamus and brainstem passing through the external segment of the globus pallidus (GPe) and the subthalamic nucleus (STN) before looping back to the internal segment of the globus pallidus (Gpi) [41] is responsible for the termination of movement (regulated by striatal dopamine D2 receptors resulting in inhibition of the disinhibition) (**Figure 11**).

The main centers of the brain's motivation and reward systems include: the medial forebrain bundle (Ach), the ventral tegmental area (DA), the nucleus accumbens (95% of neurons are GABAergic medium spiny neurons with D1 or D2 receptors [42]; 1–2% of the remaining interneurons are large aspiny cholinergic or GABAergic), the septum, the amygdala, the prefrontal cortex, and certain parts of the thalamus. Each of these structures participate in various aspects of behavioral response. All of these centers are interconnected and innervate the hypothalamus, informing it of the presence of incoming or potential rewards. The lateral and ventromedial nuclei of the hypothalamus are especially involved in these reward circuits. The hypothalamus then acts in turn not only on the ventral tegmental area but also on the autonomic and endocrine functions of the entire body, through the pituitary gland (**Figures 5** and **10**) [26, 37].

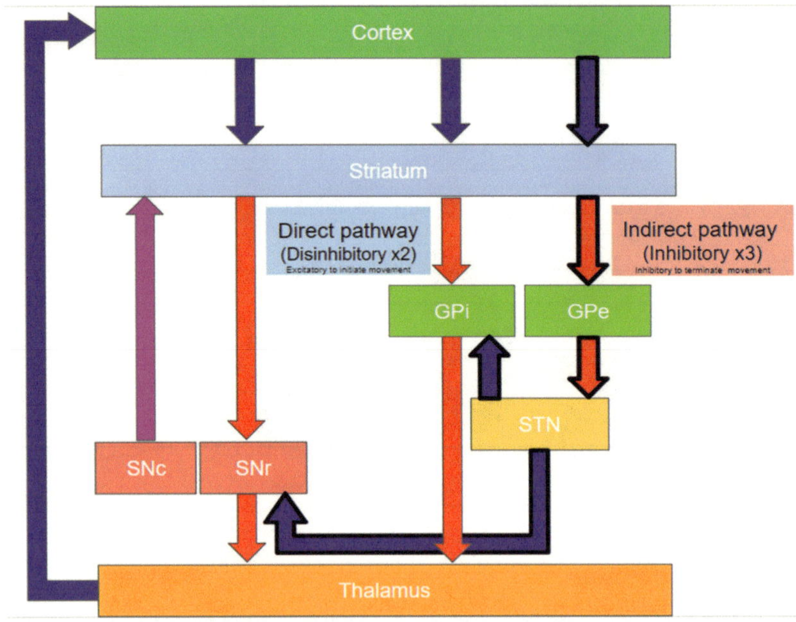

Figure 11.
Connectivity diagram demonstrating the direct, indirect and modulatory pathways in cortical-basal ganglia-thalamo-cortical multiple interactive feedback loops. Excitatory glutamatergic pathways are depicted as blue arrows, inhibitory GABAergic pathways as red arrows, and modulatory dopaminergic input as magenta arrow.

6. The primary emotional circuits

Within the limbic system, four primary emotional circuits emerge from the interaction of neocortical and subcortical structures through different neurotransmitter system projections. One of the most powerful systems (behavioral drives) is the 'pleasure-reward (joy) circuit', based on dopamine (excitation) and serotonin (inhibition) balance. The VTA through dopaminergic pathways communicates with the prefrontal cortex through sensory and motor inputs while integrating inputs from the nucleus accumbens, hypothalamic nuclei, hippocampus, and amygdala (**Figures 5** and **10**) [43–46].

The 'fear circuit' has both long and short pathways, processing information by higher brain centers and the hippocampus, through direct and indirect paths to the amygdala. This way, the complexity of the response and time to elicit actions as well can be controlled. These pathways are used to convert sensory inputs from thalamus to emotional response from the amygdala to elicit visceral responses from the hypothalamus and relay back to the ventromedial vmPFC for conscious emotional recognition (**Figure 6**) [26, 34].

The 'anger circuit' results in two forms of aggression, affective or predatory aggression. Predatory aggression is related to feeding behavior and is not accompanied by sympathetic physiological response that affective aggression is associated with. In affective aggression actions are heavily driven by the amygdala and the hypothalamus as primal emotions, but PAG and VTA neural pathways add more complex behaviors through serotoninergic and other pathways (**Figure 6**) [26, 34, 46].

Aversive, threatening, or unexpected stimuli that provoke fight or flight responses activate the brain's arousal and punishment circuits, which enable us to cope with unpleasant situations [44, 45]. The 'punishment circuit' includes various brain structures, such as the hypothalamus, the thalamus, and the periaqueductal gray matter, while secondary centers of this circuit are found in the amygdala and the hippocampus [45].

The punishment and arousal circuits by means of cholinergic and noradrenergic neurons stimulate the secretion of adrenal corticotropic hormone (ACTH), which in turn stimulates the adrenal glands to release adrenalin to prepare the body's organs for fight or flight. Interestingly, stimulation of the punishment circuit can inhibit the reward circuit (fear and punishment can drive out pleasures). The medial forebrain bundle and the periventricular system (periaqueductal gray matter) are two major systems of motivation in human beings, which encourage people to behave so as to suppress their instinctive impulses and avoid painful experiences [45, 46].

The behavioral inhibition system (BIS identified by Henri Laborit in the early 1970s) is associated with the septo-hippocampal system, the amygdala, and the basal nuclei of the hypothalamus. It receives feedback inputs from the prefrontal cortex (perceived dangers or threats) and transmits its outputs via the noradrenergic fibers of the locus coeruleus and the serotoninergic fibers of the medial raphe nuclei. Serotonin plays an important role as inhibitory neurotransmitter in mood regulation, conferring also the sense of contentment one experiences with happiness. The BIS may be excessively activated when both 'fight and flight' (BAS) seem impossible and the only remaining behavioral option is to submit passively (freeze and anxiety). Such behavioral inhibition from chronic stress can have pathological consequences on human health, resulting in neuropsychiatric and functional neurological disorders (**Figures** 5, **6**, 7 and **10**) [46].

7. Hippocampus and limbocortical networks in perception of space, time, and motion: Navigation through memory, attention, and motivation

The hippocampus is fundamentally involved in integrating spatial, temporal, and motion-related visual cues to support navigation and episodic memory, often in emotionally salient or goal-directed contexts. Its capacity to link dynamic environmental cues with internal representations is essential for behaviors driven by reward anticipation or strategic planning [47].

Spatial perception has long been associated with hippocampal place cells, which exhibit location-specific firing. While visual landmarks influence the orientation of place cell fields [47, 48], the hippocampal code is remarkably invariant to sensory modality shifts. Blind rats show preserved place cell functionality [49], and tactile or olfactory cues alone can elicit robust place fields [50, 51]. This multimodal flexibility underscores the hippocampus's reliance on motion and self-referential (idiothetic) inputs, rather than purely visual information, to build spatial maps [52–54].

In primates, spatial view cells encode where in the environment the individual is looking, independent of body position. These neurons help associate external space ("out there") with remembered objects or rewards [55, 56]. Such cells can maintain activity during recall, even without external stimuli, allowing an object or place to act as a retrieval cue for the other. These processes are central to episodic memory and involve associative binding mechanisms in the CA3 subfield, which enables pattern completion and rapid one-trial learning [57, 58].

The hippocampus operates as part of a dynamic loop with the limbocortical network. During memory formation, information flows from the neocortex to the hippocampus, marked by neocortical alpha/beta desynchronization followed by hippocampal gamma synchronization. During retrieval, this direction reverses, reflecting hippocampal-driven reinstatement of cortical patterns [59]. This bidirectional coupling ensures that temporally sequenced, multimodal experiences are both encoded and retrievable—a prerequisite for effective reward-based and goal-directed navigation.

Motion perception, especially head and eye movements, has emerged as another crucial component of hippocampal representation. Freely moving macaques display theta-phase locking of hippocampal neurons at the onset of movement, with spatial coding dominated by head direction and eye movement parameters rather than gaze location [60]. These findings extend our understanding of hippocampal coding into the domain of 3D movement through space, suggesting a multiplexed representation of direction, motion, and place that can dynamically adjust to behavioral demands [61].

Temporal sequencing, another dimension of episodic memory, is also encoded by the hippocampus. Recent theories suggest that the same attractor mechanisms responsible for spatial pattern completion also support the association of episodic events across time [62]. This aligns with findings that dorsal CA1 neurons can encode sequences of distance, head angle, and allocentric position in task-specific ways [63]. These cells multiplex their responses depending on task demands, enabling the hippocampus to construct and recall episodes as temporally organized patterns.

Furthermore, emotional and motivational contexts modulate hippocampal activity. Certain spatial view neurons respond selectively to reward locations, linking spatial representation directly with behavioral drives [55, 56]. This highlights the role of the hippocampus in integrating motivational salience with episodic memory, ensuring that memory supports not only navigation but also adaptive goal pursuit.

In conclusion, the hippocampus serves as a nexus where space, time, and movement information from multiple sensory modalities converge with motivation, attention, and episodic memory [62, 63]. Through its integration of multimodal inputs, dynamic feedback with the neocortex, and specialized mechanisms for associative learning, the hippocampus enables organisms like humans to navigate in space and time not only the physical environment but also through episodic memories and emotional experiences, rewards and goals, expectancy and uncertainty, through a more abstract representation of the social environment and the self (**Figure 4**).

8. Limbocortical networks in perception of psychosocial space, flow of time, and sense of self: Navigation through semantics, emotions, and behavior

Semantic cognition arises from the integration of information across various sensory modalities (visual, auditory, tactile, olfactory, etc.) in a network that binds modality-specific information into multi-modal or amodal concepts and is multiplexed with emotional, language, and introspective systems through higher association cortices and the widely distributed limbocortical network [64]. For example, in the ventral visual stream, there is a hierarchical and feature-sensitive organization in category-specific modules like the parahippocampal place area (PPA) selectively responsive to images of places [65] and the fusiform face area (FFA) specific for face perception [66]. Although rapid categorical go/no-go (animal/nonanimal) responses can be driven by lower-level cues through early attentional and sensorimotor integration mechanisms (already from the lateral occipital complex) [67], the PPA and

FFA respond to mid-level visual categorical features (based on texture and contour arrangements), while high-level semantic content contributes to more detailed or multi-modal object recognition [68]. Core modality-specific hubs (e.g., auditory or visual association cortex) then feed into convergence zones, primarily located in the anterior temporal lobe (ATL) and middle temporal gyrus, angular gyrus (AG), and supramarginal gyrus (parietal lobe), areas responsible for combining perceptual features into coherent conceptual knowledge (**Figure 2**) [64, 69].

Language functions, which rely on regions such as Wernicke's (receptive) area connected through the arcuate fasciculus to Broca's (productive) area and dorsolateral prefrontal cortex (DLPFC), interface with the semantic system via shared fronto-temporal (uncinate fasciculus) and frontoparietal networks (superior longitudinal fasciculus), enabling naming, comprehension, and contextual use of meaning [70]. Semantics is further contextualized and retrieved through episodic memory systems, engaging the hippocampus, medial prefrontal cortex (mPFC), and posterior cingulate cortex. Semantic memory relies more on the ATL, AG, mPFC, DLPFC, and the anterior cingulate cortex (ACC)—all integrated with the hippocampus through the default mode network and semantic control networks (salience network) (**Figure 5**) [64, 69, 70].

The neocortex enables the higher-level processing of complex emotions (anxiety, depression, love, happiness), and underlying cognitive processes can be paired with different stimuli, allowing humans to create conditional and unconditional contexts for action and behavior [71]. For example, anxiety can be seen as fear without a specific target (a state of increased arousal and fear through enhanced noradrenergic and reduced GABAergic, serotoninergic and dopaminergic effects). On the other hand, pleasure driven by continuous dopamine release (impulse response) may heighten arousal through the noradrenergic system but does not necessarily result in happiness unless a state of emotional contentment, regulated by serotonin, is achieved (**Figure 10**) [26, 37, 46].

The evolved neocortex bestows humans with distinct traits, such as the ability to learn from memories of the past, imagine, predict, and anticipate the future. Human imagination and ability for flexible social networking on a large scale allows humans to plan, handle abstract concepts, and effectively manipulate the ambient environment (the present). Anticipation of the future is shaped by experiences from the past, with constant input of new stimuli and output of responses weighed against memories and experiences, social context, norms, and cultural customs (**Figure 11**) [72, 73].

This casts a different perspective into how human perception of space, time, and motion is deeply intertwined with such emotional and cognitive processes, giving rise to more abstract representations of the outer/inner environments through psychosocial space, flow of time, and a sense of self. As we continuously process past experiences and anticipate future events, our sense of 'present' becomes a superposition of instantaneous emotional states, often interfering or conflicting with each other. This complex interplay of emotions and cognition defines our personal perception of space and flow of time, influencing behavior, thoughts, and affect. Unlike other species, humans are uniquely aware of their mortality, which influences daily life by eliciting emotional states like faith, hope, spirituality, or religiousness, against the awe, fear, and anxiety of the unknown and the supernatural (**Figure 12**) [26, 32–34].

Overactive dopaminergic and glutamatergic brain systems and reduced inhibitory GABAergic control systems can lead to behaviors of addiction, gambling, (impulse control disorders), hallucination, psychosis, anxiety, and hyperkinetic movement

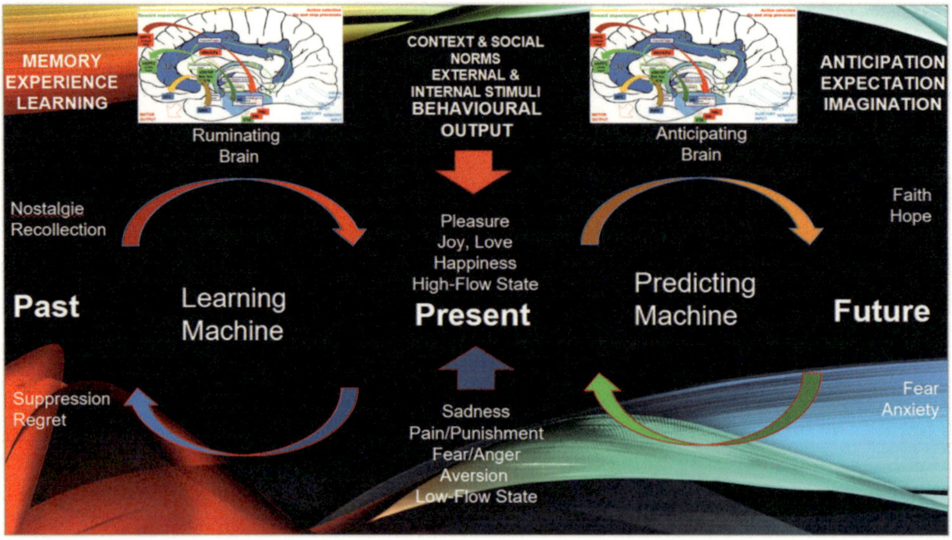

Figure 12.
The human brain as a learning and predicting machine and the implications for cognitive, affective and behavioral neuropsychiatric disorders. Human perception of 'relative space-time' dependent on high or low flow emotional states. Superposition of emotional states generated by large-scale integration of limbo-cortical networks (hippocampal function crucial in episodic memory formation through encoding of location, time and context of events during active exploration of the environment and the self).

disorders, while reduced dopaminergic and cholinergic input is associated with a slowing of movement (bradykinesia) and thought processes (bradyphrenia) as seen in Parkinson's disease and Lewy-Body dementia. Disturbances in these systems can thus result in paranoia, hallucinations, and delusions, illustrating the intricate relationship between emotional states, cognitive processes, and motor functions (thought processes are integrated with movement and e-motional circuits) (**Figure 11**) [37, 71].

9. Functional neurological, psychiatric and post-traumatic stress disorders

Psychodynamic models of conversion or functional neurological disorder (FND) [74] propose that subconscious conflicts manifest with somatic symptoms as a defense mechanism to suppress these conflicts and protect the individual from anxiety and emotional distress [75–77], thus avoiding overwhelming responses [78]. Patients may reenact subconscious memories of adverse life events and patterns of previous stress responses (fight or flight or freeze) with physical symptoms and abnormal behaviors to new conflicts or traumatic events, as a coping mechanism to emotional dysregulation [74].

Functional MRI studies have shown that patients with FND exhibit different patterns of regional brain activity compared to healthy controls during the recall of traumatic events. These differences include altered activation in the prefrontal cortex and hippocampus, with some studies finding a correlation between these brain activities and the severity of the symptoms [79, 80]. Additionally, hypersensitive responses of the amygdala to fear stimuli, coupled with abnormal self-focused attention (depersonalization during injury or panic), may contribute to sensations or movements perceived as involuntary symptoms (altered sense of self-control) [74].

The pathophysiology of FND can be conceptualized by the Bayesian principles of predictive coding and active inference in information processing [81]. The brain constantly generates predictions about sensory inputs based on prior experiences. These predictions are then updated by incoming sensory information (predictive coding). The brain tries then to minimize prediction errors by either adjusting its predictions (perceptual inference) or acting on the environment (active inference) (**Figure 12**) [81].

In FND, there is a disruption in this predictive processing [82] and an imbalance in the integration of sensory data and top-down predictions, resulting in distortions in perception, sense of agency, and motor control [83]. The symptoms of FND therefore can be viewed as a result of the brain's inaccurate predictions about bodily states and motor actions [74, 81].

In cases of heightened sensitivity to emotional or interoceptive signals, the brain may generate predictions that are overly influenced by these signals, leading to impaired processing of emotional and sensory information. Moreover, neuroimaging findings have identified altered activities in the limbic and salience networks [80], as well as in cortical regions involved in predictive processing and emotional regulation [84, 85].

In post-traumatic stress disorder (PTSD) [85], it is proposed that overactive and hyperconnected SN destabilizes intrinsically weakly connected and hypoactive DMN and FPN networks. Alternations in networks such as increased posterior SN connectivity to the posterior insula (PI) may result in raised sensitivity to stimuli and potential threats that contribute to avoidance and hypervigilance in PTSD patients. Hyperactivation in the AI is linked with re-experiencing traumatic memories (**Figure 3**) [86].

The SN with a low threshold for perceived saliency is not able to efficiently regulate the DMN and FPN switching. The impairment of cognitive control over salience processing in PTSD may be reflected in the reduced insular functional connectivity in the ACC and the supplementary motor region. The FPN and the DMN are also weakly interconnected and hypoactive, which causes narrowed cognition and incapacity for top-down SN regulation in the FPN as well as dissociation and fear generalization in the DMN (**Figure 3**) [71].

Therapeutic interventions aim to recalibrate the brain's predictive models. Cognitive behavioral therapy (CBT) [87] focuses on challenging and changing cognitive and emotional distortions (such as thoughts, beliefs, and attitudes), along with their associated behaviors, to improve emotional regulation and develop effective coping strategies and emotional resilience for managing current and future challenges [88].

Cognitive behavioral therapy (CBT), sensory grounding techniques, and a range of mindfulness, desensitization and memory reprogramming techniques such as Emotional Freedom Technique (EFT), Matrix Reeimprinting, Thought Field, Eye Movement Desensitization and Reprocessing (EMDR), Targeted Memory Reprogramming (TMR), and breathing techniques help individuals to reconnect with themselves and the environment in order to process more accurately sensory or interoceptive input, minimize perceptual distortions and top-down prediction errors, and/or consciously reprogram painful memories and negative thoughts [89, 90].

Mindfulness techniques and sensory grounding and breathing exercises can also help recover motor and autonomic control, improve cardiorespiratory synchronization (heart rate variability), and importantly resynchronize brain waves in a more relaxing/receptive alpha vs. theta mode, working against anxiety [90]. EEG studies show an increase in alpha and a decrease in theta power [91], while an fMRI study highlighted increased activity in cortical (prefrontal, motor, and parietal cortices) and subcortical (pons, thalamus, sub-parabrachial nucleus, periaqueductal gray, and hypothalamus) structures [92]. Sleep hygiene is also very important. Anxiolytics and antidepressants and/or pain-threshold or emotion regulation drugs may shortly be used as adjuncts.

Implementing and combining the above techniques can help modify maladaptive beliefs and expectations, adjust the brain's predictive processing, restore emotional balance and flow, reduce symptom severity, and improve self-agency (**Figure 12**) [90, 92].

Author details

Nick Tsarouchas[1*], Nicholas Tsarouchas[2] and Constantin Tsarouchas[3]

1 Department of Clinical Neurophysiology, East Kent Hospitals University NHS Foundation Trust, King's College Hospital London, UK

2 Department of Clinical Neurosciences, University of Cambridge, UK

3 Department of Science, Langton Star Centre SLBS, UK

*Address all correspondence to: nick_tsarouchas@yahoo.com

References

[1] Tsarouchas N. Clinical neurophysiology of epileptogenic networks. In: Neurophysiology - Networks, Plasticity, Pathophysiology and Behavior. London, UK: IntechOpen; 2022. DOI: 10.5772/intechopen.104952

[2] Ross MH, Pawlina W. Histology: A Text and Atlas. 7th ed. Philadelphia, PA: Wolters Kluwer Health; 2016. pp. 356-403

[3] Waxman SG. Clinical Neuroanatomy. 27th ed. New York, NY: McGraw-Hill Education; 2013. pp. 183-194

[4] Patestas MA, Gartner LP. A Textbook of Neuroanatomy. Malden, MA: Blackwell Publishing; 2006. pp. 398-422

[5] Weininger J et al. Papez's forgotten tract: 80 years of unreconciled findings concerning the thalamocingulate tract. Frontiers in Neuroanatomy. 2019;**13**:14

[6] Edinger L. The Anatomy of the Central Nervous System of Man and of Vertebrates in General. 5th ed. Philadelphia, Pa, USA: F.A. Davis; 1899. Edited by W. S. Hall assisted by P. L. Holland and E. P. Carlton

[7] Buzsaki G, Leung LW, Vanderwolf CH. Cellular bases of hippocampal EEG in the behaving rat. Brain Research. 1983;**287**:139-171

[8] Okonogi T, Sasaki T. Theta-range oscillations in stress-induced mental disorders as an oscillotherapeutic target. Frontiers in Behavioral Neuroscience. 2021;**15**:698-753

[9] Sigurdsson T, Duvarci S. Hippocampal-prefrontal interactions in cognition, behavior and psychiatric disease. Frontiers in Systems Neuroscience. 2016;**9**:190

[10] Mocellin P, Mikulovic S. The role of the medial septum-associated networks in controlling locomotion and motivation to move. Frontiers in Neural Circuits. 2021;**15**:699-798

[11] Bressler SL, Menon V. Large-scale brain networks in cognition: Emerging methods and principles. Trends in Cognitive Sciences. 2010;**14**(6):277-290

[12] Anderson RJ et al. Repetitive transcranial magnetic stimulation for treatment of resistant depression: Re-establishing connections. Clinical Neurophysiology. 2016;**127**:3394-3405

[13] Menon V. The triple network model, insight and large-scale brain organization in autism. Biological Psychiatry. 2018;**84**:236-238

[14] Menon V, Palaniyappan L, Supekar K. Integrative brain network and salience models of psychopathology and cognitive dysfunction in schizophrenia. Biological Psychiatry. 2022;**94**(2):108-120

[15] Banovac I, Sedmak D, Judaš M, Petanjek Z. Von economo neurons - Primate-specific or commonplace in the mammalian brain? Frontiers in Neural Circuits. 2021;**15**:714611

[16] Chong JSX, Ng GJP, Lee SC, Zhou J. Salience network connectivity in the insula is associated with individual differences in interoceptive accuracy. Brain Structure and Function. 2017;**222**:1635-1644

[17] Seeley WW. The salience network: A neural system for perceiving and responding to homeostatic demands.

The Journal of Neuroscience. 2019;**39**:9878-9882

[18] Catani M et al. A revised limbic system model for memory, emotion and behaviour. Neuroscience and Biobehavioral Reviews. 2013;**37**(8):1724-1737

[19] Anderson P, Morris R, Amaral DG, Bliss TVP, O'Keefe J, editors. The Hippocampus Book. 1st ed. New York: Oxford University Press; 2006. ISBN 978-0-19-510027-3

[20] Schlichting ML, Gumus M, Zhu T, Mack ML. The structure of hippocampal circuitry relates to rapid category learning in humans. Hippocampus. 2021;**31**(11):1179-1190

[21] Scharfman HE, Myers CE. Hilar mossy cells of the dentate gyrus: A historical perspective. Frontiers in Neural Circuits. 2013;**9**(6):106

[22] Schultz SR, Rolls ET. Analysis of information transmission in the Schaffer collaterals. Hippocampus. 1999;**9**(5):582-598

[23] Schlingloff D, Káli S, Freund TF, Hájos N, Gulyás AI. Mechanisms of sharp wave initiation and ripple generation. The Journal of Neuroscience. 2014;**34**(34):11385-11398

[24] Müller C, Remy S. Septo-hippocampal interaction. Cell and Tissue Research. 2018;**373**(3):565-575

[25] Rolls ET. The cingulate cortex and limbic systems for action, emotion, and memory. Handbook of Clinical Neurology. 2019;**166**:23-37

[26] Šimić G, Tkalčić M, Vukić V, Mulc D, et al. Understanding emotions: Origins and roles of the amygdala. Biomolecules. 2021;**11**:823

[27] Mancall E, Brock D, Gray H. Gray's Clinical Neuroanatomy: The Anatomic Basis for Clinical Neuroscience. Philadelphia: Elsevier/Saunders; 2011

[28] Haines DE, Mihailoff GA, Cunningham W, Schenk M, et al. Fundamental Neuroscience for Basic and Clinical Applications. Philadelphia, PA: Elsevier; 2018

[29] Gu S, Wang F, Patel NP, Bourgeois JA, Huang JH. A model for basic emotions using observations of behavior in drosophila. Frontiers in Psychology. 2019;**10**:781

[30] George DT, Ameli R, Koob GF. Periaqueductal Gray sheds light on dark areas of psychopathology. Trends in Neurosciences. 2019;**42**(5):349-360

[31] Brandão ML, Lovick TA. Role of the dorsal periaqueductal gray in posttraumatic stress disorder: Mediation by dopamine and neurokinin. Translational Psychiatry. 2019;**9**:232

[32] Andrea S, de Sousa R. Emotion. In: Zalta EN, editor. The Stanford Encyclopedia of Philosophy (Summer 2021 Edition). Available from: https://plato.stanford.edu/archives/sum2021/entries/emotion/

[33] Russell J. A circumplex model of affect. Journal of Personality and Social Psychology. 1980;**39**(6):1161-1178

[34] Hartley CA, Phelps EA. Changing fear: The neurocircuitry of emotion regulation. Neuropsychopharmacology. 2010;**35**(1):136-146

[35] MacLean PD. The Triune Brain in Evolution: Role in Paleocerebral Functions. New York: Plenum Press; 1990

[36] Panksepp J. Affective neuroscience of the emotional BrainMind: Evolutionary

perspectives and implications for understanding depression. Dialogues in Clinical Neuroscience. 2010;**12**(4):533-545

[37] Macpherson T, Hikida T. Role of basal ganglia neurocircuitry in the pathology of psychiatric disorders. Psychiatry and Clinical Neurosciences. 2019;**73**(6):289-301

[38] Haber SN. The primate basal ganglia: Parallel and integrative networks. Journal of Chemical Neuroanatomy. 2003;**26**:317-330

[39] Mink JW. The basal ganglia: Focused selection and inhibition of competing motor programs. Progress in Neurobiology. 1996;**50**:381-425

[40] Alexander GE, Crutcher MD. Functional architecture of basal ganglia circuits: Neural substrates of parallel processing. Trends in Neurosciences. 1990;**13**:266-271

[41] Alexander GE, at al. Parallel organization of functionally segregated circuits linking basal ganglia and cortex. Annual Review of Neuroscience. 1986;**9**:357-381

[42] Kupchik YM et al. Coding the direct/indirect pathways by D1 and D2 receptors is not valid for accumbens projections. Nature Neuroscience. 2015;**18**:1230-1232

[43] Wise RA. Dopamine, learning and motivation. Nature Reviews Neuroscience. 2004;**5**(6):483-494

[44] Aston-Jones G, Cohen JD. An integrative theory of locus coeruleus-norepinephrine function: Adaptive gain and optimal performance. Annual Review of Neuroscience. 2005;**28**:403-450

[45] Morrow JD, Dworkin SI. Serotonin and the regulation of mood: A review of the neurochemical basis of depression. Biological Psychiatry. 1999;**46**(5):686-694

[46] Gray JA. The behavioral inhibition system and the behavioral activation system: A revised model. Journal of Research in Personality. 1994;**28**(4):225-232

[47] Muller RU, Kubie JL. The effects of changes in the environment on the spatial firing of hippocampal complex-spike cells. Journal of Neuroscience. 1987;**7**(7):1951-1968

[48] Acharya L, Aghajan ZM, Vuong C, Moore JJ, Mehta MR. Causal influence of visual cues on hippocampal directional selectivity. Cell. 2016;**164**(1-2):197-207

[49] Poucet B, Lenck-Santini PP, et al. Place cells, spatial representation and navigation in blind rats. Journal of Physiology-Paris. 2003;**97**(4-6):613-620

[50] Royer S, Buzsáki G. Delta oscillations in the hippocampus during behavior: Coordination of multiple theta modules. PLoS One. 2012;7(9):e44827

[51] Ruiz N, Axel R, Datta SR. A wiring logic for olfactory behavior. Nature. 2021;**596**(7871):184-190

[52] Eichenbaum H et al. The hippocampus, memory, and place cells: Is it spatial memory or a memory space? Neuron. 1999;**23**(2):209-226

[53] Knierim JJ et al. Hippocampal place cells: Parallel input streams, subregional processing, and implications for episodic memory. Hippocampus. 2006;**16**(9):755-764

[54] Ravassard P et al. Multisensory control of hippocampal spatiotemporal selectivity. Science. 2013;**340**(6138):1342-1346

[55] Rolls ET et al. Information about spatial view in an ensemble of primate hippocampal cells. Journal of Neurophysiology. 1998;**79**(4):1797-1813

[56] Rolls ET. The primate hippocampus and episodic memory. In: Dere E, Easton A, Nadel L, Huston JP, editors. Handbook of Behavioral Neuroscience. Vol. 18. Amsterdam, The Netherlands: Elsevier; 2008. pp. 417-462. ISBN 978 0 444 53174 2

[57] Rolls ET. Mechanisms for pattern completion and pattern separation in the hippocampus. Frontiers in Systems Neuroscience. 2013;**7**:74

[58] Rolls ET, Zhang C, Feng J. Hippocampal storage and recall of neocortical "what"-"where" representations. Hippocampus. Nov 2024;**34**(11):608-624

[59] Griffiths BJ, Parish G, et al. Directional coupling of slow and fast hippocampal gamma with neocortical alpha/beta oscillations in human episodic memory. Proceedings of the National Academy of Sciences. 2019;**116**(43):21834-21842

[60] Mao D et al. Spatial representations in macaque hippocampal formation during free navigation. Neuron. 2021;**109**(21):3597-3611

[61] Jacobs J et al. Direct recordings of grid-like neuronal activity in human spatial navigation. Nature Neuroscience. 2013;**16**(9):1188-1190

[62] Rolls ET, Treves A. A theory of hippocampal function: New developments. Progress in Neurobiology. Jul 2024;**238**:102636

[63] Moore JJ et al. Linking hippocampal multiplexed tuning, Hebbian plasticity and navigation. Nature. 2021;**599**:442-448

[64] Lambon Ralph MA et al. The neural and computational bases of semantic cognition. Nature Reviews Neuroscience. 2017;**18**(1):42-55

[65] Epstein R, Kanwisher N. A cortical representation of the local visual environment. Neuron. 1998;**21**(2):373-383

[66] Kanwisher N et al. The fusiform face area: A module in human extrastriate cortex specialized for face perception. Journal of Neuroscience. 1997;**17**(11):4302-4311

[67] Tsarouchas N et al. Effects of moderate hypobaric hypoxia on evoked categorical visuocognitive responses. Clinical Neurophysiology. 2008;**119**(7):1475-1485

[68] Coggan DD et al. Selectivity for mid-level properties of faces and places in the fusiform face area and parahippocampal place area. The European Journal of Neuroscience. 2019;**49**(12):1587-1596

[69] Binder JR et al. Where is the semantic system? A critical review and meta-analysis of 120 functional neuroimaging studies. Cerebral Cortex. 2009;**19**(12):2767-2796

[70] Jung JY, Lambon Ralph MA. Distinct but cooperating brain networks supporting semantic cognition. Cerebral Cortex. 2023;**33**(5):2539-2553

[71] Schimmelpfennig J et al. The role of the salience network in cognitive and affective deficits. Frontiers in Human Neuroscience. 2023;**17**:1133367

[72] Rakic P. Evolution of the neocortex: A perspective from developmental biology. Nature Reviews. Neuroscience. 2009;**10**(10):724-735

[73] Schacter DL et al. The future of memory: Remembering, imagining, and the brain. Neuron. 2012;**76**(4):677-694

[74] Mavroudis I et al. Understanding functional neurological disorder: Recent insights and diagnostic challenges. International Journal of Molecular Sciences. 2024;**25**(8):4470

[75] Stone J et al. Conversion disorder: Current problems and potential solutions for DSM-5. Journal of Psychosomatic Research. 2011;**71**:369-376

[76] Stone J. Functional symptoms in neurology: Management. Journal of Neurology, Neurosurgery, and Psychiatry. 2005;**76**:i13-i21

[77] Abbey SE. The American Psychiatric Publishing Textbook of Psychosomatic Medicine. Arlington, VA, USA: American Psychiatric Publishing, Inc.; 2005. Somatization and somatoform disorders

[78] Gabbard GO. Gabbard's Treatments of Psychiatric Disorders. Washington, DC, USA: American Psychiatric Pub; 2007

[79] Aybek S et al. Neural correlates of recall of life events in conversion disorder. JAMA Psychiatry. 2014;**71**:52

[80] Diez I et al. Corticolimbic fast-tracking: Enhanced multimodal integration in functional neurological disorder. Journal of Neurology, Neurosurgery, and Psychiatry. 2019;**90**:929-938

[81] Edwards MJ, Adams RA, Brown H, Parees I, Friston KJ. A Bayesian account of "hysteria". Brain. 2012;**135**:3495-3512

[82] Friston KJ, Daunizeau J, Kilner J, Kiebel SJ. Action and behavior: A free-energy formulation. Biological Cybernetics. 2010;**102**:227-260

[83] Cojan Y, Waber L, Carruzzo A, Vuilleumier P. Motor inhibition in hysterical conversion paralysis. NeuroImage. 2009;**47**:1026-1037

[84] Nachev P et al. Volition and conflict in human medial frontal cortex. Current Biology. 2005;**15**:122-128

[85] Lebois LAM et al. Deconstructing dissociation: A triple network model of trauma-related dissociation and its subtypes. Neuropsychopharmacology. 2022;**47**(13):2261-2270

[86] Nicholson AA et al. Classifying heterogeneous presentations of PTSD via the default mode, central executive and salience networks with machine learning. Neuroimage: Clinical. 2020;**27**:102262

[87] Beck JS. Cognitive Behavior Therapy: Basics and beyond. 2nd ed. New York: The Guilford Press; 2011. pp. 19-20

[88] Field TA, Beeson ET, Jones LK. The new ABCs: A practitioner's guide to neuroscience-informed cognitive-behavior therapy. Journal of Mental Health Counseling. 2015;**37**(3):206-220

[89] Benjamin CL et al. History of cognitive-behavioral therapy in youth. Child and Adolescent Psychiatric Clinics of North America. 2011;**20**(2):179-189

[90] Zaccaro A et al. How breath-control can change your life: A systematic review on psycho-physiological correlates of slow breathing. Frontiers in Human Neuroscience. 2018;**12**:353

[91] Sinha M et al. Impact of altered breathing patterns on interaction of EEG and heart rate variability. Annals of Neurosciences. 2020;**27**(2):67-74

[92] Perez DL et al. Neuroimaging in functional neurological disorder: State of the field and research agenda. Neuroimage: Clinical. 2021;**30**:102623

Section 2

Hippocampal Dysfunctions

Chapter 6

Hippocampal Vascularization Patterns and Its Role in Vascular Impairment

Fereshteh Azedi and Mohammad Taghi Joghataei

Abstract

Although there is extensive research on the hippocampus and its vital roles in memory, learning, and emotion, the vascularization patterns and vascular endothelium of the hippocampus have received comparatively less focus, especially concerning pathological conditions such as ischemia or stroke. In this review, we propose that the vascularization patterns and vascular cells of the hippocampus may significantly influence the brain's structure and function during ischemic events and strokes. Our discussion will concentrate on hippocampal stroke and highlight important aspects of hippocampal endothelial cells, including pericytes, in this context.

Keywords: hippocamp, vascular, impairment, ischemia, stroke

1. Introduction

The hippocampus plays several critical roles in brain functions [1], including memory, learning, and emotion [2]. Any impairment in this area can significantly affect essential processes within the brain [3, 4]. Understanding the structure of the hippocampus and its neuronal circuits is crucial for developing new strategies to protect this vital region [5]. Consequently, there is a wealth of prior research in this area [4, 6]. However, there remains a lack of studies focusing on the vascular supply and patterns within the hippocampus. Blood circulation in the hippocampus is particularly vulnerable to damage from stroke and cerebral ischemia, more so than in other neurological conditions [7]. This vulnerability is attributed to the distinct architecture of its layers compared to other cortical areas [8]. Additionally, previous findings indicate that blood flow and circulation in the hippocampus are lower, making it more susceptible to hippocampal strokes or infarctions than other regions of the brain [9].

Specific vascular endothelial cells in the hippocampus play crucial roles in both physiological and pathophysiological conditions [10]. The blood-brain barrier (BBB), often referred to as the neurovascular unit (NVU), consists of various components, including endothelial cells, pericytes, the basement membrane, astrocyte end-feet, and surrounding oligodendrocytes and microglia [11]. Neurovascular coupling is a process that links these components to neurons, resulting in increased blood flow to specific areas in response to heightened neuronal activity [12]. A distinctive aspect of the NVU is the close, and sometimes direct, contact between its cellular components, facilitating effective communication [13]. Blood vessels are lined with endothelial cells and pericytes. Pericytes, which are mesenchymal-derived cells originating from the brain side [14], are found in capillaries, precapillary arterioles, and postcapillary venules; however, larger vessels do not contain vascular smooth muscle cells (VSMCs) [15]. Collectively, pericytes and VSMCs are referred to as vascular mural cells (VMCs) [16].

The hippocampus is notably one of the first areas of the brain to experience blood-brain barrier (BBB) leakage. Furthermore, the degradation of the BBB is a normal part of the aging process, and this breakdown is more pronounced in patients with mild cognitive impairment (MCI). These findings may be associated with the lower number of pericytes in the human hippocampus compared to other brain regions [16]. Additionally, it is important to highlight the presence of endothelial cells with a more inflammatory profile in this area of the brain. The condition of the underlying endothelial cells and pericytes, along with reduced coverage by pericytes, may contribute to the hippocampus's vulnerability to ischemic injury [17].

2. The organization of the blood vessels in the hippocampus

The main supply to the hippocampus usually arises from the posterior circulation *via* single or multiple middle and posterior hippocampal arteries. Additionally, the collateral branches associated with the posterior cerebral artery (PCA) play a crucial role in supplying blood to the hippocampus, supplemented by contributions from the anterior choroidal artery (AChA). Erdem and his team investigated 30 fixed brain hemispheres postmortem through microscopy. Their findings indicate that the hippocampus is most likely to receive a mixed supply from the branches of the PCA and AChA, a pattern observed in 17 out of 30 hemispheres (57%) [18].

Spallazzi et al. conducted an evaluation of hippocampal vascularization patterns using high-resolution 7 Tesla time-of-flight MRA in 62 hemispheres, focusing on healthy young adults aged 19 to 34 *in vivo*. The researchers found that 31 (50%) of the hemispheres received a mixed vascular supply from both the PCA and AChA.

The most frequently observed patterns for the origin of the hippocampal arteries were primarily branches of the PCA, including the inferior temporal branches of the PCA (27–34%) and the anterior inferior temporal branch of the PCA (10–11%). The least common vascularization pattern noted was the hippocampus being solely supplied by branches of the AChA, which occurred in 3–5% of individuals [19].

Previous research indicates that the primary source of blood supply to the hippocampus is the posterior cerebral artery (PCA). The variability in the Circle of Willis leads to differences in blood flow contributions to both the PCA and the hippocampus. In smaller mammals such as cats, sheep, and gerbils, a greater portion of hippocampal blood flow generally comes from the anterior circulation, while the PCA is mainly supplied by the carotid arteries *via* the posterior communicating artery. In humans, the PCA is typically supplied by the vertebrobasilar system, making the posterior circulation the main source of blood supply to the hippocampus [20].

Conversely, around 20–30% of individuals exhibit a fetal PCA, which is characterized by a posterior communicating artery that is larger than the P1 segment of the PCA or by an underdeveloped P1 segment. This results in the anterior circulation supplying the majority of the blood flow to the PCA. As a result, the differences in how the anterior and posterior circulations contribute to the supply of the distal branches of the PCA that nourish the hippocampus are clear (**Figure 1**) [21].

DOI: http://dx.doi.org/10.5772/intechopen.1011628

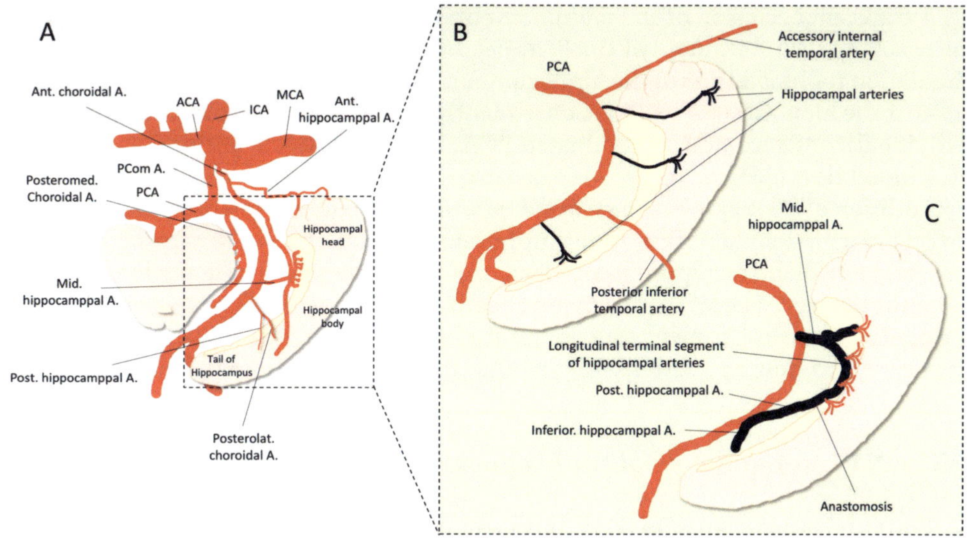

Figure 1.
Blood supply to the hippocampal region. Illustrations of the macrovascular supply of the hippocampus, including an anatomical variation of the hippocampal arterial supply. A: The variation of the vascular supply of the hippocampus as described by Erdem et al. B: The general macrovascular framework of the mesial temporal lobe. ACA: anterior cerebral artery, ICA: internal carotid artery, MCA: middle cerebral artery, PcomA: posterior communicating artery, PCA: posterior cerebral artery, A: artery.

2.1 Vascular supply in the hippocampus compared to the neocortex under physiological and pathological states

The neocortex is organized into six horizontal layers of neurons, while the hippocampus has three layers, with densely packed large pyramidal neuron cell bodies in its middle layer [22].

The activity patterns of large groups of hippocampal pyramidal neurons, known as place cells, differ from those in cortical brain regions. The energy demands in the active hippocampus are likely lower than those in the active cortex, and the mechanisms that align neuronal metabolic needs with corresponding increases in local blood flow may vary from those in other, more extensively researched cortical areas [23].

Research has thoroughly mapped the microvasculature of the rodent brain, consistently showing that the hippocampus has a lower density of blood vessels compared to other brain regions. Studies indicate that the hippocampus exhibits the lowest vascular density, which impacts oxygen diffusion due to its fewer, more evenly spaced microvessels compared to the corpus callosum [18].

While there is a reduction in vascular density, it is thought that the metabolic needs of the hippocampus continue to be adequately met, likely due to a decrease in the number of spatially organized neurons in the cortical regions. Given the notable decline in capillary density, the increased distance between microvessels, and the densely packed pyramidal neurons, it seems that the hippocampus may struggle to maintain adequate perfusion under pathological conditions [24]. Even minor reductions in blood flow to the hippocampus can lead to significant impacts on neuronal activity, memory, and cognitive functions due to issues such as capillary rarefaction and hyper constriction [25].

A transient occlusion of the middle cerebral artery (tMCAO) occurs in gerbils and mice lacking the P1 segment of the PCA, leading to a greater reliance on the anterior circulation for blood flow to the hippocampus. This can result in infarction in specific areas of the hippocampal region. Consequently, in cases of cerebral ischemic stroke in individuals with an anterior-dominated PCA, it is essential to identify the source of PCA blood flow [26].

Additionally, a major blockage in the carotid system or middle cerebral artery (MCA) can hinder blood flow to the hippocampus, leading to ischemia and memory loss after a stroke. The hippocampus is particularly susceptible to hypoxic and ischemic damage. Therefore, to support healthy memory and cognitive function, it is essential to ensure proper perfusion of the hippocampus, which encompasses both baseline blood flow and activity-related fluctuations in blood flow [10, 27].

3. The NVU components of the hippocampus

The NVU is made up of several components, including endothelial cells, pericytes, the basement membrane, astrocyte end-feet, and the surrounding oligodendrocytes and microglia.

3.1 Vascular endothelial cells

The endothelium forms a continuous layer across various vascular levels, including arteries, precapillary vessels, capillaries, postcapillary venules, and veins. Mural cells are also present in different segments of the vasculature, with smooth muscle cells (SMCs) found in arterioles and venules and pericytes located in capillaries [28]. The perivascular space is defined by the vascular and astroglial membranes, which merge, resulting in their disappearance [12]. Alterations at the cellular and molecular levels in endothelial cells within the cerebrovascular system are recognized as key factors contributing to neuropathological disorders [29].

3.2 Pericytes

Pericytes are crucial for the cerebrovascular system, playing a significant role in maintaining cerebrovascular homeostasis [16]. Endothelial cells affect how pericytes regulate the integrity of the blood-brain barrier, angiogenesis, and hemodynamic responses in brain microvessels [15]. Furthermore, pericytes share characteristics with immune cells, including their responses to inflammatory stimuli, antigen presentation, and regulation of fibrosis. Their phagocytic ability enables pericytes to eliminate harmful substances like amyloid-β (Aβ) peptides from perivascular regions. In a mouse model of amyloidosis, a deficiency in pericytes caused by Pdgfrb haploinsufficiency impairs Aβ clearance, resulting in increased accumulation of Aβ in the brain [30].

Pericytes play a role similar to that of mural cells in the capillary endothelium, precapillary arterioles, and postcapillary venules. Their functions extend beyond regulating blood flow; they also participate in paracrine signaling during angiogenesis and phagocytosis. The function of the blood-brain barrier is significantly influenced by pericytes [31].

It is not clear how other important cellular parts of the neurovascular unit, like pericytes, are regulated in cognitively stable stroke survivors or those who develop poststroke depression (PSD) and vertebral artery dissection (VAD). The breakdown of the hippocampal BBB is the cause of ischemic injury, which is a common occurrence for capillary pericytes. Previous studies have employed PDGF receptor immunoreactivity to monitor pericyte coverage in various conditions, but the lack of more reliable markers has prevented greater characterization of pericytes [32]. Notch3, ANG1, and VEGF are other important signaling that have important roles in preserving the BBB integrity (**Figure 2A**) [29, 33].

Previous research indicates that reduced PDGFB-PDGFRb signaling results in a deficiency of pericytes, disrupting homeostasis and affecting tight junctions and basement membrane proteins [25]. This degradation of the blood-brain barrier (BBB) leads to increased fluid flow and a loss of selectivity for proteins and macromolecules. Neurotoxins like thrombin and fibrin can cross the BBB, contributing to neurodegeneration. The passage of serum proteins such as albumin and IgG across the BBB causes edema. Additionally, microvascular degradation and pericapillary edema diminish capillary blood flow, resulting in hypoxia (**Figure 2B**) [34].

Besides, age-associated dementia disorders are associated with a loss of capillary pericytes in the hippocampus, which is mostly specific to the CA1 region [2]. Pericyte cell loss is probably linked to the age-related breakdown of the neurovascular unit of the hippocampus, which negatively impacts BBB function. The bilateral common carotid artery stenosis (BCAS) model of chronic cerebral hypoperfusion replicated these findings, and tissue volume loss was also associated with them. BCAS mice exposed to full-time environmental enrichment (EE) showed remarkable restoration of both CA1 structure volume and capillary density, as well as pericyte numbers. Changes in tissue perfusion and local cellular requirements influence the responses of capillary pericyte cells, which can be revived through appropriate interventions [35].

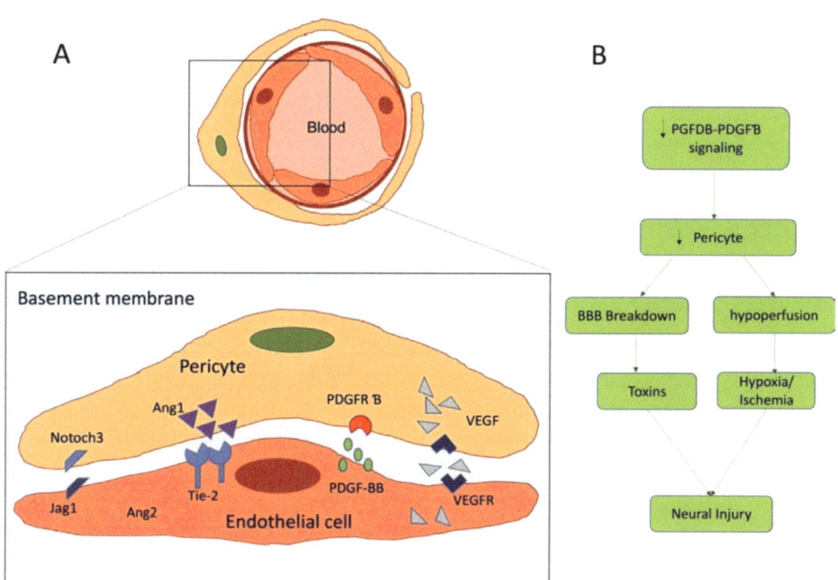

Figure 2.
A: pericytes communicating with endothelial cells, including key signaling pathways (e.g., PDGF-BB, Notch3, ANG1, and VEGF). B: The diagram illustrates that a decrease in PDGFB-PDGFRb signaling results in the loss of pericytes. This deficiency in pericytes leads to a breakdown of the blood-brain barrier (BBB) and reduced blood flow, which ultimately contributes to neuronal injury.

Likewise, it is well established that in physiological conditions, hippocampal mural cells exhibit reduced levels of ion channels and skeletal muscle actin (Acta1). Moreover, endothelial cells in the hippocampus show decreased levels of prostaglandin E synthase (Ptges) and Kir 2.1, an inwardly rectifying potassium channel responsible for transmitting vasodilatory signals from capillaries to arterioles. As a result, the hippocampus seems to be especially susceptible to disruptions in the BBB due to variations in the structural mechanisms of pericytes and neurovascular coupling, which stem from the diverse gene expression of endothelial cells and pericytes in different regions [36]. This results in diminished communication between endothelial cells and pericytes, such as through prostaglandins, which impacts their capacity to regulate cerebral blood flow [37].

3.3 The NVU components in the hippocampus versus the cortex

Cholinergic neurons originating from the basal forebrain innervate the neurovascular unit (NVU) in both the cortex and hippocampus. The hippocampus, in particular, exhibits greater cholinergic interaction with perivascular astrocytes in capillaries, along with a thicker basement membrane in veins compared to the cortex. Furthermore, research indicates that astrocytes in the hippocampus experience more pronounced age-related changes in gene expression than those in the cortex. Additionally, prior studies suggest regional variations in the composition and function of vascular cells, such as endothelial cells and pericytes, between the cortex and hippocampus. Microglia, the brain's resident immune cells, also contribute to the NVU and may be implicated in neurodegenerative diseases. Research has shown a reduction in microglial coverage within the NVU in Alzheimer's disease in both the hippocampus and cortex, with more significant changes observed in the cortex (**Figure 3**).

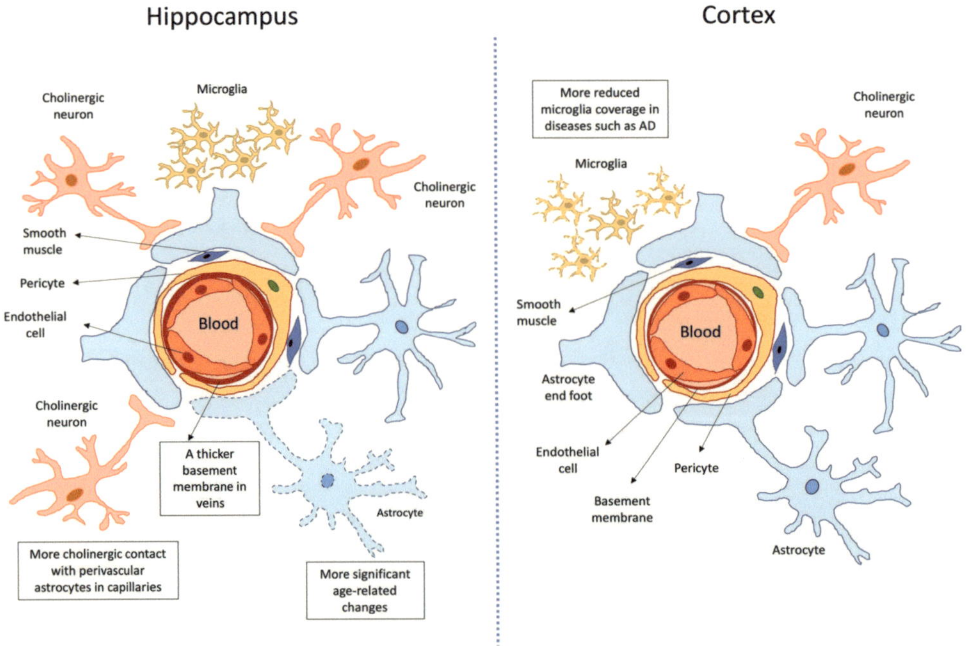

Figure 3.
The NVU components in the hippocampus versus the cortex.

4. Future directions

Gaining a deeper understanding of the mechanisms behind stroke, mild cognitive impairment (MCI), and age-related dementias associated with vascular issues is vital for progressing both basic science and clinical research. Identifying potential therapeutic targets plays a key role in this effort. One promising target is the vasculature of the hippocampus, particularly the function of arterioles and the blood-brain barrier (BBB). This region may offer significant therapeutic opportunities for addressing stroke and other neurovascular diseases [38].

Diagnosing conditions that impact the hippocampus can be difficult due to the similarity of their clinical symptoms. Consequently, imaging findings are essential for achieving an accurate diagnosis. Future research employing advanced imaging techniques and analyses is needed to establish a clear link between variations in hippocampal blood flow and differences in macrovascular anatomy among individuals. There is an urgent need to enhance the detection and understanding of vascular abnormalities at the micro-level, where critical vascular nourishment and cellular metabolic changes occur. Mapping the vasculature of the hippocampus has immediate implications for comprehending the effects of normal aging and the underlying causes of various neurovascular diseases [39].

Research on the vascularization of the hippocampus has traditionally depended on imaging techniques such as conventional computed tomography (CT) and magnetic resonance imaging (MRI), which provide limited resolution. To obtain higher resolution, researchers have turned to methods like light microscopy, electron microscopy, and a combination of injection and corrosion techniques with scanning electron microscopy. However, these advanced approaches do not preserve the samples [40].

Recently, there have been significant advancements in nondestructive imaging techniques that improve visualization at both macro and micro scales through the use of synchrotron radiation. A prominent technique is Hierarchical Phase-Contrast Tomography (HiP-CT). Looking ahead, HiP-CT aims to enhance *in vivo* medical imaging by utilizing synchrotron data as a reference to train super-resolution algorithms for integration into standard imaging machines. These developments have the potential to not only enrich our understanding of micro-anatomy but also aid in surgical guidance and deepen our insights into hippocampal pathologies [41].

5. Conclusions

This comprehensive review examines our current understanding of vascular functionality in the hippocampus, hemodynamic processes in this region, and the role of the blood-brain barrier. It emphasizes characteristics that differentiate the hippocampus from other cerebrovascular areas, which increase its susceptibility to hypoxic or ischemic damage. By studying hippocampal blood vessel development in living subjects, along with perfusion and clinical data, we can begin to analyze how differences in hippocampal vascularization among individuals relate to the interplay between vascular and degenerative diseases in this brain region. Furthermore, our findings may provide valuable insights into the neurovascular mapping and angiographic patterns of the hippocampus, as well as their implications for related research areas, such as studies on micro- and macro-vasculature in the hippocampus.

Conflict of interest

The authors declare no conflict of interest.

Author details

Fereshteh Azedi[1,2] and Mohammad Taghi Joghataei[1,2]*

1 Cellular and Molecular Research Center, Iran University of Medical Sciences, Iran

2 Department of Neuroscience, Faculty of Advanced Technologies in Medicine, Iran University of Medical Sciences, Tehran, Iran

*Address all correspondence to: mt.joghataei@yahoo.com

References

[1] Johnson AC. Hippocampal vascular supply and its role in vascular cognitive impairment. Stroke. 2023;**54**(3):673-685

[2] Uemura MT, Maki T, Ihara M, Lee VMY, Trojanowski JQ. Brain microvascular Pericytes in vascular cognitive impairment and dementia. Frontiers in Aging Neuroscience. 2020;**12**:80

[3] Azarpazhooh MR, Hachinski V. Vascular cognitive impairment: A preventable component of dementia. Handbook of Clinical Neurology. 2019;**167**:377-391

[4] Gemmell E, Bosomworth H, Allan L, Hall R, Khundakar A, Oakley AE, et al. Hippocampal neuronal atrophy and cognitive function in delayed poststroke and aging-related dementias. Stroke. 2011;**43**(3):808-814

[5] Perosa V, Priester A, Ziegler G, Cardenas-Blanco A, Dobisch L, Spallazzi M, et al. Hippocampal vascular reserve associated with cognitive performance and hippocampal volume. Brain. 2020;**143**(2):622-634

[6] Sachdev PS, Chen X, Joscelyne A, Wen W, Altendorf A, Brodaty H. Hippocampal size and dementia in stroke patients: The Sydney Stroke Study. Journal of the Neurological Sciences. 2007;**260**(1-2):71-77

[7] Ding R, Hase Y, Ameen-Ali KE, Ndung'u M, Stevenson W, Barsby J, et al. Loss of capillary pericytes and the blood-brain barrier in white matter in poststroke and vascular dementias and Alzheimer's disease. Brain Pathology. 2020;**30**(6):1087-1101

[8] Fein G, Di Sclafani V, Tanabe J, Cardenas V, Weiner MW, Jagust WJ, et al. Hippocampal and cortical atrophy predict dementia in subcortical ischemic vascular disease. Neurology. 2000;**55**(11):1626-1635

[9] Vikner T, Eklund A, Karalija N, Malm J, Riklund K, Lindenberger U, et al. Cerebral arterial pulsatility is linked to hippocampal microvascular function and episodic memory in healthy older adults. Journal of Cerebral Blood Flow and Metabolism. 2021;**41**(7):1778-1790

[10] Toth P, Tarantini S, Csiszar A, Ungvari Z. Functional vascular contributions to cognitive impairment and dementia: Mechanisms and consequences of cerebral autoregulatory dysfunction, endothelial impairment, and neurovascular uncoupling in aging. American Journal of Physiology. Heart and Circulatory Physiology. 2016;**312**(1):H1-H20

[11] Burke MJ, Nelson L, Slade JY, Oakley AE, Khundakar AA, Kalaria RN. Morphometry of the hippocampal microvasculature in post-stroke and age-related dementias. Neuropathology and Applied Neurobiology. 2013;**40**(3):284-295

[12] Kirabali T, Rust R, Rigotti S, Siccoli A, Nitsch RM, Kulic L. Distinct changes in all major components of the neurovascular unit across different neuropathological stages of Alzheimer's disease. Brain Pathology. 2020;**30**(6):1056-1070

[13] Berthiaume AA, Hartmann DA, Majesky MW, Bhat NR, Shih AY. Pericyte structural remodeling in cerebrovascular health and homeostasis. Frontiers in Aging Neuroscience. 2018;**10**:210

[14] Jackson S, ElAli A, Virgintino D, Gilbert MR. Blood-brain barrier pericyte

importance in malignant gliomas: What we can learn from stroke and Alzheimer's disease. Neuro-Oncology. 2017;**19**(9):1173-1182

[15] Winkler EA, Birk H, Burkhardt JK, Chen X, Yue JK, Guo D, et al. Reductions in brain pericytes are associated with arteriovenous malformation vascular instability. Journal of Neurosurgery. 2018;**129**(6):1464-1474

[16] Beard DJ, Brown LS, Sutherland BA. The rise of pericytes in neurovascular research. Journal of Cerebral Blood Flow and Metabolism. 2020;**40**(12):2366-2373

[17] Ding R, Hase Y, Burke M, Foster V, Stevenson W, Polvikoski T, et al. Loss with ageing but preservation of frontal cortical capillary pericytes in post-stroke dementia, vascular dementia and Alzheimer's disease. Acta Neuropathologica Communications. 2021;**9**(1):130

[18] Erdem A, Yaargil G, Roth P. Microsurgical anatomy of the hippocampal arteries. Journal of Neurosurgery. 1993;**79**(2):256-265

[19] Spallazzi M, Dobisch L, Becke A, Berron D, Stucht D, Oeltze-Jafra S, et al. Hippocampal vascularization patterns: A high-resolution 7 Tesla time-of-flight magnetic resonance angiography study. NeuroImage: Clinical. 2018;**21**:101609

[20] Vockert N, Perosa V, Ziegler G, Schreiber F, Priester A, Spallazzi M, et al. Hippocampal vascularization patterns exert local and distant effects on brain structure but not vascular pathology in old age. Brain Communications. 2021;**3**(3):fcab127

[21] Wong WS, Tsuruda JS, Liberman RL, Chirino A, Vogt JF, Gangitano E. Color Doppler imaging of intracranial vessels in the neonate. AJR. American Journal of Roentgenology. 1989;**152**(5):1065-1070

[22] Coyle P. Vascular patterns of the rat hippocampal formation. Experimental Neurology. 1976;**52**(3):447-458

[23] Simonds GR, Truwit CL. Anatomy of the cerebral vasculature. Neuroimaging Clinics of North America. 1994;**4**(4):691-706

[24] Komiyama M. Functional anatomy of the cerebral arteries. No Shinkei Geka. 2005;**33**(3):213-224

[25] Miners JS, Schulz I, Love S. Differing associations between A-B accumulation, hypoperfusion, blood-brain barrier dysfunction and loss of PDGFRB pericyte marker in the precuneus and parietal white matter in Alzheimer's disease. Journal of Cerebral Blood Flow and Metabolism. 2017;**38**(1):103-115

[26] Stępień T, Tarka S, Chutorański D, Felczak P, Acewicz A, Wierzba-Bobrowicz T. Neurogenesis in adult human brain after hemorrhage and ischemic stroke. Folia Neuropathologica. 2019;**56**(4):293-300

[27] Kim JH, Ko PW, Lee HW, Jeong JY, Lee MG, Lee WH, et al. Astrocyte-derived lipocalin-2 mediates hippocampal damage and cognitive deficits in experimental models of vascular dementia. Glia. 2017;**65**(9):1471-1490

[28] Hase Y, Ding R, Harrison G, Hawthorne E, King A, Gettings S, et al. White matter capillaries in vascular and neurodegenerative dementias. Acta Neuropathologica Communications. 2019;**7**(1):16

[29] Lee C, Agoston DV. Vascular endothelial growth factor is involved in mediating increased de novo hippocampal neurogenesis in response to traumatic brain injury. Journal of Neurotrauma. 2009;**27**(3):541-553

[30] Hase Y, Jobson D, Cheong J, Gotama K, Maffei L, Hase M, et al. Hippocampal capillary pericytes in post-stroke and vascular dementias and Alzheimer's disease and experimental chronic cerebral hypoperfusion. Acta Neuropathologica Communications. 2024;**12**(1):29

[31] Underly RG, Levy M, Hartmann DA, Grant RI, Watson AN, Shih AY. Pericytes as inducers of rapid, matrix metalloproteinase-9-dependent capillary damage during ischemia. The Journal of Neuroscience. 2017;**37**(1):129-140

[32] Winkler EA, Sagare AP, Zlokovic BV. The pericyte: A forgotten cell type with important implications for Alzheimer's disease? Brain Pathology. 2014;**24**(4):371-386

[33] Helman AM, Murphy MP. Vascular cognitive impairment: Modeling a critical neurologic disease *in vitro* and *in vivo*. Biochimica et Biophysica Acta. 2015;**1862**(5):975-982

[34] Tayler H, Miners JS, Güzel Ö, MacLachlan R, Love S. Mediators of cerebral hypoperfusion and blood-brain barrier leakiness in Alzheimer's disease, vascular dementia and mixed dementia. Brain Pathology. 2021;**31**(4):e12935

[35] De Jong GI, Farkas E, Stienstra CM, Plass JR, Keijser JN, de la Torre JC, et al. Cerebral hypoperfusion yields capillary damage in the hippocampal CA1 area that correlates with spatial memory impairment. Neuroscience. 1999;**91**(1):203-210

[36] Kirschen GW, Kéry R, Ge S. The hippocampal neuro-Glio-vascular network: Metabolic vulnerability and potential neurogenic regeneration in disease. Brain Plasticity. 2018;**3**(2):129-144

[37] Hood RJ, Sanchez-Bezanilla S, Beard DJ, Rust R, Turner RJ, Stuckey SM, et al. Leakage beyond the primary lesion: A temporal analysis of cerebrovascular dysregulation at sites of hippocampal secondary neurodegeneration following cortical photothrombotic stroke. Journal of Neurochemistry. 2023;**167**(6):733-752

[38] Scher AI, Xu Y, Korf ES, Hartley SW, Witter MP, Scheltens P, et al. Hippocampal morphometry in population-based incident Alzheimer's disease and vascular dementia: The HAAS. Journal of Neurology, Neurosurgery, and Psychiatry. 2010;**82**(4):373-376

[39] Buch S, Chen Y, Jella P, Ge Y, Haacke E. Vascular mapping of the human hippocampus using ferumoxytol-enhanced MRI. NeuroImage. 2022;**15**(250):118957

[40] Li C, Buch S, Sun Z, Muccio M, Jiang L, Chen Y, et al. In vivo mapping of hippocampal venous vasculature and oxygenation using susceptibility imaging at 7T. NeuroImage. 2024;**1**(291):120597

[41] Bellier A, Tafforeau P, Bouziane A, Angelloz-Nicoud T, Lee P, Walsh C. Micro to macro scale anatomical analysis of the human hippocampal arteries with synchrotron hierarchical phase-contrast tomography. Surgical and Radiologic Anatomy. 2024;**46**(11):1753-1760

Chapter 7

Effects of Radiotherapy on the Hippocampus and Strategies to Minimize Neurotoxicity

Prateek Mehra, Julia Malone and Shawn Malone

Abstract

Radiotherapy and Radiosurgery are routinely used in the management of malignant and benign brain tumors. In addition, radiosurgery is used to treat select benign conditions such as Arteriovenous Malformations and Trigeminal Neuralgia. Radiotherapy can cause important late side effects on the brain including neurocognitive toxicity. The neurotoxicity is in part related to effects of radiation on the hippocampus. Improvements in radiotherapy techniques have resulted in reduced neurotoxicity. These treatment strategies have included hippocampus avoidance intensity modulated radiotherapy (IMRT) and proton therapy. In addition, radiosurgery is an effective strategy to treat select primary and secondary brain tumors and helps to minimize late side effects of radiation.

Keywords: radiotherapy, radiosurgery, hippocampus, neurocognitive toxicity, hippocampal sparing techniques

1. Introduction

The hippocampus is known to be integral to many neurocognitive functions in the brain. Chiefly, it is related to memory consolidation, learning, attention and sensory information processing. The hippocampus forms a part of several important brain circuits such as Papez circuit and the trisynaptic circuit. It also receives input and output signals from the entorhinal and prefrontal cortices [1]. Brain radiotherapy for benign and malignant tumors can have important functional side effects on the hippocampus. There are a number of evolving strategies to help minimize neurocognitive effects of radiotherapy.

2. Role of radiation therapy and radiosurgery treatment

Radiotherapy is an important part of treatment for malignant and benign primary brain tumors and brain metastases [2, 3]. Radiotherapy is also used to treat other benign conditions such as arteriovenous malformations and Trigeminal Neuralgia [4, 5]. Some of the more common uses of brain radiation are radiation treatment are for post-op cavities in high grade gliomas and radiotherapy and radiosurgical treatment of brain metastases [2, 3].

Radiotherapy is routinely used in high grade gliomas following surgical debulking. The BTSG 69-01 [6] and 1981 SGSG [7] studies both demonstrated an improvement in survival with adjuvant radiotherapy as compared to supportive care in patients with glioblastoma. Addition of Temozolomide chemotherapy to adjuvant radiotherapy further improves survival (Stupp et al.) [8]. Anaplastic gliomas and low grade gliomas are also treated using combination radiation and chemotherapy as shown by RTOG 9802 [9], EORTC 22845 [10], RTOG 9402 [11] and CATNON [12] studies. Gliomas are typically infiltrative tumors, hence the target area for radiation includes the tumor bed with a margin. This margin can range from 0.5 cm to 2.0 cm depending on the aggressiveness of the cancer, volume of treatment and the performance status of the patient [13, 14].

Brain metastases are routinely managed with radiotherapy and radiosurgery treatment. Surgery is indicated in select patients with brain metastases including those with solitary metastases, or tumors causing marked mass effect [3]. In patients treated with surgery, adjuvant radiotherapy or radiosurgery are used to treat the surgical bed. Management strategies for brain metastases vary by patients age, performance level, type of cancer, extent of extracranial disease and number and location of brain metastases [3].

Radiosurgery is also an effective method of treatment of benign brain lesions such as meningiomas [15], acoustic neuromas [16], pituitary adenomas [17] and arteriovenous malformations [4]. In addition, functional conditions such as trigeminal neuralgia can be treated effectively with radiosurgery [5]. RTOG 0539 study showed improvements in progression-free survival local control rates after surgery in patients with all grades of meningiomas [18]. Maruyama and colleagues showed an 88% decrease in risk of hemorrhage after AVM obliteration through Gamma Knife radiosurgery [19]. The International Stereotactic Radiosurgery Society published a systematic review of 65 studies which showed 80–87% freedom from pain through radiosurgery for patients with trigeminal neuralgia [5]. Regis et al. from the Timone Hospital, Marseille published their research on acoustic neuromas, comparing surgical treatment versus radiosurgery with Gamma Knife. They found that radiosurgery resulted in better hearing preservation, less facial nerve damage and shorter hospital stay as compared to open surgical approach [20].

3. Side effects of radiation

Radiation treatment can lead to acute, subacute and chronic side effects. In the short period after radiotherapy, there can be cerebral edema resulting in headaches, nausea, vomiting and worsening of pre-treatment neurological deficits. In the subacute and chronic timeline, there is a small risk of radionecrosis due to death of tissue surrounding the original radiation target [21]. In addition, radiotherapy can result in functional impairment such as memory loss and neurocognitive changes due to damage to the hippocampus, prefrontal and frontal regions.

One of the many ways through which radiation change can manifest in the brain is volume loss. Decrease in gray matter, white matter and whole brain volumes have been observed in both adults and in children [22–24]. Cortical thinning has been repeatedly observed in children specifically [25]. Nagtegaal et al. evaluated the change in volume of multiple brain sub-structures and found a decrease in volume of amygdala, hippocampus, nucleus accumbens, globus pallidus, thalamus and putamen [26]. Only the caudate nucleus seemed to show no change in volume after treatment. Cerebellar atrophy has also been observed in multiple studies [27, 28]. Vascular changes have also been recorded, specifically decreasing fractional anisotropy, increasing mean diffusivity and increasing radial diffusivity [29–31]. These changes tend to indicate increased cerebral edema and demyelination.

Radiation can lead to neurotoxicity in a variety of manners. Radiation results in oxidative stress leading to DNA damage and mitotic death of neurons. Neuroinflammation of glial cells and decreased hippocampal neurogenic function are related to loss of hippocampal function apart from the oxidative stress that radiation puts on all brain cells [32]. Seibert et al. carried out a longitudinal study in which they measured the hippocampal volume before and one year after partial brain radiotherapy for primary brain tumors [33]. They correlated the mean hippocampal dose against the hippocampal volume change after one year. Hippocampal volume loss was strongly dependent on the mean dose received by the hippocampus. There was significant volume loss after 40Gy or higher mean dose whereas no such loss seen with lower mean dose (< 10Gy).

4. Hippocampal avoidance during whole brain radiation

RTOG 0933 study evaluated the benefit of Hippocampal Avoidance in patients receiving whole brain radiotherapy. In the trial, Gondi evaluated cognitive function and quality of life at baseline and at 2, 4 and 6 months after Hippocampal-Avoidance Whole Brain Radiotherapy (HA-WBRT) radiotherapy [34]. HA-WBRT was carried out by first contouring the bilateral hippocampi and then ensuring that they received less than 9Gy to the entire volume and maximum dose did not exceed 16Gy. The patients were assessed with the Hopkins Verbal Learning Test - Revised Delayed Recall (HVLT-R DR). The assessment was compared against historical controls who had undergone WBRT without any hippocampal sparing and had been assessed using the same HVLT-R DR. The mean relative decline in HVLT-R DR scores was 7% for the HA-WBRT group, which was significantly less than the 30% which was seen on average in the non-hippocampal sparing historical cohort. This study outlined the importance of minimizing radiation dose to the hippocampus to maintain neurocognitive functioning.

5. Role of Memantine in patients treated with radiotherapy

Another strategy to preserve neurocognitive function in patients treated with radiation is the use of Memantine. Memantine is a N-methyl-D-aspartate receptor (NMDAR) antagonist. It has been shown to reduce neurotoxicity in Alzheimer's disease and modulate the activity of glutamate in the brain [35]. Glutamate is one of brain's excitatory neurotransmitters. While there are many hypotheses on the molecular mechanisms of neurotoxicity due to radiation, one of the most popular is the ischemia-hypoxia cascade leading to increased glutamate levels inside the brain. This leads to excessive activation of NMDAR. These receptors are critical to maintaining synaptic plasticity integral to memory and learning. Over-activation of NMDARs results in calcium influx in neuronal cells, leading to excitotoxicity and cell death [36].

Brown and colleagues carried out a phase III randomized controlled trial that investigated the role of memantine as a possible neuroprotective agent in patients receiving whole brain radiotherapy [37]. The investigators divided the 554 patients into two arms - one receiving Memantine with escalating dose over 24 weeks and the other receiving placebo. Patients were treated with 37.5Gy over 15 fractions and were assessed for neurocognitive functioning through multiple tests including the Hopkins Verbal Learning Test - Revised (HVLT-R), Trail Making Test Parts A and B (TMT-A / TMT-B) and Controlled Oral Word Association (COWA). Tests were carried out at baseline, 8, 16 24 and 52 weeks. The Memantine treatment arm had a significantly longer time to cognitive decline and the probability of cognitive failure at 24 weeks was lower with memantine than with placebo. This study confirmed the benefit of Memantine as a neuroprotective agent.

The NRG Oncology CC001 study built upon these concepts even further [38]. This study compared the neurotoxicity of HA-WBRT versus WBRT with both arms receiving Memantine. They recruited 518 patients who were randomly assigned to either arm. The neurocognitive functioning was tested through HVLT-R and TMT-A / TMT-B at baseline and at 2, 4, 6 and 12 months after whole brain radiotherapy. Risk of cognitive failure was lower when both HA-WBRT and Memantine were used. There was less decline in executive function at 4 months (23.3% for HA-WBRT vs. 40.4% for WBRT). In addition, there was less decline in learning and memory at 6 months (11.5% vs. 24.7% and 16.4% vs. 33.3%). Survival and intracranial progression rates were comparable indicating that decreasing the dose to the hippocampus did not lead to higher chance of relapse.

6. Evolution of radiotherapy techniques

For most cancers such as gliomas, radiotherapy is delivered using high energy photons on a linear accelerator or LINAC. On a LINAC, electrons are accelerated under high voltage and strike a tungsten target to produce high energy x-ray or photons. The radiation beam is modulated or shaped to ensure maximum radiation coverage of the target tissue whereas the dose to the other organs is minimized. The beam is modulated with multi-leaf collimators (MLCs) in a radiotherapy technique called Intensity Modulated Radiotherapy (IMRT). An advancement of IMRT is Volumetric Modulated Arc Therapy (VMAT) in which the beam is continuously modulated as the machine rotates around the patient. VMAT is an efficient method to deliver highly conformal radiation doses to target tissues while minimizing the dose to normal tissues. An integral part of modern radiotherapy techniques is to use on line image guidance (Imager Guided Radiotherapy or IGRT) to ensure accurate delivery of the treatment to the intended target [39].

7. Radiosurgery for brain lesions

Stereotactic Radiotherapy (SRT) or Stereotactic Radiosurgery (SRS) is a method of delivering high dose radiation in 1 to 5 treatment fractions to small intracranial target lesions [39]. Radiosurgery is used to treat brain metastases and many benign tumors such as acoustic neuromas, meningiomas and pituitary tumors. It is also used to treat AVMs and Trigeminal Neuralgia. The target lesion is localized using a stereotactic coordinate system and stereotactic principals. With SRT there is a very rapid fall-off in radiation dose; therefore, the surrounding brain tissue (including the hippocampus) receives negligible radiation dose. Minimizing dose of radiation to adjacent normal brain tissue helps minimize the risk of late radiation sequelae.

SRS is an effective method of controlling brain metastases. The use and efficacy of SRS has reduced the need for whole brain radiotherapy in many patients with intracranial metastases. SRS allows for very low doses of radiation to the hippocampi. In a phase 3 randomized trial Brown et al. compared the neurocognitive decline in patients who underwent stereotactic radiosurgery (SRS) versus those who underwent WBRT and SRS [40]. They found that patients receiving SRS alone had less cognitive deterioration at 3 months and the data did not point to any worsening of survival because of the omission of WBRT. The investigators recommended that for patients with 1–3 metastases, SRS alone is the preferred treatment strategy compared to WBRT. Similar results were obtained by Chang et al. when they carried out a similar prospective clinical trial [41].

Burgess performed a dosimetric study to assess whether hippocampal dose can be decreased further in patients treated with stereotactic radiosurgery [42]. Sixty patients with brain metastases historically treated with SRS were re-planned to minimize hippocampal dose while ensuring maintenance of target coverage. The maximum, minimum, mean and dose to 40% of hippocampus were compared between the original plans (in which hippocampal sparing was not performed) against SRS plans in which hippocampal sparing had been performed. This technique resulted in further reductions in hippocampal dose: a decrease in minimum dose by 35%, maximum dose by 55%, mean dose by 52% and dose to 40% of hippocampus by 50%. The further reduction in hippocampal dose using SRS with hippocampal sparing should help further preserve neurocognitive function in patients with brain metastases. Similar principles can be applied to other patients treated with SRS or IMRT radiation to the brain.

8. Proton beam radiotherapy

Technology continues to advance. Radiotherapy has mostly been carried out through photons (high energy x-rays) in the modern radiotherapy era. Proton therapy is quickly becoming the preferred method of treatment for certain patient populations, e.g. children and young adults with brain tumors. Proton therapy provides a favorable dose distribution due to the Bragg peak effect which results in minimal exit radiation dose beyond the target lesion [43]. Proton therapy machines can be used to treat irregular targets with very tight treatment margins. Dosimetric studies have compared hippocampal dose when radiotherapy was carried out through Volumetric Modulated Arc Therapy (VMAT) versus Intensity Modulated Proton Therapy (IMPT). IMPT allowed for significantly reduced dose to the hippocampus, with mean dose reducing from 13.7Gy with VMAT to 5.4Gy with IMPT in pediatric patients and 11.7Gy to 4.4Gy in adult patients [44]. Through advanced techniques including IMRT, SRS and proton therapy risks of neurocognitive dysfunction have been minimized compared to historic radiotherapy treatments.

Author details

Prateek Mehra, Julia Malone and Shawn Malone*
The Ottawa Hospital, Ottawa, Canada

*Address all correspondence to: shawnmalone89@gmail.com

References

[1] Jing R, Cai Q, Li W. In: Zhang X, editor. Hippocampus - Cytoarchitecture and Diseases. IntechOpen; 2022. DOI: 10.5772/intechopen.95716

[2] Jiang T, Nam DH, Ram Z, et al. Clinical practice guidelines for the management of adult diffuse gliomas. Cancer Letters. 2021;**499**:60-72. DOI: 10.1016/j.canlet.2020.10.050

[3] Vogelbaum MA, Brown PD, Messersmith H, et al. Treatment for brain metastases: ASCO-SNO-ASTRO guideline [published correction appears in J Clin Oncol. 2022 Apr 20;40(12):1392. doi: 10.1200/JCO.22.00593]. Journal of Clinical Oncology. 2022;**40**(5):492-516. DOI: 10.1200/JCO.21.02314

[4] Graffeo CS, Sahgal A, De Salles A, et al. Stereotactic radiosurgery for Spetzler-Martin grade I and II arteriovenous malformations: International Society of Stereotactic Radiosurgery (ISRS) practice guideline. Neurosurgery. 2020;**87**(3):442-452. DOI: 10.1093/neuros/nyaa004

[5] Tuleasca C, Régis J, Sahgal A, et al. Stereotactic radiosurgery for trigeminal neuralgia: A systematic review. Journal of Neurosurgery. 2019;**130**(3):733-757. DOI: 10.3171/2017.9.JNS17545

[6] Walker MD, Alexander E Jr, Hunt WE, et al. Evaluation of BCNU and/or radiotherapy in the treatment of anaplastic gliomas. A cooperative clinical trial. Journal of Neurosurgery. 1978;**49**(3):333-343. DOI: 10.3171/jns.1978.49.3.0333

[7] Kristiansen K, Hagen S, Kollevold T, et al. Combined modality therapy of operated astrocytomas grade III and IV. Confirmation of the value of postoperative irradiation and lack of potentiation of bleomycin on survival time: A prospective multicenter trial of the Scandinavian glioblastoma study group. Cancer. 1981;**47**(4):649-652. DOI: 10.1002/1097-0142(19810215)47:4<649::aid-cncr2820470405>3.0.co;2-w

[8] Stupp R, Mason WP, van den Bent MJ, et al. Radiotherapy plus concomitant and adjuvant temozolomide for glioblastoma. The New England Journal of Medicine. 2005;**352**(10):987-996. DOI: 10.1056/NEJMoa043330

[9] Shaw EG, Wang M, Coons SW, et al. Randomized trial of radiation therapy plus procarbazine, lomustine, and vincristine chemotherapy for supratentorial adult low-grade glioma: Initial results of RTOG 9802. Journal of Clinical Oncology. 2012;**30**(25):3065-3070. DOI: 10.1200/JCO.2011.35.8598

[10] van den Bent MJ, Afra D, de Witte O, et al. Long-term efficacy of early versus delayed radiotherapy for low-grade astrocytoma and oligodendroglioma in adults: The EORTC 22845 randomised trial [published correction appears in Lancet. 2006 Jun 3;367(9525):1818]. Lancet. 2005;**366**(9490):985-990. DOI: 10.1016/S0140-6736(05)67070-5

[11] Cairncross G, Wang M, Shaw E, et al. Phase III trial of chemoradiotherapy for anaplastic oligodendroglioma: Long-term results of RTOG 9402. Journal of Clinical Oncology. 2013;**31**(3):337-343. DOI: 10.1200/JCO.2012.43.2674

[12] van den Bent MJ, Tesileanu CMS, Wick W, et al. Adjuvant and concurrent temozolomide for 1p/19q non-co-deleted anaplastic glioma (CATNON; EORTC study 26053-22054): Second interim

analysis of a randomised, open-label, phase 3 study. The Lancet Oncology. 2021;**22**(6):813-823. DOI: 10.1016/S1470-2045(21)00090-5

[13] Halasz LM, Attia A, Bradfield L, et al. Radiation therapy for IDH-mutant grade 2 and grade 3 diffuse glioma: An ASTRO clinical practice guideline. Practical Radiation Oncology. 2022;**12**(5):370-386. DOI: 10.1016/j.prro.2022.05.004

[14] Niyazi M, Andratschke N, Bendszus M, et al. ESTRO-EANO guideline on target delineation and radiotherapy details for glioblastoma. Radiotherapy and Oncology. 2023;**184**:109663. DOI: 10.1016/j.radonc.2023.109663

[15] Chen WC, Perlow HK, Choudhury A, Nguyen MP, Mirchia K, Youngblood MW, et al. Radiotherapy for meningiomas. Journal of Neuro-Oncology. 2022;**160**(2):505-515. DOI: 10.1007/s11060-022-04171-9. Epub 2022 Oct 31

[16] Tsao MN, Sahgal A, Xu W, De Salles A, Hayashi M, Levivier M, et al. Stereotactic radiosurgery for vestibular schwannoma: International stereotactic radiosurgery society (ISRS) practice guideline. Journal of Radiosurgery & SBRT. 2017;**5**(1):5-24

[17] Kotecha R, Sahgal A, Rubens M, et al. Stereotactic radiosurgery for non-functioning pituitary adenomas: Meta-analysis and International stereotactic radiosurgery society practice opinion. Neuro-Oncology. 2020;**22**(3):318-332. DOI: 10.1093/neuonc/noz225

[18] Rogers CL, Won M, Vogelbaum MA, et al. High-risk meningioma: Initial outcomes from NRG Oncology/RTOG 0539. International Journal of Radiation Oncology, Biology, Physics. 2020;**106**(4):790-799. DOI: 10.1016/j.ijrobp.2019.11.028

[19] Maruyama K, Kawahara N, Shin M, et al. The risk of hemorrhage after radiosurgery for cerebral arteriovenous malformations. The New England Journal of Medicine. 2005;**352**(2):146-153. DOI: 10.1056/NEJMoa040907

[20] Régis J, Pellet W, Delsanti C, et al. Functional outcome after gamma knife surgery or microsurgery for vestibular schwannomas. Journal of Neurosurgery. 2002;**97**(5):1091-1100. DOI: 10.3171/jns.2002.97.5.1091

[21] Barisano G, Bergamaschi S, Acharya J, Rajamohan A, Gibbs W, Kim P, et al. Complications of radiotherapy and radiosurgery in the brain and spine. Neurographics (2011). 2018;**8**(3):167-187. DOI: 10.3174/ng.1700066

[22] Reddick WE, Mulhern RK, Elkin TD, Glass JO, Merchant TE, Langston JW. A hybrid neural network analysis of subtle brain volume differences in children surviving brain tumors. Magnetic Resonance Imaging. 1998;**16**(4):413-421. DOI: 10.1016/s0730-725x(98)00014-9

[23] Gommlich A, Raschke F, Wahl H, Troost EGC. Retrospective assessment of MRI-based volumetric changes of normal tissues in glioma patients following radio(chemo)therapy. Clinical and Translational Radiation Oncology. 2017;**8**:17-21. Published 2017 Nov 22. DOI: 10.1016/j.ctro.2017.11.008

[24] Prust MJ, Jafari-Khouzani K, Kalpathy-Cramer J, et al. Standard chemoradiation for glioblastoma results in progressive brain volume loss. Neurology. 2015;**85**(8):683-691. DOI: 10.1212/WNL.0000000000001861

[25] Liu AK, Marcus KJ, Fischl B, et al. Changes in cerebral cortex of children

treated for medulloblastoma. International Journal of Radiation Oncology, Biology, Physics. 2007;**68**(4):992-998. DOI: 10.1016/j.ijrobp.2007.01.034

[26] Nagtegaal SHJ, David S, Philippens MEP, Snijders TJ, Leemans A, Verhoeff JJC. Dose-dependent volume loss in subcortical deep grey matter structures after cranial radiotherapy. Clinical and Translational Radiation Oncology. 2020;**26**:35-41. Published 2020 Nov 15. DOI: 10.1016/j.ctro.2020.11.005

[27] Raschke F, Seidlitz A, Wesemann T, et al. Dose dependent cerebellar atrophy in glioma patients after radio(chemo) therapy. Radiotherapy and Oncology. 2020;**150**:262-267. DOI: 10.1016/j.radonc.2020.07.044

[28] Ailion AS, King TZ, Wang L, et al. Cerebellar atrophy in adult survivors of childhood cerebellar tumor. Journal of the International Neuropsychological Society. 2016;**22**(5):501-511. DOI: 10.1017/S1355617716000138

[29] Chawla S, Wang S, Kim S, et al. Radiation injury to the normal brain measured by 3D-echo-planar spectroscopic imaging and diffusion tensor imaging: Initial experience. Journal of Neuroimaging. 2015;**25**(1):97-104. DOI: 10.1111/jon.12070

[30] Mabbott DJ, Noseworthy MD, Bouffet E, Rockel C, Laughlin S. Diffusion tensor imaging of white matter after cranial radiation in children for medulloblastoma: Correlation with IQ. Neuro-Oncology. 2006;**8**(3):244-252. DOI: 10.1215/15228517-2006-002

[31] Connor M, Karunamuni R, McDonald C, et al. Regional susceptibility to dose-dependent white matter damage after brain radiotherapy. Radiotherapy and Oncology. 2017;**123**(2):209-217. DOI: 10.1016/j.radonc.2017.04.006

[32] Cuccurullo V, Di Stasio GD, Cascini GL, Gatta G, Bianco C. The molecular effects of ionizing radiations on brain cells: Radiation necrosis vs tumor recurrence. Diagnostics (Basel). 2019;**9**(4):127. DOI: 10.3390/diagnostics9040127

[33] Seibert TM, Karunamuni R, Bartsch H, Kaifi S, Krishnan AP, Dalia Y, et al. Radiation dose-dependent hippocampal atrophy detected with longitudinal volumetric magnetic resonance imaging. International Journal of Radiation Oncology, Biology, Physics. 2017;**97**(2):263-269. DOI: 10.1016/j.ijrobp.2016.10.035. Epub 2016 Oct 31

[34] Gondi V, Pugh SL, Tome WA, Caine C, Corn B, Kanner A, et al. Preservation of memory with conformal avoidance of the hippocampal neural stem-cell compartment during whole-brain radiotherapy for brain metastases (RTOG 0933): A phase II multi-institutional trial. Journal of Clinical Oncology. 2014;**32**(34):3810-3816. DOI: 10.1200/JCO.2014.57.2909. Epub 2014 Oct 27

[35] Rogawski MA, Wenk GL. The neuropharmacological basis for the use of memantine in the treatment of Alzheimer's disease. CNS Drug Reviews. 2003;**9**(3):275-308. DOI: 10.1111/j.1527-3458.2003.tb00254.x

[36] Chilukuri S, Burela N. Memantine for prevention of brain irradiation-induced cognitive toxicity: A tale of an underappreciated and underused intervention. JCO Global Oncology. 2020;**6**:1384-1388. DOI: 10.1200/GO.20.00342

[37] Brown PD, Pugh S, Laack NN, Wefel JS, Khuntia D, Meyers C, et al.

Memantine for the prevention of cognitive dysfunction in patients receiving whole-brain radiotherapy: A randomized, double-blind, placebo-controlled trial. Neuro-Oncology. 2013;**15**(10):1429-1437. DOI: 10.1093/neuonc/not114. Epub 2013 Aug 16

[38] Brown PD, Gondi V, Pugh S, Tome WA, Wefel JS, Armstrong TS, et al. Hippocampal avoidance during whole-brain radiotherapy plus Memantine for patients with brain metastases: Phase III trial NRG Oncology CC001. Journal of Clinical Oncology. 2020;**38**(10):1019-1029. DOI: 10.1200/JCO.19.02767. Epub 2020 Feb 14

[39] Gardner SJ, Kim J, Chetty IJ. Modern radiation therapy planning and delivery. Hematology/Oncology Clinics of North America. 2019;**33**(6):947-962. DOI: 10.1016/j.hoc.2019.08.005

[40] Brown PD, Jaeckle K, Ballman KV, Farace E, Cerhan JH, Anderson SK, et al. Effect of radiosurgery alone vs radiosurgery with whole brain radiation therapy on cognitive function in patients with 1 to 3 brain metastases: A randomized clinical trial. JAMA. 2016;**316**(4):401-409. DOI: 10.1001/jama.2016.9839. Erratum in: JAMA. 2018 Aug 7;320(5):510. doi: 10.1001/jama.2018.9890

[41] Chang EL, Wefel JS, Hess KR, Allen PK, Lang FF, Kornguth DG, et al. Neurocognition in patients with brain metastases treated with radiosurgery or radiosurgery plus whole-brain irradiation: A randomised controlled trial. The Lancet Oncology. 2009;**10**(11):1037-1044. DOI: 10.1016/S1470-2045(09)70263-3. Epub 2009 Oct 2

[42] Burgess L, Nair V, Gratton J, Doody J, Chang L, Malone S. Stereotactic radiosurgery optimization with hippocampal-sparing in patients treated for brain metastases. Physics and Imaging in Radiation Oncology. 2021;**17**:106-110. DOI: 10.1016/j.phro.2021.02.001

[43] Liu H, Chang JY. Proton therapy in clinical practice. Chinese Journal of Cancer. 2011;**30**(5):315-326. DOI: 10.5732/cjc.010.10529

[44] Stoker J, Vora S, Patel A, Grosshans D, Brown PD, Vern-Gross T, et al. Advantages of intensity modulated proton therapy during hippocampal avoidance whole brain radiation therapy. Physics and Imaging in Radiation Oncology. 2018;**8**:28-32. DOI: 10.1016/j.phro.2018.11.001

Chapter 8

Fetal Alcohol Exposure and Hippocampal Dysfunction in the Vervet Monkey

Alexandra Haddad, Amari Eubanks, Annalia Burke-Carreno, Anthony Okeh, Banuja Munasinghe, Maria Sneed, Roberta Palmour, Maurice Ptito and Mark W. Burke

Abstract

Exposure to ethanol *in utero* is recognized as a leading cause of preventable developmental disorder. Children with fetal alcohol syndrome disorders (FASD) display behavioral and intellectual impairments that strongly implicate the hippocampus, an area essential for learning and memory. Small animal models indicate the third trimester equivalent as a critical period for hippocampal damage. We have developed a non-human primate model where dams voluntarily and naturally consume alcohol in a minimally stress environment. We have found even low-moderate fetal alcohol exposure (FAE) leads to reduced neuronal populations in the hippocampus, along with reduced immature neuronal population and stem cell activity. This model provides a platform in which to test potential therapeutic interventions to minimize the effects of fetal alcohol exposure.

Keywords: hippocampus, fetal alcohol exposure, plasticity, development, perineuronal net

1. Introduction

The reported detrimental consequences of alcohol consumption during pregnancy can be traced back to the 1700's with the Royal College of Physicians of London describing children of alcoholic mothers as "weak and feeble" [1]. The link between the toxic effects of alcohol consumption and pregnancy would later appear in the literature at the end of the nineteenth century [1]. The clinical term of fetal alcohol syndrome (FAS) was finally introduced in 1973 and attributed to heavy maternal drinking, with physical and neurobehavioral anomalies [2–4]. However, there is a continuum of fetal alcohol exposure (FAE) deficits termed fetal alcohol spectrum disorder (FASD), an umbrella term to include FAS, partial fetal alcohol syndrome, alcohol-related neurodevelopmental disorder and alcohol-relate birth defects [5]. In the absence of the characteristic craniofacial dysmorphology which is evident in FAS, diagnosing FASD remains a challenge, typically relying on maternal self-reporting and the presence of neurobehavioral deficits [6].

The prevalence of FASD is estimated to be between 1 and 4% of live births [7], however 14% of women report consuming ethanol during pregnancy and 5% binge drinking [8, 9]. Amongst children in foster care or adopted children, it is estimated that the prevalence could be 10–15 times higher than in the general population [10]. Currently there is no laboratory test that can identify and quantify prenatal alcohol use over a protracted period. Recently there has been an emphasis to identify unique signatures of ethanol exposure by assessing biomarkers of ethanol consumption such as phosphatidylethanol (PEth), fatty acid ethyl esters (FAEES), or ethyl glucuronide (EtG) in newborn dried blood spots, that has revealed exposure rates between 8 and 15.5% [11–13]. There is also a postnatal risk score assessment that has recently been developed that may have clinical potential in identifying children that have been exposed to prenatal ethanol [14]. The inability to accurately diagnose FASD leads to under- and mis-diagnoses [15] which may contribute to the public misconception that prenatal alcohol exposure, even moderate drinking, does not impact the developing fetus [5, 16].

Fetal alcohol exposure (FAE) at moderate levels, negatively affects neurodevelopment and behavior that can have life-long consequences on the affected children [17, 18]. Clinical and animal models suggest the involvement of multiple brain regions that contribute to cognitive, executive and behavioral manifestations of fetal alcohol exposure [17, 19]. While it is recognized that the developing brain is more susceptible to injury than the adult brain [20], *the hippocampus is generally regarded as an area particularly vulnerability to insult* [21, 22]. The hippocampus, which is involved with learning, memory, spatial navigation, social memory, and emotional regulation [21, 23–26], has been consistently implicated the pathogenesis associated with FAE [27]. This chapter aims to review clinical and preclinical animal model evidence that links FAE to hippocampal dysfunction. It focuses on characterizing structural and functional alterations within the hippocampus, elucidating molecular and cellular mechanisms underlying these effects, and identifying emerging biomarkers that may serve as early indicators of FAE-related neurodevelopmental impairments. The goal is to clarify how prenatal alcohol exposure disrupts fetal brain maturation, with particular emphasis on memory-related neural circuits.

2. Neuropsychological and long-term effects of fetal alcohol exposure

Imaging studies show a broad array of structural and functional anomalies associated with fetal alcohol exposure. Gray matter alterations in the frontal, temporal, parietal and occipital lobes have been shown along with global cortical thickness reductions [28]. Hippocampal volume [29–32] and deformities have also been detected along with agenesis of hippocampal commissure [28] and are associated with deficits in verbal and nonverbal memory [29] and spatial navigation [33]. Morphological alterations within the hippocampus, specifically thinner and less curvature of the CA1 and subiculum, are associated with lower IQ in FAE [34]. These morphological changes were not, however, associated with overall cognitive functioning, although there is an association with right hippocampal thinning and deficits in episodic memory [34]. While there are a multitude of structural changes reported in FASD [28], a specific pattern of alterations that could act as a biomarker for FASD remains elusive. However, bilateral hippocampi, along with bilateral putamen and right pallidum volumes in MRIs have shown to be consistently reduced in FAE and combined could potentially be used help discriminate FAE/FASD from control subjects [32]. Default mode network analysis also shows reduced functional connectivity between the medial prefrontal cortex and hippocampus along with other limbic regions which is associated with decreased cognitive control and attention [35]. Children exposed prenatally to alcohol experience exhibit a multitude of damaging neuropsychological effects that are present from early infancy and follow them throughout their adult years that either directly involve the hippocampus or hippocampal network.

Children diagnosed with FASD report significantly lower performance on spelling, writing, arithmetic, and overall IQ [36]. FASD children show visual-motor integration deficiencies, such as problems explaining local versus global characteristics in a context of visual stimuli and spatial learning and memory [37, 38]. Children exposed prenatally to alcohol show deficits in hippocampal-dependent learning, such as impairment in place learning and spared cued-navigation [38]. Deficits in virtual spatial navigation in FASD children has further been linked to reduced hippocampal volume [33]. This deficit in spatial learning navigation is comparable to the impairments seen in rodents prenatally exposed to ethanol and rodents with hippocampal damage [39]. Children exposed to alcohol prenatally show planning and problem-solving deficiencies, as well as difficulty inhibiting responses to stimuli [40]. Difficulties with abstract thinking as well as with maintaining and manipulating information in working memory is common in pediatric FASD patients [40]. Impairment in immediate memory, immediate delayed recall, retrospective and prospective memory are also prevalent [36, 41].

Impairment to executive functioning in those prenatally exposed to alcohol cause severe problems in attention, planning, strategy use, and working memory [42]. Prenatal alcohol exposure later affects an individual's problem-solving abilities, as they struggle to form and shift through concepts and think analytically [43]. Children exposed to prenatal alcohol have significant deficits in verbal abilities and general intellectual abilities, as well as in executive functioning, visual spatial ability, mood regulation, attention, and poorer impulse control [44]. This tends to lead to deficits in adaptive functioning (e.g. activities for daily living and social functioning), such as communication and social interaction skills, social judgment abilities, practical problem-solving skills and socialization skills [17, 37]. Patients with FASD have major difficulties with adaptive behaviors that render adverse life outcomes more common, as over half of these adolescents will experience disruptive school experiences, trouble with the law, confinement (e.g. detention, jail, prison, or psychiatric/inpatient setting), and many will have involvement in repeated inappropriate sexual behaviors and alcohol/drug problems [45].

While the neuropsychological assessments indicate disturbances within the hippocampal circuitry [38], the ability correlate maternal alcohol consumption, including quantity, pattern and timing, to neuropsychological complications remains complicated due to the reliance of maternal self-reporting [46, 47]. Animal models have been essential in our understanding of the pathogenesis of FAE these models can control for the pattern, timing, quantity and poly-drug use and prescription medications that can impact the developing brain.

3. Small animal models of fetal alcohol exposure

Clinical as well as animal studies have demonstrated that there is a continuum of neurological impacts of FAE that include, but not limited to, hippocampal-related behavioral, molecular, anatomical and physiological alterations. Rodents like mice and rats are the most commonly employed as models of FAE that have consistently demonstrated cognitive deficits, growth retardation, craniofacial abnormalities, and physical impairments mimicking human conditions [48].

Rodent models have provided invaluable insights on the effects of prenatal ethanol exposure on hippocampus-related behavior, structure, and function in controlled experimental settings. However, species choice, method, timing and duration of alcohol exposure, and method of alcohol exposure influence hippocampal-related outcomes (**Table 1**) [27, 48]. Similar to clinical aspects of FAE, learning, memory and spatial memory in rodents are related to hippocampal function [39]. Behaviorally, fear and spatial memory are affected by binge-like gestational exposure [82] and during the third trimester equivalent (post-natal days 1–10) [83]. Following more moderate alcohol exposure, object discrimination is normal [84], spatial location learning and retention has been shown to be normal [84, 85], and male rats have deficits in working memory in particular with processing spatial information [84], with reduced anxiety-like behavior [85].

Fetal alcohol exposure induces the generation of ROS, resulting in oxidative stress and activation of inflammatory pathways in the hippocampus, which may lead to damage or dysfunction [86–88]. Microglia activation has been reported following binge-like post-natal exposure that is accompanied by elevated cytokines like interleukin-1 beta and tumor necrosis factor-alpha [71, 88] despite reduced microglia population [65]. While there are reports of an overall reduced microglia population, there is evidence of elevated microglia activation in the pro-inflammatory phase that lasts well into adulthood [56]. Although elevated inflammation has been reported with post-natal ethanol exposure, it does not necessitate accompanying hippocampal neuronal loss [71], but may affect long-term myelination, plasticity and neurogenesis [56, 89].

Hippocampal plasticity is key to learning and memory, but it is also a feature of vulnerability. In rodents exposed to alcohol during the first trimester equivalent, AMPA-synaptic currents are disrupted in the hippocampus resulting in decreased object recognition [90]. Synaptic plasticity includes LTP and LTD, both responsible for forming functional neural circuits in the hippocampus. Prenatal alcohol exposure may interfere with those plasticity mechanisms responsible for altered synaptic connectivity that will ultimately lead to flawed function in memory. Alteration of these mechanisms during sensitive developmental periods, especially during early life, has extended consequences on hippocampal-related network cognitive functions of the brain. Synaptic plasticity in the form of long-term potentiation is also affected, but is dependent on developmental timing, dosage and method of alcohol exposure [27]. Heavy-binge-like exposure in the third trimester equivalent tends to decrease long-term potentiation (LTP) in the CA1 region [91–93], whereas gestational and moderate post-natal exposure have less of an effect on LTP [94]. Within the dentate gyrus, LTP has been reported to be reduced following second trimester equivalent, with only minor alterations in the first- or third-trimester equivalence [95]. Likewise, there is a gender-specific impairment of LTP and long-term depression (LTD) in the dentate gyrus following oral ethanol administration throughout gestation [96].

Species	Alcohol Exposure*	Exposure Type**	BEC mg/dl	Measurement	Results	Reference
SD Rats	E1-20	Intragastric	420	Neuronal population	CA1, CA3, DG ns	[49]
SD Rats	E10-20	Intragastric	311	Neuronal population	CA1, CA3 ns	[50]
SD Rats	E1-20	Intragastric	314	Neuronal population	CA1, CA3 ns	[50]
SD Rats	E5-21	Intragastric	289	Neuronal Morphology	Decreased dendritic arborization CA1-3 DG	[51]
SD Rats	P4-9	Intragastric	359	Neuronal population	CA1, CA3 Decrease	[50]
SD Rats	E1-20 + P4-9	Intragastric	335	Neuronal population	CA1, CA3 Decrease	[50]
SD Rats	E1-20	Oral Diet	184	Stem Cell Proliferation	BrdU at PND95 ns	[52]
SD Rats	E1-22, P4-10	Intragastric	140-210	Stem Cell Proliferation/ Immature Neurons	No difference BRDU, Ki-67; Inc. in maturational marker NeuroD	[53]
SD Rats	E1-20	Oral Diet	100	Immature Neurons	Decreased in aged animals	[54]
SD Rats	E0-21	Oral Diet	144	Immature neurons	Reduced in females	[55]
SD Rats	E6-P21	Oral Diet		Neural Progenitor Cells and Activated Microglia	Decrease in NPC; Elevated activated microglia; Elevated calbindin neurons	[56, 57]
SD Rats	G11-20	Intragastric	216	Gene Expression	Sex-specific disregulation in proline, alaninine and citrulline biosynthesis and xenobiotic matabolism	[58]
Long Evans Rats	E1-10	Intragastric	298	Neuronal Population	CA1, CA3, DG ns	[59]
Long Evans Rats	E11-22	Intragastric	322	Neuronal population	CA1, CA3, DG ns	[59]
Long Evans Rats	P2-10	Intragastric	370	Neuronal population	CA1 Decreased CA3, DG ns	[59]

Species	Alcohol Exposure*	Exposure Type**	BEC mg/dl	Measurement	Results	Reference
Long Evans Rats	E1-22 + P2-10	Intragastric	378	Neuronal population	CA1 Decreased CA3, DG ns	[59]
Long Evans Rats	E6-21 + P4-12	Intragastric	339	Neuronal population	CA1 Decreased CA3, DG ns	[60]
Long-Evans Rats	P4-9	Intragastric	328	Immature Neuron Morphology	Decreased dendritic morphology of immature neurons	[61]
Long-Evans Rats	P4-10	Intragastric	315	Immature neurons	Long-term reduction in DG immature neuronal population	[62]
Long-Evans Rats	P4-9	Intragastric	330	Stem Cell Proliferation	BrdU on PND 42 or 72 ns	[63]
Long-Evans Rats	E1-21	Oral	60	Parvalbumin interneurons	CA3 reduction in males; DG reduction in females	[64]
Long-Evans Rats	P4-9	Intragastric	359	Microglia population	CA1-3, DG Decreased number of microglia; increased pro-inflammatory cytokines and anti-inflammatory TGF-ß	[65]
Long-Evans Rats	G0-20	Oral	44-110	Gene Expression	Downregulation of pathways involved in cell adhesion, immune response and toxin metabolism	[66]
Lewis Rats	P4-9	Intragastric	265	Neuronal population	CA1 Decrease DG, CA3 ns	[67]
Wistar Rats	E7-21	Intragastric	245	Behavior, Immature and Mature Neurons	Deficits spatial learning; lower DG neurons; normal pyramidal and immature neuronal populations	[68]
Wistar Rats	E7-21	Intragastric	246	Morphology	Spine density and synaptic proteins ns	[69]
Wistar Rats	P10-15	Vapor chamber	432	Neuronal population	CA1-3 DG ns Hilus Dec	[70]
Wistar Rats	P3-5	Vapor chamber	500	Neuronal population/ Inflammation	CA1-3, DG-ns Elevated cytokine expression; Elevated GFAP expression	[71]

Species	Alcohol Exposure*	Exposure Type**	BEC mg/dl	Measurement	Results	Reference
C57BL/6 Mice	E0-P21	Oral	121	Proliferating progenitors	No effect on progenitors	[72]
C57BL/6 Mice	E7-16	Intragastric	184	Proliferation	Ki-67 unchanged Decreased DCX+ immature neurons	[73]
C57BL/6 Mice	P4-10	Intragastric	326	Immature Neurons	No effect on immature DG neurons; Dec mature DG neurons indicating differentiation inhibition	[74]
C57BL/6 Mice	P2-8	Intraperitoneal	NA: Binge-like	Dendritic Morphology CA1	Impaired object recognition and spatial memory; reduced dendritic arborization complexity and spine density	[75]
C57BL/6 Mice	P2-7	Vapor Chamber	≈239 (44-52 mM)	Dendritic Morphology	Increased density, complexity, length, number of ends and nodes in dendrites; possibly regulated by astrocytes	[76]
C57BL/6 Venus-VGAT mice	P2-9	Vapor Chamber	297	Interneurons	Decreased	[77]
NestinCreER^{T2}: tdTomato bitransgenic mice	P3-15	Vapor Chamber	160	Neurogenesis	No change in total number or survival	[78]
C57BL/6 Mice	E8-12	Intragastric	NA	Gene Expression	Pathway analysis shows developmental gene and calcium signaling pathway alteration	[79]
C57BL/6 Mice	P4-9	Intragastric	401	Gene Expression	Induced pathways of ribosome biogenesis; inhibited transcriptomes of inhibitory interneurons	[80]

**Rodent neurodevelopment is substantially shorter than that of humans and non-human primates. Embryonic/fetal development lasts 19-21 days (E0-21) and rats and mice are born prematurely at the equivalence to the beginning of the third trimester (P0) compared to humans and non-human primates. The first 10 days (P0-10) of life are considered the third-trimester equivalence [81].*
***Methods of ethanol administration vary across experiments each with their advantages and limitations. Injections involving subcutaneous or intraperitoneal produce rapid increase in blood ethanol content (BEC); Inhalation via vapor chamber is a rapid method that reliably introduces alcohol to the animal without the stress of intubation, but does not have a control equivalent; Intragastric intubation delivers alcohol directly to the stomach with a syringe allowing a rapid binge-like exposure, but it is labor-intensive, invasive and can lead to high mortality rates; Oral route is provided in a liquid ethanol solution as either its main or only food source with pair-red control groups as a an isovolumetric and isocaloric equivalence for the alcohol consumption [48].*

Table 1.
Hippocampal neuronal populations following prenatal ethanol exposure.

Early models of FAE reported mossy fiber alterations in the hippocampus highlighting the vulnerability of this region [97]. Subsequent models over the past 40-years have been used to elucidate the extent and timing of neuronal loss. Repeated intragastric binge-like exposure (blood alcohol concentration < 250 mg/dl) in rats indicate a critical period of the third-trimester equivalent for alcohol-induced neuronal loss primarily affecting the CA1 region [50, 59, 60, 98]. However, inconsistencies exist regarding timing and extent of neuronal loss, potentially due to species differences and the route of administration (see **Table 1**). While the most consistent data indicate a particular vulnerability of the CA1 region, neuronal numbers in other regions like the CA2-3 and dentate gyrus are either unchanged [59, 60, 68, 71, 99] or decreased [50] following third trimester equivalent exposure. Morphological changes to hippocampal neurons in the form of decreased arborization have also been reported following chronic binge-like exposure during the first two trimester [51] and third trimester equivalents [61]. Stem cell proliferation markers (e.g. BrdU and Ki-67) in the dentate gyrus are reported to remain unchanged given varying concentrations, duration and timing of exposure in rodents [53, 54, 62, 72, 73, 100]. However, evidence suggests that despite the lack of changes in stem cell proliferation, the early neuron maturational marker NeuroD is upregulated in the dentate gyrus and could serve as a potential compensatory mechanism in adolescent subjects [53]. A subsequent loss of immature neurons (e.g. doublecortin-positive) has been reported at a later time point in aged animals [54, 62], indicating long-term consequences of FAE on hippocampal learning and memory capacity [62]. The loss of interneurons [77], particularly parvalbumin positive interneurons [64] is significant as they play an essential role in the perineuronal network underlying development and memory consolidation, both of which are disrupted in fetal alcohol exposure [101, 102].

Small animal model systems provide an efficient and accessible method of investigating the timing, dosage and neuropathogenic mechanisms of fetal alcohol exposure. While rodent models show specific alterations within the hippocampus, they also show potential circuity alterations within the reuniens nucleus, a key thalamic interface between the medial prefrontal cortex and hippocampus [103, 104], which leads to impaired oscillatory synchrony between these areas [105]. Rodent studies also suggest potential sex differences in FAE with males displaying a reduced hippocampal neuronal survival and LTP [27, 106], females expressing an elevated hippocampal immune response [107] and females performing better on hippocampal-dependent behaviors than males [86, 108]. There are, however, limitations to rodent models, primarily due to the abbreviated gestational and maturation periods. Embryonic/fetal development lasts 19-21 days (E0-21) and birth (P0) is the equivalent to the beginning of the third trimester in humans and non-human primates. The first 10 days (P0-10) of life are considered the third-trimester equivalence [81]. This shortened developmental period limits the exposure time and the artificial administration of ethanol complicate extrapolation to the clinical condition. Likewise, the binge-like exposure commonly used in rodent studies does not recapitulate the pattern seen in the clinical setting [109].

4. Non-human primate model of fetal alcohol exposure

Since rodent neuroanatomical and developmental findings do not fully translate to humans, non-human primate models have been developed to reduce variability and better replicate human fetal alcohol exposure (see **Figure 1** for methodological

DOI: http://dx.doi.org/10.5772/intechopen.1014194

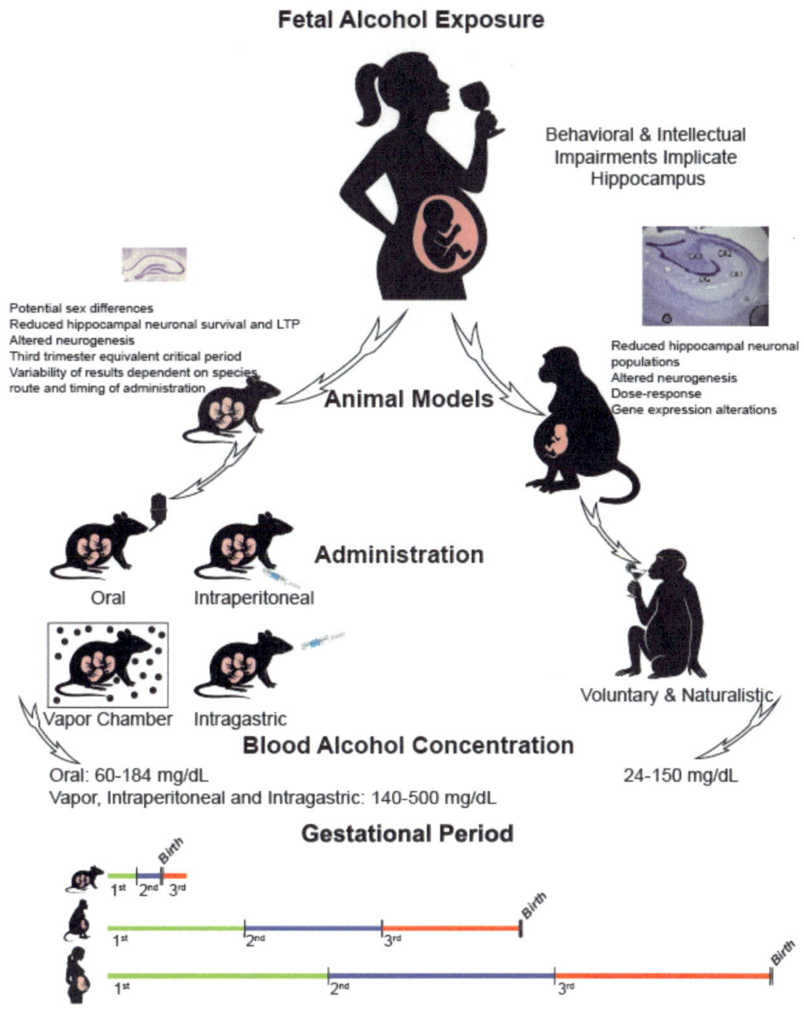

Figure 1.
Schematic Overview. Fetal alcohol exposure (FAE) disrupts hippocampal development, contributing to the cognitive deficits seen in the clinical setting. Animal models that can control the pattern, timing, and quantity, are essential in our understanding of the pathogenesis of FAE on the developing hippocampus. Rodent models demonstrate hippocampal alterations in behavior, structure, and function, particularly altered neuronal populations, neurogenesis and long-term potentiation (LTP). While rodent models reveal critical third-trimester vulnerability, they are limited by artificial exposure methods typically resulting a rapid rise in blood ethanol content (BEC), as well as a short gestation that restricts exposure windows and complicating translation to humans. Non-human primate models, such as our voluntary drinking vervet paradigm, more closely replicates human patterns and extended development, revealing dose-dependent neuronal loss, impaired neurogenesis, and altered gene expression in the hippocampus.

overview [110]. Naturalistic FAE models in non-human primates allows dams to voluntarily consume moderate levels of alcohol during gestion, closely modeling the consumption patterns seen in the clinical setting [19, 109, 111–115]. In the rhesus monkey model, subjects voluntarily consumed 0.6 g/kg/day alcohol solution in early gestation (E0-50), second-third trimester equivalent (E-50-135) or throughout gestation with blood ethanol concentration reaching ≈20-50 mg/dl. Similar to the clinical setting, moderate prenatal ethanol exposure in the rhesus monkey has shown some cognitive and behavioral impairment and reduces adaptation to stress. However, neuroanatomical evidence of ethanol-induced hippocampal damage has not been investigated [111, 112, 116, 117]. Episodic-binge-like exposure during gastrulation or throughout gestation in pig-tail macaques resulting in blood ethanol concentration of ≈230 mg/dl, likewise results in learning and memory deficits as well as visual-paired comparison performance impairment, indicative of medial temporal lobe and hippocampal dysfunction [118–120]. The episodic-binge-like model results in a neuronal a reduction in the somatosensory-motor cortices [121] and altered cell cycle of stem cell proliferation in the subgranular zone of the dentate gyrus [120].

Our group has developed a non-human primate model of FAE by taking advantage of the moderate and naturalistic drinking pattern in the vervet monkey (*Chlorocebus aethiops* sabeus) to model the exposure frequently reported FAE in human epidemiological investigations [122–125]. Our studies also take advantage of a comparable protracted developmental period in the monkey [81] by examining multiple time points from birth through early adolescence.

To develop this model, we established stable social breeding groups of 8-10 alcohol-preferring females and one male housed in their natural environment at the laboratories of the Behavioral Science Foundation (BSF), St. Kitts. The method of identifying alcohol-preferring females has previously been described [126]. Each group setting was further enriched with ropes, poles, bars, and novel objects. Subjects were fed high-protein primate chow and fresh local produce, with water available *ad libitum*. Females were trained using reinforcement to transition from their social setting into an adjoining sectioned tunnel leading to their home cage so that during drinking periods, each subject occupied an individual compartment. No sedation of any kind was required to move animals from the social group to drinking compartments thereby minimizing potential stress. The individual compartments enabled precise monitoring of subsequent alcohol consumption. Additionally, females were trained to present their leg for phlebotomy without anesthesia [109, 113].

The social breeding groups were behaviorally monitored for reproductive activity and females examined twice weekly to determine pregnancy. At approximately gestational day 100 (range 75–117 days; calculated retrospectively from birth) of a 165-day gestation period, pregnant females would enter the sectioned tunnel for 4 hours, four times per week. They were provided access to a 10% v/v solution of ethanol in a calibrated drinking bottle (or an isocaloric sucrose mixture for control subjects) with water concurrently available. After the drinking period, dams were allowed to return to their social group in the main enclosure. Alcohol availability remained restricted for the remainder of gestation. To ensure infants did not receive additional alcohol exposure through breast milk, alcohol availability ceased upon parturition. Following parturition, maternal alcohol consumption was calculated based on the total volume of ethanol consumed and expressed as g/kg body weight/drinking day, as well as total exposure (g/kg) over the gestational period (**Table 2**) [19]. At the end of the drinking period, blood (1 ml, saphenous vein) was drawn without anesthesia during weeks 2, 4, 6, and 8 of exposure to measure of blood ethanol level (alcohol dehydrogenase method, Sigma). None of the offspring produced in this manner had facial dysmorphology (**Figure 2**) [113]. Our naturalistic and voluntary consumption model yielded blood alcohol concentrations of ≈90 mg/dl (range 43–132 mg/dl) similar to those found in women after 2–5 standard drinks [123]. These values are considerably lower than those achieved in most rodent studies (**Table 1**). However, the total number of exposure days was higher, with our monkeys having been exposed for ≈38 days spanning the latter part of the second trimester through parturition.

Animal #	Sex	Alc or Suc started[a]	Average Alc (g/kg/day)[b]	Total Alc exposure (g)	Average BEC[c]	Age at sacrifice
O1808-3-2	f	87	1.46	68.9	61	30 d
O2898-5	m	96	2.64	103.13	112	18 d
O3245-3	f	76	2.82	149.5	121	4 d
O3307-3	f	94	3.17	126.87	132	35 d
O5011-4	m	82	1.97	82.81	72	15 d
O5154-2	m	112	2.09	64.82	95	1 d
		91 ± 13	2.36 ± .63	99.33 ± 33.7	98.8 ± 28	17.1 ± 14
O3065-8	m	94	2.98	122.13	125	5 mos
O3066-6	m	80	2.57	123.30	118	4.5 mos
O3327-4	m	95	2.16	86.37	77	5 mos
O5330-4	m	112	2.23	71.63	86	5.2 mos
O5399-1	m	106	2.48	86.75	109	5.4 mos
		97 ± 12	2.48 ± .33	98 ± 23.3	103 ± 21	5 ± .3
O2762-5	m	117	1.01	24.35	43	24 mos
O5066-1	m	109	1.49	63.9	65	24 mos
O5106-1	m	109	1.79	59.2	72	24 mos
O5332-1	f	106	2.19	76.5	91	24 mos
O3082-3	f	115	1.79	48.3	76	24 mos
O5219-1	m	103	2.45	88.3	121	22 mos
O3295-3	m	95	2.63	107.0	132	21 mos
O5011-3	m	77	2.81	135.1	118	24 mos
O3295-2	m	75	2.82	143.9	97	24 mos
O3307-2	f	111	2.64	81.8	105	24 mos
O3327-2	m	113	2.77	85.73	104	22 mos
O3327-1	m	115	2.98	89.4	120	21 mos
		103.75 ± 14	2.28 ± .63	83.62 ± 33.7	95.3 ± 27	23.2 ± 1.3

[a]*Day of gestation alcohol or sucrose treatment started out of a 165-day gestation period.*
[b]*Ethanol (g/kg) ingested by the dam over the entire drinking period.*
[c]*BEC mg/dl average blood ethanol content (BEC) measured on 3–4 occasions at the end of a 4 h exposure [19, 109, 114].*

Table 2.
Subject profile.

Both control and FAE, were group-housed with their mothers until the age of 6-months, then transferred to a nursery setting for an additional 6-months. At 1-year of age, all subjects were moved into large social outdoor enclosures forming peer groups of 12 animals. We histologically examined the hippocampi of subjects at several time points during the post-natal period ranging from birth until 2-years of age, a period of extensive dendritic and axonal maturation of pyramidal neurons in the hippocampus of non-human primates [127, 128] as well as active neurogenesis [129, 130]. Using design-based stereology, we previously reported a significant

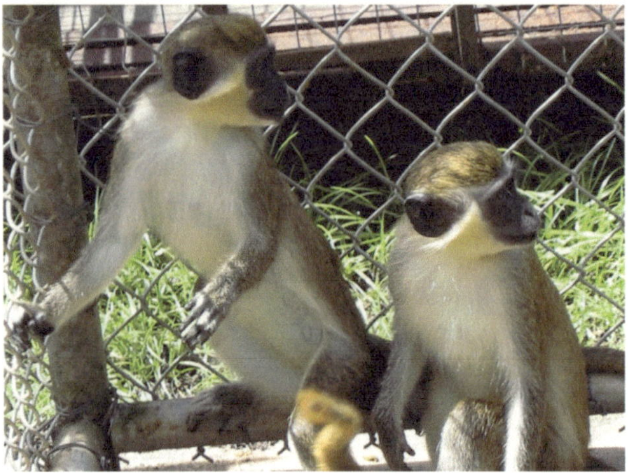

Figure 2.
Subjects. Vervet monkeys were exposed to moderate levels of ethanol during the third trimester of gestation. Socially housed female vervet monkeys voluntarily drank a range of 1.0–4.0 g/kg ethanol/day or isocaloric sucrose (control) four times a week during the last 2-months of gestation. Offspring were housed in their natural environment in social groups. None of the offspring showed craniofacial dysmorphology. Subject on the left is FAE subject and the subject on the right is an age-matched control subject.

neuronal reduction of neuronal populations within the CA1-3 fields of the hippocampus at birth, 5-months and at 2-years of age (**Figure 3**) [109]. Over time, we were able to expand the 2-year-old subject pool to include subjects with lower and higher ethanol exposure than our original study. We found significant negative correlation between daily ethanol exposure and both neuronal population and regional volume throughout the CA1-3 fields. However, only in the CA1 was there a significant negative correlation between blood ethanol concentration (BEC) and neuronal population (**Figure 4**) [19]. Similarly, we found a significant negative correlation between the number of immature neurons, indicated by doublecortin immunoreactivity (DCX+ neurons) in the dentate gyrus and both daily ethanol exposure and average BEC, but

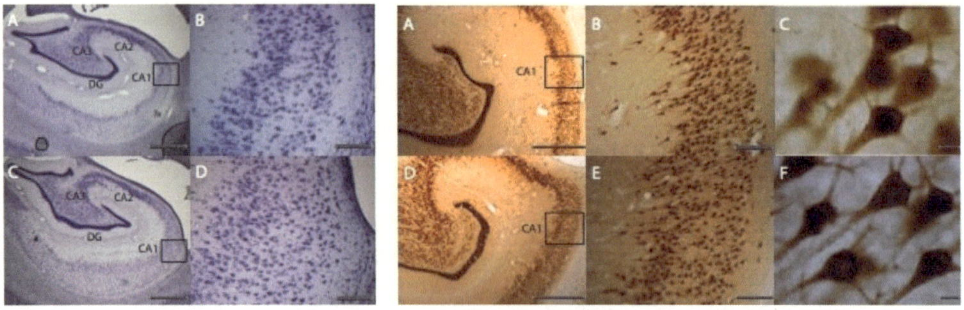

Figure 3.
Reduced Hippocampal Neuronal Population. Cresyl violet stained sections (Left panels A-D) were used for design-based stereology estimation of neuronal populations for all subjects and immunostained NeuN sections (right panel A-F), a putative marker for mature neurons, are used to illustrate neuronal reductions. FAE subjects display significant reduction in hippocampal neuronal population across the CA1-3 subregions (left panels A and B and right panels A-C) compared to control subjects (C and D left panels and D-F right panels). Leftmost sections of each panel are taken at 2.5x magnification (scale bar = 1 mm), midsections are taken from the CA1 region (inset box) at 10x magnification (scale bar = 100 μm), and right-hand images C and F are at 100x magnification (scale bar = 10 μm).

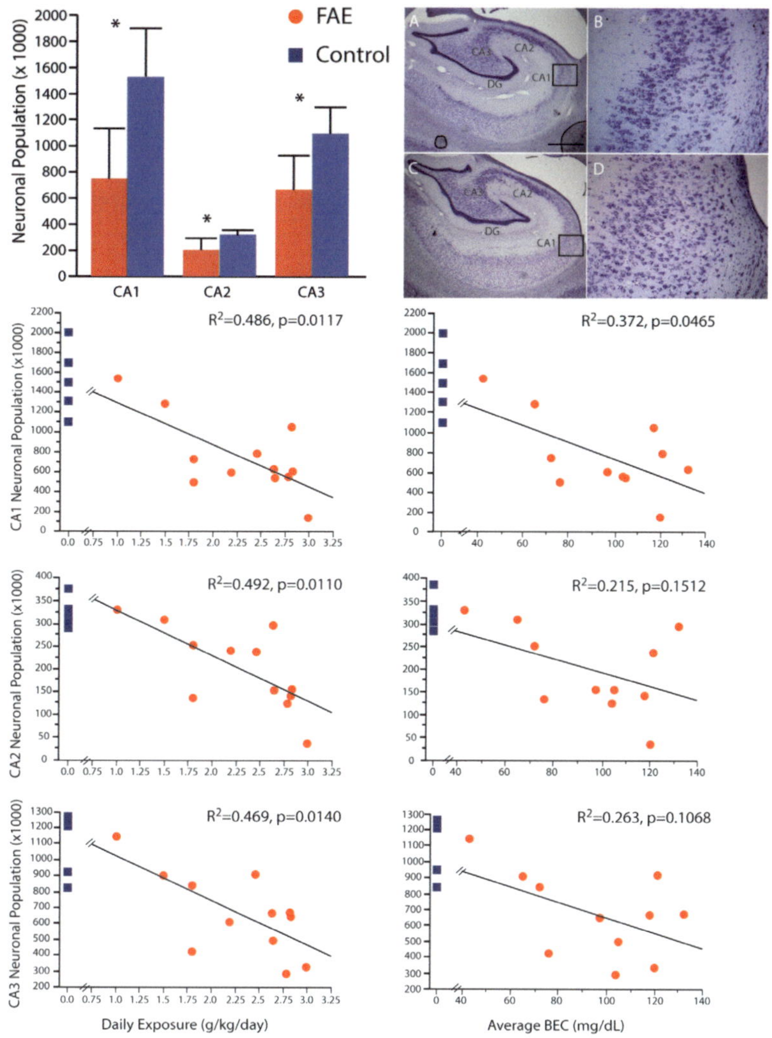

Figure 4.
*Dose Response. FAE subjects have significantly lower neuronal populations in the CA1-3 fields of the hippocampus even with the inclusion of subjects with lower alcohol exposure (top left panel). Cresyl violet stained sections from the hippocampus of FAE (A, B) and control (C, D) subjects show a fragmented and meager populated pyramidal layer. *p < 0.05 FAE vs. control. (A, C) scale bar = 1 mm (2.5x magnification); (B, D) are taken from the CA1 region (inset from A, C) scale bar = 100 µm (10x magnification). There was a significant negative correlation between daily ethanol exposure and neuronal populations throughout the CA1-3 regions and a negative correlation between BEC and neuronal population only in the CA1 region [19].*

not total exposure (**Figure 5**) [19]. Moreover, we found fewer actively proliferating stem cells at the neonatal period, as indicated by Ki-67 immunoreactivity, in both the granular and the hilus regions compared to controls. However, by the 2-years of age no differences were observed between FAE and control subjects (**Figure 6**) [114]. The pattern of immature neuron and active proliferation in this model differs from that reported in small animal models where some studies suggest lack of changes [63, 68, 72–74], decreased in these populations [56, 73], or a delayed/adult-onset decrease [54]. These reported differences may be due to alcohol exposure, differential BEC or species variation.

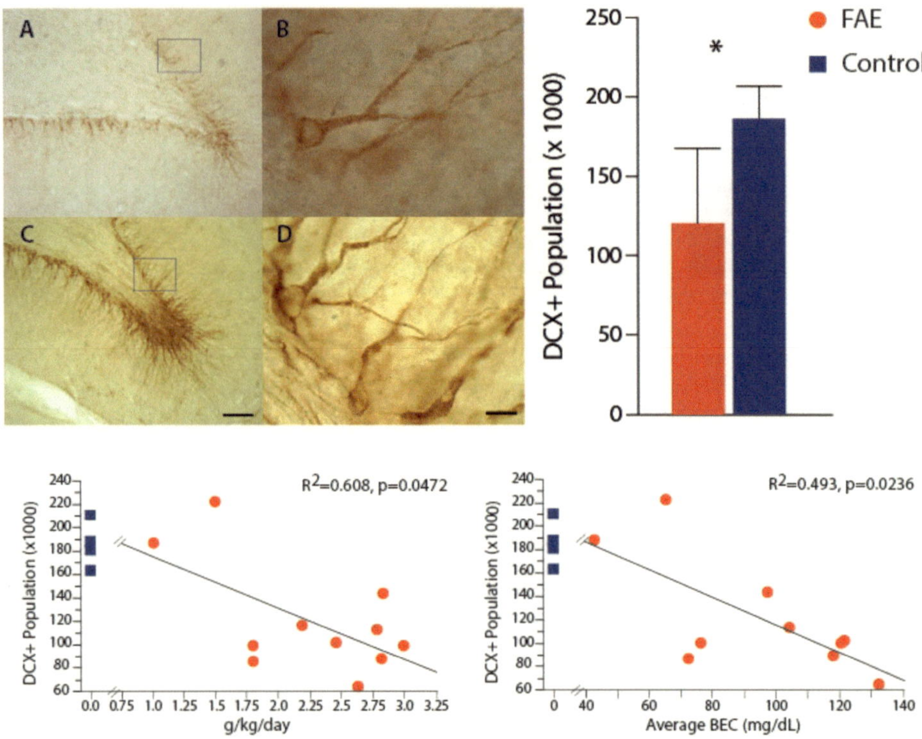

Figure 5.
*Reduced Immature Neuronal Population. There is a reduction in doublecortin-positive (DCX+) neurons in the dentate gyrus in FAE subjects (A, B) vs. control (C, D) subjects. The number of DCX+ neurons were negatively correlated with daily ethanol exposure and average BEC, but not total exposure. *p < 0.05. (A, C) scale bar = 100 μm; (B, D) scale bar = 10 μm [19].*

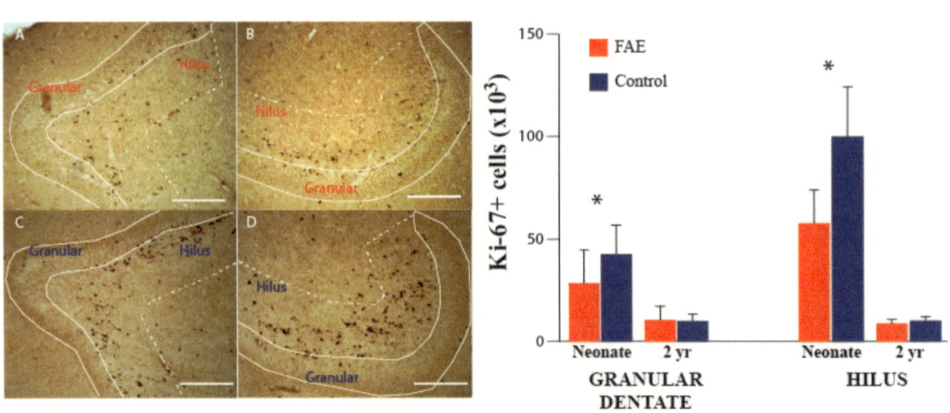

Figure 6.
*Reduced Cell Proliferation. FAE subjects (A and B) show a significant reduction of Ki-67 positive cells, a marker for actively proliferating cells, in the granular layer of the dentate gyrus and hilus region as compared to control subjects (C and D). Images taken at 10x magnification; scale bar = 200 μm. There was significant reduction in Ki-67+ cells from the neonatal time point to the age of 2-years for both groups, but no difference between groups. *p < 0.05 [114].*

DOI: http://dx.doi.org/10.5772/intechopen.1014194

Like the CA fields in non-human primates, the dentate gyrus undergoes substantial postnatal development [127, 128, 131–136]. Unlike the CA fields though neurogenesis of granule cells is considerably prolonged extending to the early postnatal period [132]. In primates up to 30% of granule cells destined for the dentate gyrus are formed in the first 3 months of life [132, 136] compared to at least 85% being produced postnatally in the rodent [137]. In control subjects the 30% increase in the granule cell layer volume from birth to 2 years parallels the neuronal population increase reported in other non-human primate species [136].

Fetal alcohol exposure in the vervet monkey alters the number of multiple genetic markers and protein levels within the hippocampus. At the mRNA level, gene expression changes are observed in pathways related to neurogenesis, synaptic function and microglia-mediated neuroprotection. These molecular alterations likely underlie the structural and functional deficits in the hippocampus and may serve as potential targets for therapeutic intervention [138].

With an estimated 122 distinct types of neurons in the hippocampus, it is one of the most complex regions of the brain [139]. We are just beginning to scratch the surface of the diversity of these populations of neurons which includes perineural nets (PNNs) which are thought to play a role in memory consolidation and development [101, 102, 140, 141]. PNNs are extracellular matrix assemblies of molecules including chondroitin sulfate proteoglycans, hyaluronan, tenascin-R, and link proteins. These components form a mesh-like machinery around neurons, particularly those arising from parvalbumin positive (PV+) interneurons. PNNs play an extremely important role in the functional maturation of the PV+ interneurons, especially in the hippocampus, where their assembly promotes the inhibitory performance of these interneurons in memory-related circuits. PNNs help maintain the excitatory-inhibitory balance in neural circuits by stabilizing PV+ interneurons. This stabilization ensures that only the most active neurons participate in memory engrams, a crucial process for forming sparse and precise engrams for memory recall. Moreover, maturation of PNNs around PV+ interneurons indicates closure of the critical periods of plasticity in the brain, marking a transition from a highly flexible developmental state to a much more consolidated and adult-like function in both sensory and cognitive systems [102]. Understanding how PNNs interact with various types of hippocampal neurons, particularly under pathological conditions like FAE, may reveal new avenues for therapeutic interventions.

5. Conclusions

Given the paucity of neuroanatomical data in clinical cases of FASD, we must rely on animal models to understand the neurobiology of this disorder. While rodent models exist, only non-human primates can accurately model the CNS developmental and social behavior in FASD. To address the limitations from small animal studies, we developed naturalistic model of maternal ethanol consumption by the Old-World monkey, the closest to human on the cladistic tree. This model allows for systematic and quantitative hippocampal analysis of changes in response to levels of alcohol consumption frequently encountered in a social context (**Figure 7**). These changes are compatible with observed behavioral alterations (Palmour, unpublished observations) and are consistent with the human clinical data [142]. The period of alcohol

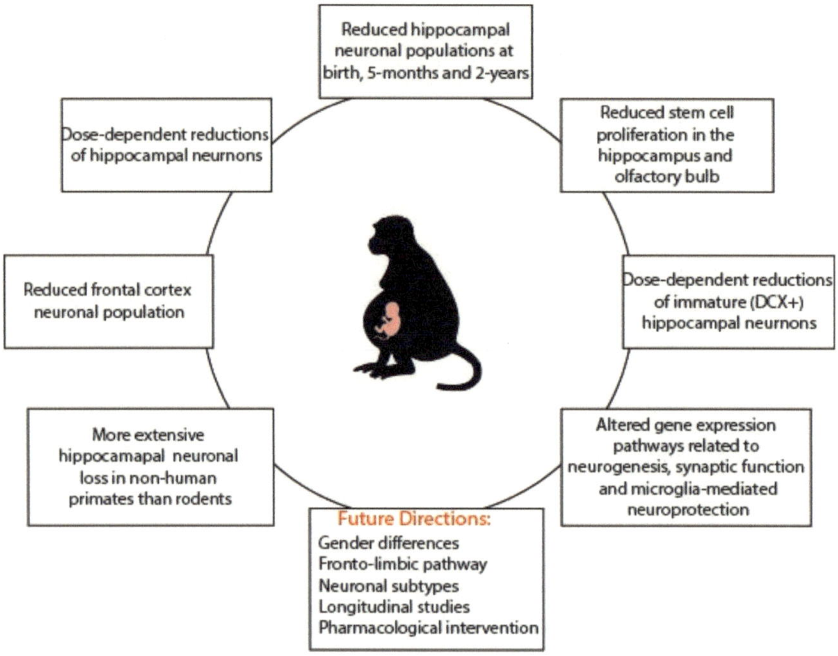

Figure 7.
Vervet FAE Model Results Overview. Our voluntary and naturalistic non-human primate model of FAE has shown disruptions in hippocampal development. Specifically, this model has shown deficits in neuronal populations and stem cell proliferation at multiple time points in the hippocampus. There is a dose-dependent reduction in pyramidal neurons and immature hippocampal neurons. There is altered gene expression related to hippocampal development. Deficits in our model extend to the frontal cortex suggesting a frontal-hippocampal network disruption that may contribute to the limbic and executive functioning deficits seen in the clinical setting. Future directions within this model include exploring gender differences, further exploring alterations in the fronto-limbic pathway and pharmacological interventions to minimize the impact of FAE.

exposure is also a contributing factor and is a consequence of phylogenetic developmental differences between rats and monkeys. Our series of studies corroborates rodent literature suggesting that the third trimester is a critical period for ethanol-induced neuronal loss in the hippocampus, however the extent of loss is much more profound and extensive in the current model.

Although the sample sizes in our current non-human primate model are insufficient to assess potential sex differences, an expanding body of literature indicates that males may be more vulnerable than females to developmental insults [143]. Males with FASD tend to have higher rates of attention deficit-hyperactivity disorder, oppositional and conduct disorders that may lead to the reported higher level of school difficulties and incarceration. Females diagnosed with FASD tend to have higher rates of anxiety, endocrine disorders and depression [144]. Rodent studies corroborate sex-related response differences to FAE, with males tending to be more susceptible to hippocampus-related behavioral alterations along with deficits in hippocampal LTP and neuronal survivability [86, 107, 108]. As we increase the number of subjects in our non-human primate model, identifying potential FAE-related sex differences in the hippocampus will be essential for understanding the full spectrum of neurodevelopmental outcomes and for developing targeted, sex-specific interventions.

Our dose-dependent study revealed a reduction of the hippocampal neuronal population, even at low levels of alcohol exposure. However, this is only a partial picture. More than just quantifying cell loss, it is essential that future studies include electrophysiological assessments of long-term potentiation and depression that may underlie synaptic plasticity. Further investigations into synaptic function and changes in protein markers might shed more light on the molecular mechanisms involved in damage resulting from fetal alcohol. This multi-focal approach is necessary for a complete understanding of how FAE disrupts hippocampal development and function.

While this chapter has focused on specific impacts of FAE on the developing hippocampus, clinical data suggests a broad range of deficits involving the hippocampal-prefrontal and limbic pathways [33, 34, 36, 37, 42, 145, 146]. Data from our model suggests that FAE also results in reduced neuronal populations in the frontal cortex [113] and altered thalamic nuclei [115]. Rodent models also show behavioral deficits in executive function [147] that correspond to damage in the reuniens, the thalamic nucleus at the interface between the medial prefrontal cortex and hippocampus [148]. Furthermore, FAE disrupts the functional interaction between the medial prefrontal cortex and hippocampus [105]. The hippocampal-prefrontal and limbic pathways are involved in working memory, cognition [149], episodic memory, goal-directed behavior [150], and emotional regulation [151], bi-directional interaction between medial prefrontal cortex and hippocampus via the reuniens thalamic nucleus is critical for working, episodic and emotional memory [152]. It would be expected that FAE-induced alterations in the hippocampus would also be accompanied by changes in other cortical and subcortical areas disrupting the hippocampal network. Additional investigations are warranted for the potential effects on hippocampal network function and cognitive outcomes at the connectivity and mechanistic levels will require both rodent and non-human primate models.

As we unravel the complexities of the hippocampus, the web of interactions and what they mean for both normal function and disease states can be understood only with a more comprehensive approach. While much remains to be understood about the mechanisms of neuronal loss in these animals, the model described here serves a valuable tool for prompt, quantitative and evolutionarily relevant evaluation of intervention strategies facilitating safe and timely clinical translation.

Author details

Alexandra Haddad[1†], Amari Eubanks[2†], Annalia Burke-Carreno[3†], Anthony Okeh[2†], Banuja Munasinghe[2†], Maria Sneed[2†], Roberta Palmour[4,5,6], Maurice Ptito[7,8,9*] and Mark W. Burke[2*]

1 Department of Psychology, Concordia University, Montréal, QC, Canada

2 Department of Physiology and Biophysics, College of Medicine, Howard University, Washington, DC, USA

3 Department of Animal Sciences University of Guelph, ON, Canada

4 Behavioural Science Foundation, St. Kitts, Saint Kitts and Nevis

5 Department of Psychiatry, Faculty of Medicine, McGill University, Montréal, QC, Canada

6 Departments of Human Genetics and Psychiatry, Faculty of Medicine, McGill University, Montréal, QC, Canada

7 Ecole d'Optométrie, Université de Montréal, Québec, Canada

8 Department of Neurology and Neurosurgery, Montreal Neurological Institute, McGill University, Quebec, Canada

9 Department of Applied Mathematics and Computer Science Visual Computing, Danish Technical University, Denmark

*Address all correspondence to: maurice.ptito@umontreal.ca and mark.burke@howard.edu

† These authors contributed equally.

References

[1] Calhoun F, Warren K. Fetal alcohol syndrome: Historical perspectives. Neuroscience and Biobehavioral Reviews. 2007;**31**(2):168-171. DOI: 10.1016/j.neubiorev.2006.06.023

[2] Jones KL, Smith DW. Recognition of the fetal alcohol syndrome in early infancy. Lancet. 1973;**302**(7836):999-1001. DOI: 10.1016/s0140-6736(73)91092-1

[3] Clarren SK, Smith DW. The fetal alcohol syndrome. The New England Journal of Medicine. 1978;**298**(19):1063-1067. DOI: 10.1056/NEJM197805112981906

[4] Jones KL, Smith DW, Hanson JW. The fetal alcohol syndrome: Clinical delineation. Annals of the New York Academy of Sciences. 1976;**273**:130-139. DOI: 10.1111/j.1749-6632.1976.tb52873.x

[5] Wozniak JR, Riley EP, Charness ME. Clinical presentation, diagnosis, and management of fetal alcohol spectrum disorder. Lancet Neurology. 2019;**18**(8):760-770. DOI: 10.1016/S1474-4422(19)30150-4

[6] Denny L, Coles S, Blitz R. Fetal alcohol syndrome and fetal alcohol spectrum disorders. American Family Physician. 2017;**96**(8):515-522

[7] May PA, Baete A, Russo J, Elliott AJ, Blankenship J, Kalberg WO, et al. Prevalence and characteristics of fetal alcohol spectrum disorders. Pediatrics. 2014;**134**(5):855-866. DOI: 10.1542/peds.2013-3319

[8] Luong J, Board A, Gosdin L, Dunkley J, Thierry JM, Pitasi M, et al. Alcohol use, screening, and brief intervention among pregnant persons - 24 U.S. jurisdictions, 2017 and 2019. MMWR. Morbidity and Mortality Weekly Report. 2023;**72**(3):55-62. DOI: 10.15585/mmwr.mm7203a2

[9] Popova S, Lange S, Probst C, Gmel G, Rehm J. Estimation of national, regional, and global prevalence of alcohol use during pregnancy and fetal alcohol syndrome: A systematic review and meta-analysis. The Lancet Global Health. 2017;**5**(3):e290-e299. DOI: 10.1016/S2214-109X(17)30021-9

[10] Bakhireva LN, Garrison L, Shrestha S, Sharkis J, Miranda R, Rogers K. Challenges of diagnosing fetal alcohol spectrum disorders in foster and adopted children. Alcohol. 2018;**67**:37-43. DOI: 10.1016/j.alcohol.2017.05.004

[11] Bakhireva LN, Sharkis J, Shrestha S, Miranda-Sohrabji TJ, Williams S, Miranda RC. Prevalence of prenatal alcohol exposure in the state of Texas as assessed by phosphatidylethanol in newborn dried blood spot specimens. Alcoholism, Clinical and Experimental Research. 2017;**41**(5):1004-1011. DOI: 10.1111/acer.13375

[12] DiBattista A, Ogrel S, MacKenzie AE, Chakraborty P. Quantitation of phosphatidylethanols in dried blood spots to determine rates of prenatal alcohol exposure in Ontario. Alcoholism, Clinical and Experimental Research. 2022;**46**(2):243-251. DOI: 10.1111/acer.14766

[13] Bager H, Christensen LP, Husby S, Bjerregaard L. Biomarkers for the detection of prenatal alcohol exposure: A review. Alcoholism, Clinical and Experimental Research. 2017;**41**(2):251-261. DOI: 10.1111/acer.13309

[14] Bernes GA, Courchesne-Krak NS, Hyland MT, Villodas MT, Coles CD, Kable JA, et al. Development and validation of a postnatal risk score that identifies children with prenatal alcohol exposure. Alcoholism, Clinical and Experimental Research. 2022;**46**(1):52-65. DOI: 10.1111/acer.14749

[15] May PA, Hasken JM, Manning MA, Hoyme HE. The challenges and pitfalls of fetal alcohol spectrum disorders prevalence studies. Alcoholism, Clinical and Experimental Research. 2021;**45**(12):2468-2470. DOI: 10.1111/acer.14735

[16] Carpita B, Migli L, Chiarantini I, Battaglini S, Montalbano C, Carmassi C, et al. Autism spectrum disorder and fetal alcohol spectrum disorder: A literature review. Brain Sciences. 2022;**12**(6):792. DOI: 10.3390/brainsci12060792

[17] Streissguth AP, O'Malley K. Neuropsychiatric implications and long-term consequences of fetal alcohol spectrum disorders. Seminars in Clinical Neuropsychiatry. 2000;**5**(3):177-190. DOI: 10.1053/scnp.2000.6729

[18] Connor PD, Sampson PD, Bookstein FL, Barr HM, Streissguth AP. Direct and indirect effects of prenatal alcohol damage on executive function. Developmental Neuropsychology. 2000;**18**(3):331-354. DOI: 10.1207/S15326942O4Connor

[19] Burke MW, Slimani H, Ptito M, Ervin FR, Palmour RM. Dose-related reduction in hippocampal neuronal populations in fetal alcohol exposed vervet monkeys. Brain Sciences. 2022;**12**(9):1117. DOI: 10.3390/brainsci12091117

[20] Costa LG, Aschner M, Vitalone A, Syversen T, Soldin OP. Developmental neuropathology of environmental agents. Annual Review of Pharmacology and Toxicology. 2004;**44**:87-110. DOI: 10.1146/annurev.pharmtox.44.101802.121424

[21] White TA, Miller SL, Sutherland AE, Allison BJ, Camm EJ. Perinatal compromise affects development, form, and function of the hippocampus part one; clinical studies. Pediatric Research. 2024;**95**(7):1698-1708. DOI: 10.1038/s41390-024-03105-7

[22] Davidson TL, Stevenson RJ. Vulnerability of the hippocampus to insults: Links to blood-brain barrier dysfunction. International Journal of Molecular Sciences. 2024;**25**(4):1991. DOI: 10.3390/ijms25041991

[23] Li Y, Shen M, Stockton ME, Zhao X. Hippocampal deficits in neurodevelopmental disorders. Neurobiology of Learning and Memory. 2019;**165**:106945. DOI: 10.1016/j.nlm.2018.10.001

[24] White TA, Miller SL, Sutherland AE, Allison BJ, Camm EJ. Perinatal compromise affects development, form, and function of the hippocampus part two; preclinical studies. Pediatric Research. 2024;**95**(7):1709-1719. DOI: 10.1038/s41390-024-03144-0

[25] Felix-Ortiz AC, Tye KM. Amygdala inputs to the ventral hippocampus bidirectionally modulate social behavior. The Journal of Neuroscience. 2014;**34**(2):586-595. DOI: 10.1523/JNEUROSCI.4257-13.2014

[26] Rubin RD, Watson PD, Duff MC, Cohen NJ. The role of the hippocampus in flexible cognition and social behavior. Frontiers in Human Neuroscience. 2014;**8**:742. DOI: 10.3389/fnhum.2014.00742

[27] Fontaine CJ, Patten AR, Sickmann HM, Helfer JL, Christie BR. Effects of pre-natal alcohol exposure on hippocampal synaptic plasticity: Sex, age and methodological considerations. Neuroscience and Biobehavioral Reviews. 2016;**64**:12-34. DOI: 10.1016/j.neubiorev.2016.02.014

[28] Nguyen VT, Chong S, Tieng QM, Mardon K, Galloway GJ, Kurniawan ND. Radiological studies of fetal alcohol spectrum disorders in humans and animal models: An updated comprehensive review. Magnetic Resonance Imaging. 2017;**43**:10-26. DOI: 10.1016/j.mri.2017.06.012

[29] Willoughby KA, Sheard ED, Nash K, Rovet J. Effects of prenatal alcohol exposure on hippocampal volume, verbal learning, and verbal and spatial recall in late childhood. Journal of the International Neuropsychological Society. 2008;**14**(6):1022-1033. DOI: 10.1017/S1355617708081368

[30] Roediger DJ, Krueger AM, de Water E, Mueller BA, Boys CA, Hendrickson TJ, et al. Hippocampal subfield abnormalities and memory functioning in children with fetal alcohol spectrum disorders. Neurotoxicology and Teratology. 2021;**83**:106944. DOI: 10.1016/j.ntt.2020.106944

[31] Dudek J, Skocic J, Sheard E, Rovet J. Hippocampal abnormalities in youth with alcohol-related neurodevelopmental disorder. Journal of the International Neuropsychological Society. 2014;**20**(2):181-191. DOI: 10.1017/S1355617713001343

[32] Gimbel BA, Roediger DJ, Anthony ME, Ernst AM, Tuominen KA, Mueller BA, et al. Normative modeling of brain MRI data identifies small subcortical volumes and associations with cognitive function in youth with fetal alcohol spectrum disorder (FASD). NeuroImage. Clinical. 2025;**45**:103722. DOI: 10.1016/j.nicl.2024.103722

[33] Dodge NC, Thomas KGF, Meintjes EM, Molteno CD, Jacobson JL, Jacobson SW. Reduced hippocampal volumes partially mediate effects of prenatal alcohol exposure on spatial navigation on a virtual water maze task in children. Alcoholism, Clinical and Experimental Research. 2020;**44**(4):844-855. DOI: 10.1111/acer.14310

[34] Gimbel BA, Wozniak JR, Mueller BA, Tuominen KA, Ernst AM, Anthony ME, et al. Regional hippocampal thinning and gyrification abnormalities and associated cognition in children with prenatal alcohol exposure. Journal of Neurodevelopmental Disorders. 2025;**17**(1):5. DOI: 10.1186/s11689-025-09595-8

[35] Alsameen MH, Candelaria-Cook FT, Cerros CM, Hill DE, Stephen JM. Altered neuronal network connectivity in children with fetal alcohol spectrum disorder and its association with inhibitory function. Alcohol, Clinical & Experimental Research (Hoboken). 2025;**49**(10):2133-2145. DOI: 10.1111/acer.70144

[36] Tamana S, Pei J, Massey D, Massey V, Rasmussen C. Neuropsychological impairments and age-related differences in children and adolescents with fetal alcohol spectrum disorders. Journal of Population Therapeutics and Clinical Pharmacology. 2014;**21**(2):e167-e180

[37] Mattson SN, Bernes GA, Doyle LR. Fetal alcohol spectrum disorders: A review of the neurobehavioral deficits associated with prenatal alcohol exposure. Alcoholism, Clinical and Experimental Research. 2019;**43**(6):1046-1062. DOI: 10.1111/acer.14040

[38] Uecker A, Nadel L. Spatial locations gone awry: Object and spatial memory deficits in children with fetal alcohol syndrome. Neuropsychologia. 1996;**34**(3):209-223. DOI: 10.1016/0028-3932(95)00096-8

[39] Harvey RE, Berkowitz LE, Hamilton DA, Clark BJ. The effects of developmental alcohol exposure on the neurobiology of spatial processing. Neuroscience and Biobehavioral Reviews. 2019;**107**:775-794. DOI: 10.1016/j.neubiorev.2019.09.018

[40] Burden MJ, Andrew C, Saint-Amour D, Meintjes EM, Molteno CD, Hoyme HE, et al. The effects of fetal alcohol syndrome on response execution and inhibition: An event-related potential study. Alcoholism, Clinical and Experimental Research. 2009;**33**(11):1994-2004. DOI: 10.1111/j.1530-0277.2009.01038.x

[41] Lewis CE, Thomas KG, Molteno CD, Kliegel M, Meintjes EM, Jacobson JL, et al. Prospective memory impairment in children with prenatal alcohol exposure. Alcoholism, Clinical and Experimental Research. 2016;**40**(5):969-978. DOI: 10.1111/acer.13045

[42] Green CR, Mihic AM, Nikkel SM, Stade BC, Rasmussen C, Munoz DP, et al. Executive function deficits in children with fetal alcohol spectrum disorders (FASD) measured using the Cambridge neuropsychological tests automated battery (CANTAB). Journal of Child Psychology and Psychiatry. 2009;**50**(6):688-697. DOI: 10.1111/j.1469-7610.2008.01990.x

[43] Mattson SN, Crocker N, Nguyen TT. Fetal alcohol spectrum disorders: Neuropsychological and behavioral features. Neuropsychology Review. 2011;**21**(2):81-101. DOI: 10.1007/s11065-011-9167-9

[44] Coles CD, Kalberg W, Kable JA, Tabachnick B, May PA, Chambers CD. Characterizing alcohol-related neurodevelopmental disorder: Prenatal alcohol exposure and the spectrum of outcomes. Alcoholism, Clinical and Experimental Research. 2020;**44**(6):1245-1260. DOI: 10.1111/acer.14325

[45] Streissguth AP, Bookstein FL, Barr HM, Sampson PD, O'Malley K, Young JK. Risk factors for adverse life outcomes in fetal alcohol syndrome and fetal alcohol effects. Journal of Developmental and Behavioral Pediatrics. 2004;**25**(4):228-238. DOI: 10.1097/00004703-200408000-00002

[46] Ernhart CB, Morrow-Tlucak M, Sokol RJ, Martier S. Underreporting of alcohol use in pregnancy. Alcoholism, Clinical and Experimental Research. 1988;**12**(4):506-511. DOI: 10.1111/j.1530-0277.1988.tb00233.x

[47] Lange S, Shield K, Koren G, Rehm J, Popova S. A comparison of the prevalence of prenatal alcohol exposure obtained via maternal self-reports versus meconium testing: A systematic literature review and meta-analysis. BMC Pregnancy and Childbirth. 2014;**14**:127. DOI: 10.1186/1471-2393-14-127

[48] Patten AR, Fontaine CJ, Christie BR. A comparison of the different animal models of fetal alcohol spectrum disorders and their use in studying complex behaviors. Frontiers in Pediatrics. 2014;**2**:93. DOI: 10.3389/fped.2014.00093

[49] Maier SE, West JR. Regional differences in cell loss associated with binge-like alcohol exposure during the first two trimesters equivalent in the rat. Alcohol. 2001;**23**(1):49-57. DOI: 10.1016/s0741-8329(00)00133-6

[50] Livy DJ, Miller EK, Maier SE, West JR. Fetal alcohol exposure and temporal vulnerability: Effects of binge-like alcohol exposure on the developing rat hippocampus. Neurotoxicology and Teratology. 2003;**25**(4):447-458. DOI: 10.1016/s0892-0362(03)00030-8

[51] Lee J, Naik V, Orzabal M, Lunde-Young R, Ramadoss J. Morphological alteration in rat hippocampal neuronal dendrites following chronic binge prenatal alcohol exposure. Brain Research. 2021;**1768**:147587. DOI: 10.1016/j.brainres.2021.147587

[52] Redila VA, Olson AK, Swann SE, Mohades G, Webber AJ, Weinberg J, et al. Hippocampal cell proliferation is reduced following prenatal ethanol exposure but can be rescued with voluntary exercise. Hippocampus. 2006;**16**(3):305-311. DOI: 10.1002/hipo.20164

[53] Gil-Mohapel J, Boehme F, Patten A, Cox A, Kainer L, Giles E, et al. Altered adult hippocampal neuronal maturation in a rat model of fetal alcohol syndrome. Brain Research. 2011;**1384**:29-41. DOI: 10.1016/j.brainres.2011.01.116

[54] Gil-Mohapel J, Titterness AK, Patten AR, Taylor S, Ratzlaff A, Ratzlaff T, et al. Prenatal ethanol exposure differentially affects hippocampal neurogenesis in the adolescent and aged brain. Neuroscience. 2014;**273**:174-188. DOI: 10.1016/j.neuroscience.2014.05.012

[55] Uban KA, Sliwowska JH, Lieblich S, Ellis LA, Yu WK, Weinberg J, et al. Prenatal alcohol exposure reduces the proportion of newly produced neurons and glia in the dentate gyrus of the hippocampus in female rats. Hormones and Behavior. 2010;**58**(5):835-843. DOI: 10.1016/j.yhbeh.2010.08.007

[56] Takahashi Y, Yamashita R, Okano H, Takashima K, Ogawa B, Ojiro R, et al. Aberrant neurogenesis and late onset suppression of synaptic plasticity as well as sustained neuroinflammation in the hippocampal dentate gyrus after developmental exposure to ethanol in rats. Toxicology. 2021;**462**:152958. DOI: 10.1016/j.tox.2021.152958

[57] Takahashi Y, Okano H, Takashima K, Ojiro R, Tang Q, Ozawa S, et al. Oral exposure to high-dose ethanol for 28 days in rats reduces neural stem cells and immediate nascent neural progenitor cells as well as FOS-expressing newborn granule cells in adult hippocampal neurogenesis. Toxicology Letters. 2022;**360**:20-32. DOI: 10.1016/j.toxlet.2022.02.006

[58] Lunde-Young R, Ramirez J, Naik V, Orzabal M, Lee J, Konganti K, et al. Hippocampal transcriptome reveals novel targets of FASD pathogenesis. Brain and Behavior: A Cognitive Neuroscience Perspective. 2019;**9**(7):e01334. DOI: 10.1002/brb3.1334

[59] Tran TD, Kelly SJ. Critical periods for ethanol-induced cell loss in the hippocampal formation. Neurotoxicology and Teratology. 2003;**25**(5):519-528. DOI: 10.1016/s0892-0362(03)00074-6

[60] Miller MW. Generation of neurons in the rat dentate gyrus and hippocampus: Effects of prenatal and postnatal treatment with ethanol. Alcoholism, Clinical and Experimental Research. 1995;**19**(6):1500-1509. DOI: 10.1111/j.1530-0277.1995.tb01014.x

[61] Boschen KE, McKeown SE, Roth TL, Klintsova AY. Impact of exercise and a complex environment on hippocampal dendritic morphology, Bdnf gene expression, and DNA methylation in male rat pups neonatally exposed to alcohol. Developmental Neurobiology. 2017;**77**(6):708-725. DOI: 10.1002/dneu.22448

[62] Klintsova AY, Helfer JL, Calizo LH, Dong WK, Goodlett CR, Greenough WT. Persistent impairment of hippocampal neurogenesis in young adult rats following early postnatal alcohol exposure. Alcoholism, Clinical and Experimental Research. 2007;**31**(12):2073-2082. DOI: 10.1111/j.1530-0277.2007.00528.x

[63] Helfer JL, Goodlett CR, Greenough WT, Klintsova AY. The effects of exercise on adolescent hippocampal neurogenesis in a rat model of binge alcohol exposure during the brain growth spurt. Brain Research. 2009;**1294**:1-11. DOI: 10.1016/j.brainres.2009.07.090

[64] Madden JT, Thompson SM, Magcalas CM, Wagner JL, Hamilton DA, Savage DD, et al. Moderate prenatal alcohol exposure reduces parvalbumin expressing GABAergic interneurons in the dorsal hippocampus of adult male and female rat offspring. Neuroscience Letters. 2020;**718**:134700. DOI: 10.1016/j.neulet.2019.134700

[65] Boschen KE, Ruggiero MJ, Klintsova AY. Neonatal binge alcohol exposure increases microglial activation in the developing rat hippocampus. Neuroscience. 2016;**324**:355-366. DOI: 10.1016/j.neuroscience.2016.03.033

[66] Khalifa A, Palu R, Perkins AE, Volz A. Prenatal alcohol exposure alters expression of genes involved in cell adhesion, immune response, and toxin metabolism in adolescent rat hippocampus. PLoS One. 2024;**19**(1):e0293425. DOI: 10.1371/journal.pone.0293425

[67] Bonthius DJ, Woodhouse J, Bonthius NE, Taggard DA, Lothman EW. Reduced seizure threshold and hippocampal cell loss in rats exposed to alcohol during the brain growth spurt. Alcoholism, Clinical and Experimental Research. 2001;**25**(1):70-82

[68] Elibol-Can B, Dursun I, Telkes I, Kilic E, Canan S, Jakubowska-Dogru E. Examination of age-dependent effects of fetal ethanol exposure on behavior, hippocampal cell counts, and doublecortin immunoreactivity in rats. Developmental Neurobiology. 2014;**74**(5):498-513. DOI: 10.1002/dneu.22143

[69] Elibol-Can B, Kilic E, Yuruker S, Jakubowska-Dogru E. Investigation into the effects of prenatal alcohol exposure on postnatal spine development and expression of synaptophysin and PSD95 in rat hippocampus. International Journal of Developmental Neuroscience. 2014;**33**:106-114. DOI: 10.1016/j.ijdevneu.2013.12.003

[70] Miki T, Harris SJ, Wilce P, Takeuchi Y, Bedi KS. Neurons in the hilus region of the rat hippocampus are depleted in number by exposure to alcohol during early postnatal life. Hippocampus. 2000;**10**(3):284-295. DOI: 10.1002/1098-1063(2000)10:3<284::AID-HIPO9>3.0.CO;2-K

[71] Topper LA, Baculis BC, Valenzuela CF. Exposure of neonatal rats to alcohol has differential effects on neuroinflammation and neuronal survival in the cerebellum and hippocampus. Journal of Neuroinflammation. 2015;**12**:160. DOI: 10.1186/s12974-015-0382-9

[72] Choi IY, Allan AM, Cunningham LA. Moderate fetal alcohol exposure impairs the neurogenic response to an enriched environment in adult mice. Alcoholism, Clinical and Experimental Research. 2005;**29**(11):2053-2062. DOI: 10.1097/01.alc.0000187037.02670.59

[73] Olateju OI, Spocter MA, Patzke N, Ihunwo AO, Manger PR. Hippocampal neurogenesis in the C57BL/6J mice at early adulthood following prenatal

alcohol exposure. Metabolic Brain Disease. 2018;**33**(2):397-410. DOI: 10.1007/s11011-017-0156-4

[74] Xu W, Li H, He C, Frank J, Chen G. Early ethanol exposure inhibits the differentiation of hippocampal dentate gyrus granule cells in a mouse model of fetal alcohol spectrum disorders. Alcoholism, Clinical and Experimental Research. 2020;**44**(5):1112-1122. DOI: 10.1111/acer.14330

[75] Cai Y, Wu JC, Huang Y, Yu XF, Liu FH, Chen ZW, et al. Impaired cognitive function and altered dendritic morphology of hippocampal neurons in a mouse model of fetal alcohol spectrum disorder. Behavioural Brain Research. 2025;**490**:115633. DOI: 10.1016/j.bbr.2025.115633

[76] Hashimoto JG, Margolies N, Zhang X, Karpf J, Song Y, Gorham N, et al. Astrocyte extracellular matrix modulates neuronal dendritic development. Glia. 2025;**73**(8):1589-1607. DOI: 10.1002/glia.70020

[77] Bird CW, Taylor DH, Pinkowski NJ, Chavez GJ, Valenzuela CF. Long-term reductions in the population of GABAergic interneurons in the mouse hippocampus following developmental ethanol exposure. Neuroscience. 2018;**383**:60-73. DOI: 10.1016/j.neuroscience.2018.05.003

[78] Gustus K, Lozano E, Newville J, Li L, Valenzuela CF, Cunningham LA. Resistance of postnatal hippocampal neurogenesis to alcohol toxicity in a third trimester-equivalent mouse model of gestational alcohol exposure. Alcoholism, Clinical and Experimental Research. 2019;**43**(12):2504-2513. DOI: 10.1111/acer.14207

[79] Mandal C, Park KS, Jung KH, Chai YG. Ethanol-related alterations in gene expression patterns in the developing murine hippocampus. Acta Biochimica et Biophysica Sinica (Shanghai). 2015;**47**(8):581-587. DOI: 10.1093/abbs/gmv050

[80] Pinson MR, Holloway KN, Douglas JC, Kane CJM, Miranda RC, Drew PD. Divergent and overlapping hippocampal and cerebellar transcriptome responses following developmental ethanol exposure during the secondary neurogenic period. Alcoholism, Clinical and Experimental Research. 2021;**45**(7):1408-1423. DOI: 10.1111/acer.14633

[81] Clancy B, Darlington RB, Finlay BL. Translating developmental time across mammalian species. Neuroscience. 2001;**105**(1):7-17. DOI: 10.1016/s0306-4522(01)00171-3

[82] Tunc-Ozcan E, Wert SL, Lim PH, Ferreira A, Redei EE. Hippocampus-dependent memory and allele-specific gene expression in adult offspring of alcohol-consuming dams after neonatal treatment with thyroxin or metformin. Molecular Psychiatry. 2018;**23**(7):1643-1651. DOI: 10.1038/mp.2017.129

[83] Toosi A, Shajiee H, Khaksari M, Vaezi G, Hojati V. Obestatin improve spatial memory impairment in a rat model of fetal alcohol spectrum disorders via inhibiting apoptosis and neuroinflammation. Neuropeptides. 2019;**74**:88-94. DOI: 10.1016/j.npep.2019.01.001

[84] Sanchez LM, Acosta G, Cushing SD, Johnson SA, Turner SM, Davies S, et al. The effects of moderate prenatal alcohol exposure on performance in object and spatial discrimination tasks by adult male rats. Behavioural Brain Research. 2025;**478**:115324. DOI: 10.1016/j.bbr.2024.115324

[85] Acosta G, Rico KT, Madden JT, LaCour A, Wang E, Sanchez LM, et al. The effects of moderate prenatal alcohol exposure on performance in hippocampal-sensitive spatial memory and anxiety tasks by adult male and female rat offspring. Alcohol. 2024;**121**:75-86. DOI: 10.1016/j.alcohol.2024.08.002

[86] Uguz AC, Okan A, Doganyigit Z, Yilmaz S, Ates S, Arikan Soylemez ES, et al. Evaluation of TRPM2 channel-mediated autophagic signaling pathway in hippocampus and cortex tissues of rat offspring following prenatal exposure to elevated alcohol levels. Environmental Toxicology. 2025;**40**(2):222-244. DOI: 10.1002/tox.24427

[87] Chater-Diehl EJ, Laufer BI, Castellani CA, Alberry BL, Singh SM. Alteration of gene expression, DNA methylation, and histone methylation in free radical scavenging networks in adult mouse hippocampus following fetal alcohol exposure. PLoS One. 2016;**11**(5):e0154836. DOI: 10.1371/journal.pone.0154836

[88] Drew PD, Johnson JW, Douglas JC, Phelan KD, Kane CJ. Pioglitazone blocks ethanol induction of microglial activation and immune responses in the hippocampus, cerebellum, and cerebral cortex in a mouse model of fetal alcohol spectrum disorders. Alcoholism, Clinical and Experimental Research. 2015;**39**(3):445-454. DOI: 10.1111/acer.12639

[89] Niedzwiedz-Massey VM, Douglas JC, Rafferty T, Wight PA, Kane CJM, Drew PD. Ethanol modulation of hippocampal neuroinflammation, myelination, and neurodevelopment in a postnatal mouse model of fetal alcohol spectrum disorders. Neurotoxicology and Teratology. 2021;**87**:107015. DOI: 10.1016/j.ntt.2021.107015

[90] Curti L, Rizzi B, Mottarlini F, Bigagli E, Ilari A, Costa A, et al. Prenatal ethanol exposure impairs hippocampal plasticity and cognition in adolescent mice. Progress in Neuro-Psychopharmacology & Biological Psychiatry. 2025;**136**:111174. DOI: 10.1016/j.pnpbp.2024.111174

[91] Puglia MP, Valenzuela CF. Repeated third trimester-equivalent ethanol exposure inhibits long-term potentiation in the hippocampal CA1 region of neonatal rats. Alcohol. 2010;**44**(3):283-290. DOI: 10.1016/j.alcohol.2010.03.001

[92] Kervern M, Silvestre de Ferron B, Alaux-Cantin S, Fedorenko O, Antol J, Naassila M, et al. Aberrant NMDA-dependent LTD after perinatal ethanol exposure in young adult rat hippocampus. Hippocampus. 2015;**25**(8):912-923. DOI: 10.1002/hipo.22414

[93] Plaza-Briceno W, Estay SF, de la Fuente-Ortega E, Gutierrez C, Sanchez G, Hidalgo C, et al. N-methyl-d-aspartate receptor modulation by nicotinamide adenine dinucleotide phosphate oxidase type 2 drives synaptic plasticity and spatial memory impairments in rats exposed pre- and postnatally to ethanol. Antioxidants & Redox Signaling. 2020;**32**(9):602-617. DOI: 10.1089/ars.2019.7787

[94] Krahl SE, Berman RF, Hannigan JH. Electrophysiology of hippocampal CA1 neurons after prenatal ethanol exposure. Alcohol. 1999;**17**(2):125-131. DOI: 10.1016/s0741-8329(98)00043-3

[95] Helfer JL, White ER, Christie BR. Enhanced deficits in long-term potentiation in the adult dentate gyrus with 2nd trimester ethanol consumption. PLoS One. 2012;**7**(12):e51344. DOI: 10.1371/journal.pone.0051344

[96] Fontaine CJ, Pinar C, Yang W, Pang AF, Suesser KE, Choi JSJ, et al. Impaired bidirectional synaptic plasticity in juvenile offspring following prenatal ethanol exposure. Alcoholism, Clinical and Experimental Research. 2019;**43**(10):2153-2166. DOI: 10.1111/acer.14170

[97] West JR, Hodges-Savola CA. Permanent hippocampal mossy fiber hyperdevelopment following prenatal ethanol exposure. Neurobehavioral Toxicology and Teratology. 1983;**5**(1):139-150

[98] Maier RV. Ethanol abuse and the trauma patient. Surgical Infections. 2001;**2**(2):133-141; discussion 141-134. DOI: 10.1089/109629601750469456

[99] Bonthius DJ, Pantazis NJ, Karacay B, Bonthius NE, Taggard DA, Lothman EW. Alcohol exposure during the brain growth spurt promotes hippocampal seizures, rapid kindling, and spreading depression. Alcoholism, Clinical and Experimental Research. 2001;**25**(5):734-745

[100] Hamilton GF, Murawski NJ, St. Cyr SA, Jablonski SA, Schiffino FL, Stanton ME, et al. Neonatal alcohol exposure disrupts hippocampal neurogenesis and contextual fear conditioning in adult rats. Brain Research. 2011;**1412**:88-101. DOI: 10.1016/j.brainres.2011.07.027

[101] Xia F, Richards BA, Tran MM, Josselyn SA, Takehara-Nishiuchi K, Frankland PW. Parvalbumin-positive interneurons mediate neocortical-hippocampal interactions that are necessary for memory consolidation. eLife. 2017;**6**:e27868. DOI: 10.7554/eLife.27868

[102] Ramsaran AI, Wang Y, Golbabaei A, Aleshin S, de Snoo ML, Yeung BA, et al. A shift in the mechanisms controlling hippocampal engram formation during brain maturation. Science. 2023;**380**(6644):543-551. DOI: 10.1126/science.ade6530

[103] Gursky ZH, Klintsova AY. Rat model of late gestational alcohol exposure produces similar life-long changes in thalamic nucleus reuniens following moderate- versus high-dose insult. Alcohol and Alcoholism. 2022;**57**(4):413-420. DOI: 10.1093/alcalc/agac008

[104] Smith IF, Gursky ZH, Klintsova AY. Representation of prefrontal axonal efferents in the thalamic nucleus reuniens in a rodent model of fetal alcohol exposure during third trimester. Frontiers in Behavioral Neuroscience. 2022;**16**:993601. DOI: 10.3389/fnbeh.2022.993601

[105] Rosenblum HL, Kim S, Stout JJ, Klintsova AY, Griffin AL. Choice behaviors and prefrontal-hippocampal coupling are disrupted in a rat model of fetal alcohol spectrum disorders. The Journal of Neuroscience. 2025;**45**(10):e1241242025. DOI: 10.1523/JNEUROSCI.1241-24.2025

[106] Sickmann HM, Patten AR, Morch K, Sawchuk S, Zhang C, Parton R, et al. Prenatal ethanol exposure has sex-specific effects on hippocampal long-term potentiation. Hippocampus. 2014;**24**(1):54-64. DOI: 10.1002/hipo.22203

[107] Ruggiero MJ, Boschen KE, Roth TL, Klintsova AY. Sex differences in early postnatal microglial colonization of the developing rat hippocampus following a single-day alcohol exposure. Journal of Neuroimmune Pharmacology. 2018;**13**(2):189-203. DOI: 10.1007/s11481-017-9774-1

[108] Ieraci A, Herrera DG. Early postnatal ethanol exposure in mice

induces sex-dependent memory impairment and reduction of hippocampal NMDA-R2B expression in adulthood. Neuroscience. 2020;**427**:105-115. DOI: 10.1016/j.neuroscience.2019.11.045

[109] Burke MW, Ptito M, Ervin FR, Palmour RM. Hippocampal neuron populations are reduced in vervet monkeys with fetal alcohol exposure. Developmental Psychobiology. 2015;**57**(4):470-485. DOI: 10.1002/dev.21311

[110] Schneider ML, Moore CF, Adkins MM. The effects of prenatal alcohol exposure on behavior: Rodent and primate studies. Neuropsychology Review. 2011;**21**(2):186-203. DOI: 10.1007/s11065-011-9168-8

[111] Schneider ML, Moore CF, Becker EF. Timing of moderate alcohol exposure during pregnancy and neonatal outcome in rhesus monkeys (*Macaca mulatta*). Alcoholism, Clinical and Experimental Research. 2001;**25**(8):1238-1245

[112] Schneider ML, Moore CF, Kraemer GW. Moderate alcohol during pregnancy: Learning and behavior in adolescent rhesus monkeys. Alcoholism, Clinical and Experimental Research. 2001;**25**(9):1383-1392

[113] Burke MW, Palmour RM, Ervin FR, Ptito M. Neuronal reduction in frontal cortex of primates after prenatal alcohol exposure. Neuroreport. 2009;**20**(1):13-17. DOI: 10.1097/WNR.0b013e32831b449c

[114] Burke MW, Inyatkin A, Ptito M, Ervin FR, Palmour RM. Prenatal alcohol exposure affects progenitor cell numbers in olfactory bulbs and dentate gyrus of vervet monkeys. Brain Sciences. 2016;**6**(4):52. DOI: 10.3390/brainsci6040052

[115] Papia MF, Burke MW, Zangenehpour S, Palmour RM, Ervin FR, Ptito M. Reduced soma size of the M-neurons in the lateral geniculate nucleus following foetal alcohol exposure in non-human primates. Experimental Brain Research. 2010;**205**(2):263-271. DOI: 10.1007/s00221-010-2364-6

[116] Schneider ML, Moore CF, Kraemer GW. Moderate level alcohol during pregnancy, prenatal stress, or both and limbic-hypothalamic-pituitary-adrenocortical axis response to stress in rhesus monkeys. Child Development. 2004;**75**(1):96-109. DOI: 10.1111/j.1467-8624.2004.00656.x

[117] Schneider ML, Larson JA, Rypstat CW, Resch LM, Roberts A, Moore CF. Moderate-level prenatal alcohol exposure enhances acoustic startle magnitude and disrupts prepulse inhibition in adult rhesus monkeys. Alcoholism, Clinical and Experimental Research. 2013;**37**(10):1729-1736. DOI: 10.1111/acer.12151

[118] Clarren SK, Astley SJ, Bowden DM, Lai H, Milam AH, Rudeen PK, et al. Neuroanatomic and neurochemical abnormalities in nonhuman primate infants exposed to weekly doses of ethanol during gestation. Alcoholism, Clinical and Experimental Research. 1990;**14**(5):674-683. DOI: 10.1111/j.1530-0277.1990.tb01226.x

[119] Clarren SK, Astley SJ, Gunderson VM, Spellman D. Cognitive and behavioral deficits in nonhuman primates associated with very early embryonic binge exposures to ethanol. The Journal of Pediatrics. 1992;**121**(5 Pt. 1):789-796. DOI: 10.1016/s0022-3476(05)81917-1

[120] Fedorchak AV, Miller MW. Episodic prenatal exposure to ethanol affects postnatal neurogenesis In the

macaque dentate gyrus and visual recognition memory. International Journal of Developmental Neuroscience. 2019;**79**:65-75. DOI: 10.1016/j.ijdevneu.2019.10.005

[121] Miller MW. Exposure to ethanol during gastrulation alters somatosensory-motor cortices and the underlying white matter in the macaque. Cerebral Cortex. 2007;**17**(12):2961-2971. DOI: 10.1093/cercor/bhm024

[122] Eckardt MJ, File SE, Gessa GL, Grant KA, Guerri C, Hoffman PL, et al. Effects of moderate alcohol consumption on the central nervous system. Alcoholism, Clinical and Experimental Research. 1998;**22**(5):998-1040. DOI: 10.1111/j.1530-0277.1998.tb03695.x

[123] Ebrahim SH, Luman ET, Floyd RL, Murphy CC, Bennett EM, Boyle CA. Alcohol consumption by pregnant women in the United States during 1988-1995. Obstetrics and Gynecology. 1998;**92**(2):187-192. DOI: 10.1016/s0029-7844(98)00205-1

[124] Colvin L, Payne J, Parsons D, Kurinczuk JJ, Bower C. Alcohol consumption during pregnancy in nonindigenous west Australian women. Alcoholism, Clinical and Experimental Research. 2007;**31**(2):276-284. DOI: 10.1111/j.1530-0277.2006.00303.x

[125] Gosdin LK, Deputy NP, Kim SY, Dang EP, Denny CH. Alcohol consumption and binge drinking during pregnancy among adults aged 18-49 years - United States, 2018-2020. MMWR. Morbidity and Mortality Weekly Report. 2022;**71**(1):10-13. DOI: 10.15585/mmwr.mm7101a2

[126] Ervin FR, Palmour RM, Young SN, Guzman-Flores C, Juarez J. Voluntary consumption of beverage alcohol by vervet monkeys: Population screening, descriptive behavior and biochemical measures. Pharmacology, Biochemistry, and Behavior. 1990;**36**(2):367-373. DOI: 10.1016/0091-3057(90)90417-g

[127] Seress L, Ribak CE. Postnatal development and synaptic connections of hilar mossy cells in the hippocampal dentate gyrus of rhesus monkeys. The Journal of Comparative Neurology. 1995;**355**(1):93-110. DOI: 10.1002/cne.903550111

[128] Seress L, Ribak CE. Postnatal development of CA3 pyramidal neurons and their afferents in the Ammon's horn of rhesus monkeys. Hippocampus. 1995;**5**(3):217-231. DOI: 10.1002/hipo.450050308

[129] Favre G, Banta Lavenex P, Lavenex P. miRNA regulation of gene expression: A predictive bioinformatics analysis in the postnatally developing monkey hippocampus. PLoS One. 2012;**7**(8):e43435. DOI: 10.1371/journal.pone.0043435

[130] Jabes A, Lavenex PB, Amaral DG, Lavenex P. Quantitative analysis of postnatal neurogenesis and neuron number in the macaque monkey dentate gyrus. The European Journal of Neuroscience. 2010;**31**(2):273-285. DOI: 10.1111/j.1460-9568.2009.07061.x

[131] Rakic P, Nowakowski RS. The time of origin of neurons in the hippocampal region of the rhesus monkey. The Journal of Comparative Neurology. 1981;**196**(1):99-128. DOI: 10.1002/cne.901960109

[132] Nowakowski RS, Rakic P. The site of origin and route and rate of migration of neurons to the hippocampal region of the rhesus monkey. The Journal of Comparative Neurology. 1981;**196**(1):129-154. DOI: 10.1002/cne.901960110

[133] Duffy CJ, Rakic P. Differentiation of granule cell dendrites in the dentate gyrus of the rhesus monkey: A quantitative golgi study. The Journal of Comparative Neurology. 1983;**214**(2):224-237. DOI: 10.1002/cne.902140210

[134] Eckenhoff MF, Rakic P. Radial organization of the hippocampal dentate gyrus: A golgi, ultrastructural, and immunocytochemical analysis in the developing rhesus monkey. The Journal of Comparative Neurology. 1984;**223**(1):1-21. DOI: 10.1002/cne.902230102

[135] Seress L, Abraham H, Tornoczky T, Kosztolanyi G. Cell formation in the human hippocampal formation from mid-gestation to the late postnatal period. Neuroscience. 2001;**105**(4):831-843. DOI: 10.1016/s0306-4522(01)00156-7

[136] Lavenex P, Banta Lavenex P, Amaral DG. Postnatal development of the primate hippocampal formation. Developmental Neuroscience. 2007;**29**(1-2):179-192. DOI: 10.1159/000096222

[137] Bayer SA, Altman J. Hippocampal development in the rat: Cytogenesis and morphogenesis examined with autoradiography and low-level X-irradiation. The Journal of Comparative Neurology. 1974;**158**(1):55-79. DOI: 10.1002/cne.901580105

[138] Gillis RF, Palmour RM. miRNA expression analysis of the hippocampus in a vervet monkey model of fetal alcohol spectrum disorder reveals a potential role in global mRNA downregulation. Brain Sciences. 2023;**13**(6):934. DOI: 10.3390/brainsci13060934

[139] Wheeler DW, White CM, Rees CL, Komendantov AO, Hamilton DJ, Ascoli GA. Hippocampome.org: A knowledge base of neuron types in the rodent hippocampus. eLife. 2015;**4**:e09960. DOI: 10.7554/eLife.09960

[140] Morrison DJ, Rashid AJ, Yiu AP, Yan C, Frankland PW, Josselyn SA. Parvalbumin interneurons constrain the size of the lateral amygdala engram. Neurobiology of Learning and Memory. 2016;**135**:91-99. DOI: 10.1016/j.nlm.2016.07.007

[141] Ko SY, Frankland PW. Neurogenesis-dependent transformation of hippocampal engrams. Neuroscience Letters. 2021;**762**:136176. DOI: 10.1016/j.neulet.2021.136176

[142] Kodituwakku PW. Defining the behavioral phenotype in children with fetal alcohol spectrum disorders: A review. Neuroscience and Biobehavioral Reviews. 2007;**31**(2):192-201. DOI: 10.1016/j.neubiorev.2006.06.020

[143] DiPietro JA, Voegtline KM. The gestational foundation of sex differences in development and vulnerability. Neuroscience. 2017;**342**:4-20. DOI: 10.1016/j.neuroscience.2015.07.068

[144] Flannigan K, Poole N, Cook J, Unsworth K. Sex-related differences among individuals assessed for fetal alcohol spectrum disorder in Canada. Alcohol, Clinical & Experimental Research (Hoboken). 2023;**47**(3):613-623. DOI: 10.1111/acer.15017

[145] Doyle LR, Glass L, Wozniak JR, Kable JA, Riley EP, Coles CD, et al. Relation between oppositional/conduct behaviors and executive function among youth with histories of heavy prenatal alcohol exposure. Alcoholism, Clinical and Experimental Research. 2019;**43**(6):1135-1144. DOI: 10.1111/acer.14036

[146] Alsameen MH, Candelaria-Cook FT, Cerros CM, Hill DE, Stephen JM. Altered neuronal network connectivity

in children with fetal alcohol spectrum disorder and its association with inhibitory function. Alcohol, Clinical & Experimental Research (Hoboken). 2025;**49**(10):2133-2145. DOI: 10.1111/acer.70144

[147] Gursky ZH, Savage LM, Klintsova AY. Executive functioning-specific behavioral impairments in a rat model of human third trimester binge drinking implicate prefrontal-thalamo-hippocampal circuitry in fetal alcohol spectrum disorders. Behavioural Brain Research. 2021;**405**:113208. DOI: 10.1016/j.bbr.2021.113208

[148] Gursky ZH, Klintsova AY. Changes in representation of thalamic projection neurons within prefrontal-thalamic-hippocampal circuitry in a rat model of third trimester binge drinking. Brain Sciences. 2021;**11**(3):323. DOI: 10.3390/brainsci11030323

[149] Bahner F, Demanuele C, Schweiger J, Gerchen MF, Zamoscik V, Ueltzhoffer K, et al. Hippocampal-dorsolateral prefrontal coupling as a species-conserved cognitive mechanism: A human translational imaging study. Neuropsychopharmacology. 2015;**40**(7):1674-1681. DOI: 10.1038/npp.2015.13

[150] Numan R. A prefrontal-hippocampal comparator for goal-directed behavior: The intentional self and episodic memory. Frontiers in Behavioral Neuroscience. 2015;**9**:323. DOI: 10.3389/fnbeh.2015.00323

[151] Zhu Y, Gao H, Tong L, Li Z, Wang L, Zhang C, et al. Emotion regulation of hippocampus using real-time fMRI neurofeedback in healthy human. Frontiers in Human Neuroscience. 2019;**13**:242. DOI: 10.3389/fnhum.2019.00242

[152] Jin J, Maren S. Prefrontal-hippocampal interactions in memory and emotion. Frontiers in Systems Neuroscience. 2015;**9**:170. DOI: 10.3389/fnsys.2015.00170

Chapter 9

Anterior Temporal Lobectomy for Surgical Management of Temporal Lobe Epilepsy

Serdar Ercan

Abstract

Anterior temporal lobectomy (ATL) is a surgical procedure used in the treatment of medically refractory temporal lobe epilepsy (TLE). It is a method used to improve the quality of life of patients who do not respond to medical treatments at the desired level. The temporal lobe, especially the mesial structures, is a region where epileptogenic foci are common. Therefore, ATL plays a critical role in the surgical management of epilepsy. ATL is also applied in cases other than epilepsy, such as temporal lobe tumors, vascular malformations, and other pathologies where resection of the anterior temporal lobe is deemed necessary. Before deciding on ATL, a comprehensive evaluation, including detailed clinical assessment, neuroimaging, and electrophysiological studies, is required to ensure precise localization of the epileptogenic zone and minimize postoperative deficits. Surgical technique in ATL usually involves resection of the anterior part of the temporal lobe, which includes the amygdala and hippocampus. Dissection must be performed very carefully to preserve critical neurovascular structures, and intraoperative neuromonitoring must be used to minimize complications during resection. The success of ATL depends on the surgeon's knowledge of the complex temporal lobe anatomy and surgical experience. Despite the clinical success of ATL, its potential complications require extensive preoperative evaluation and postoperative management. Common complications include neurocognitive deficits, visual field defects, and psychiatric symptoms. This chapter aims to provide a comprehensive overview of the indications, surgical technique, and potential complications of ATL.

Keywords: anterior temporal lobectomy, temporal lobe epilepsy, surgical technique, anatomy, complication

1. Introduction

Anterior temporal lobectomy (ATL) is a major surgical intervention used primarily in the treatment of medically refractory temporal lobe epilepsy (TLE). This procedure usually involves resection of the anterior portion of the temporal lobe, including critical structures such as the hippocampus and amygdala that are involved in the pathophysiology of epilepsy. The historical development of ATL dates back to the twentieth century. With the contribution of significant advances in surgical techniques and neuroimaging, it has been accepted as one of the main treatment methods for TLE. The temporal lobe plays a crucial role in various cognitive and emotional processes. Minimizing surgical risks and optimizing patient outcomes requires a comprehensive understanding of the complex anatomical structures of this region and their interconnections. The advent of advanced imaging modalities such as magnetic resonance imaging (MRI) and positron emission tomography (PET) has increased the sensitivity and safety of ATL by improving preoperative planning and intraoperative navigation.

Despite its effectiveness, ATL also has potential complications, including cognitive impairments and neuropsychiatric sequelae. Therefore, careful patient selection and comprehensive preoperative evaluation are crucial in achieving positive results.

2. Indications for anterior temporal lobectomy

Anterior temporal lobectomy is a procedure that may be performed for the following medical conditions [1–4].

Refractory Temporal Lobe Epilepsy: Temporal lobe epilepsy is the most common form of focal epilepsy, characterized by seizures originating in the temporal lobe. These seizures often involve mesial temporal structures, including the hippocampus, amygdala, and parahippocampal gyrus. Patients with TLE typically experience complex partial seizures that may secondarily generalize. Despite optimal treatment with antiepileptic drugs, approximately 30–40% of patients continue to have seizures. These patients who do not respond to drug treatment are classified as having refractory epilepsy. ATL offers a potential treatment by eliminating the epileptogenic zone.

Mesial temporal sclerosis: Mesial temporal sclerosis (MTS), also known as hippocampal sclerosis, is a common pathological finding in TLE patients. MTS is characterized by neuronal loss and gliosis in the hippocampus, leading to a hyperexcitable state that predisposes to seizures. Patients with MTS often have a history of febrile seizures in childhood. When these patients reach adulthood, they present with epilepsy that is difficult to treat. MTS can typically be detected through high-resolution MRI, which shows hippocampal atrophy and increased signal intensity on T2-weighted images. ATL is very effective in patients with MTS, as resection of the sclerotic hippocampus significantly reduces seizures.

Temporal lobe tumors: Some benign and low-grade malignant tumors in the temporal lobe can cause refractory epilepsy. These include gangliogliomas, dysembryoplastic neuroepithelial tumors (DNETs), and low-grade astrocytomas. These tumors often disrupt the normal architecture of the temporal lobe, creating a focal point for seizure activity. Surgical resection of the tumor, together with the surrounding epileptogenic cortex, can provide seizure control and prevent tumor progression. ATL may be indicated when the tumor is located in the anterior temporal lobe and is associated with persistent seizures. Preoperative imaging, including MRI and PET, is essential to define tumor margins and plan the surgical approach.

Cortical dysplasia: Focal cortical dysplasia (FCD) is a congenital malformation of cortical development that can cause refractory epilepsy. In FCD, there is abnormal neuronal organization that leads to overstimulation. Patients with FCD often present with early-onset epilepsy that is resistant to antiepileptic drugs. Diagnosis of FCD is typically made with MRI, which can show cortical thickening, gray-white matter junction blurring, and other structural abnormalities. If the dysplastic lesion is localized in the anterior temporal lobe and there are very frequent seizures, ATL can be applied. Intraoperative electrocorticography (ECoG) can be used to identify and resect the epileptogenic cortex.

Encephalitis: Chronic encephalitis, such as Rasmussen encephalitis, can lead to progressive neurological deterioration and refractory epilepsy. Rasmussen encephalitis is a rare, chronic inflammatory disease that typically affects one hemisphere of the brain, leading to unilateral cortical atrophy and incurable seizures. Patients with Rasmussen encephalitis often present with hemiparesis, cognitive decline, and focal seizures. In cases where the anterior temporal lobe is predominantly affected, ATL controls seizures and improves the patient's quality of life. The diagnosis must be supported by the clinical picture, MRI findings of progressive cortical atrophy, and sometimes brain biopsy.

Vascular malformations: Arteriovenous malformations (AVMs) and cavernous angiomas in the temporal lobe may be among the causes of refractory epilepsy. These vascular malformations can lead to recurrent seizures due to abnormal blood flow and resulting gliosis. AVMs are formed by the fusion of abnormal blood vessels, while cavernous angiomas are clusters of enlarged capillaries. Both conditions can be visualized with MRI and angiography. Surgical removal of the malformation along with the epileptogenic cortex may provide seizure control. ATL may be indicated if the vascular malformation is located in the anterior temporal lobe and is associated with persistent seizures. In preoperative planning, detailed imaging should be performed to evaluate vascular anatomy and possible surgical risks.

Traumatic brain injury: Post-traumatic epilepsy (PTE) can develop as a result of traumatic brain injury, especially in cases where the temporal lobe is affected. Patients with PTE may experience recurrent seizures that are refractory to medical treatment. The temporal lobe is particularly susceptible to injury due to its location and the presence of bony structures in the skull. In cases where the primary focus of seizure activity is the anterior temporal lobe, anterior temporal lobectomy may be considered to achieve seizure control and improve the patient's quality of life. A history of head trauma, seizure semiology, and imaging findings of post-traumatic changes such as gliosis, encephalomalacia, or hemosiderin deposits should suggest PTE.

3. Patient selection

The following criteria should be taken as a basis for selecting patients who are likely to benefit from ATL [1, 3, 4].

Diagnosis of temporal lobe epilepsy: The patient must have a confirmed diagnosis of TLE, which is characterized by seizures originating from the temporal lobe. To make this diagnosis, clinical history, seizure semiology, and electroencephalography (EEG) findings must be used.

Medically refractory seizures: The patient must have seizures refractory to medical treatment, defined as failure to control seizures with at least two appropriate antiepileptic drugs at therapeutic doses. This criterion ensures that surgery is only considered for patients who have exhausted medical treatment options.

Localization of seizure focus: There should be clear evidence from video-EEG monitoring and neuroimaging (MRI, PET, Single Photon Emission Computed Tomography (SPECT)) showing a unilateral, well-defined epileptogenic zone within the temporal lobe. Correct localization is crucial for the success of ATL, as it allows targeted resection of the seizure focus.

Neuropsychological evaluation: A comprehensive neuropsychological assessment is necessary to determine baseline cognitive function and predict potential postoperative cognitive outcomes. This evaluation includes tests of memory, language, executive functions, and other cognitive domains. The results help identify patients who may be at risk of severe cognitive decline following surgery.

Psychiatric evaluation: A comprehensive psychiatric evaluation is necessary to identify any psychiatric comorbidities that may affect surgical outcomes or postoperative compliance. Conditions such as depression, anxiety, and psychosis should be carefully evaluated and managed before and after surgery.

A comprehensive evaluation and preliminary preparation should be made in determining suitable candidates for ATL.

- *Video-EEG monitoring*: Continuous EEG and video recording to capture and analyze seizure activity helps in precise localization of the epileptogenic zone. Video-EEG monitoring is usually done in an epilepsy monitoring unit and may require inpatient observation for several days.

- *Magnetic Resonance Imaging (MRI)*: High-resolution MRI is used to identify structural abnormalities such as hippocampal sclerosis, tumors, cortical dysplasia, and other lesions. Advanced MRI techniques such as volumetric analysis and diffusion tensor imaging can provide additional information about the integrity of white matter tracts and the extent of structural damage.

- *Positron Emission Tomography (PET)*: PET imaging is used to detect areas of hypometabolism associated with the seizure focus. Fluorodeoxyglucose (FDG)-PET is the most widely used method that provides functional information about glucose metabolism in the brain.

- *Single Photon Emission Computed Tomography (SPECT)*: Ictal and interictal SPECT imaging is used to localize areas of altered cerebral blood flow associated with seizure activity. Ictal SPECT performed during a seizure can provide valuable information about the seizure onset site.

- *Neuropsychological tests*: Comprehensive evaluation of cognitive functions, including memory, language, and executive functions, will be helpful to establish a baseline and predict postoperative changes. Specific tests may include the Wechsler Adult Intelligence Scale (WAIS), the California Verbal Learning Test (CVLT), and the Boston Naming Test (BNT).

- *Wada test (intracarotid amobarbital procedure)*: The Wada test is used to evaluate language and memory functions in each hemisphere to assess the risk of deficits after surgery. During the test, amobarbital is injected into the internal carotid artery to temporarily numb one hemisphere, allowing the function of the opposite hemisphere to be assessed.

Specific patient populations and clinical scenarios require additional considerations. Pediatric patients with TLE may benefit from early surgical intervention to prevent developmental delays and cognitive decline. During the evaluation process for children, age-appropriate neuropsychological tests and the effect of surgery on brain development should be taken into consideration [5–7]. Age alone should not be a contraindication to ATL. However, comorbidities and general health status need to be carefully evaluated. Elderly patients may be at higher risk of postoperative complications and cognitive decline, requiring a comprehensive risk-benefit analysis [1, 8].

Selection of ATL candidates should involve a multidisciplinary team consisting of epileptologists, neurosurgeons, neuropsychologists, neuroradiologists, and psychiatrists. This collaborative approach provides a comprehensive assessment of each patient's suitability for surgery and helps optimize surgical outcomes.

4. Anatomy and physiology of the anterior temporal lobectomy

4.1 Related brain structures

The anterior temporal lobe is a complex region located in the anterior part of the temporal lobe. It contains several subregions, each of which contributes uniquely to its overall function. Key structures within the ATL include:

Temporal pole: This is the most anterior part of the temporal lobe. It is involved in higher-level semantic processing and social cognition. The temporal pole integrates sensory inputs to form complex representations of objects and concepts and plays an important role in understanding and producing language as well as social interactions.

Perirhinal cortex: The perirhinal cortex, located medial to the ATL, is necessary for object recognition and memory. It combines sensory information from a variety of modalities to create detailed representations of objects, enabling objects to be identified and distinguished even under changing conditions.

Entorhinal cortex: Located adjacent to the perirhinal cortex, the entorhinal cortex serves as an important input and output center for the hippocampus. It is critical for memory formation and spatial navigation by acting as a gateway for information entering and exiting the hippocampus. This region also plays a role in processing temporal sequences and encoding episodic memories.

Amygdala: Although primarily associated with the medial temporal lobe, anterior portions of the amygdala extend into the ATL. The amygdala is crucial for emotional processing, especially in the formation and retrieval of emotional memories. It also plays a role in regulating social behavior and responses to emotional stimuli.

Hippocampus: Although primarily a medial temporal structure, anterior portions of the hippocampus are involved in episodic memory and spatial navigation. The hippocampus works closely with the entorhinal cortex to encode, store, and retrieve memories and navigate in space.

4.2 Functional effects of these structures

The ATL is an integral part of various cognitive and emotional processes, and each subregion contributes to different functional areas:

Semantic memory: ATL, especially the temporal polarity, is essential for the storage and retrieval of semantic information, which includes facts, concepts, and the meanings of words. Damage to this area, as seen in semantic dementia, causes profound deficits in the understanding and use of language and concepts. Patients with semantic dementia exhibit a striking impairment in semantic knowledge while preserving other cognitive abilities.

Object recognition: The perirhinal cortex is vital for recognizing and distinguishing objects. It combines sensory information to form complex representations, allowing objects to be identified even if they are partially hidden or viewed from different angles. This region is crucial for visual perception and memory, and dysfunction can lead to difficulties in recognizing familiar objects.

Memory and navigation: The entorhinal cortex and hippocampus work together to support episodic memory and spatial navigation. The entorhinal cortex acts as a gateway for information entering and exiting the hippocampus, facilitating the encoding and retrieval of memories. It also plays a role in processing temporal sequences and spatial contexts necessary for navigating environments.

Emotional processing: The anterior parts of the amygdala within the ATL are crucial for processing emotions, especially fear and pleasure. This region helps form emotional memories and influences social behavior by modulating responses to emotional stimuli. The amygdala's role in emotional processing is critical for survival, as it helps individuals respond appropriately to threats and rewards.

Social cognition: Temporal polarity is also associated with social cognition, including the ability to understand and predict the behavior and intentions of others. This function is critical for effective social interactions and empathy. Temporal polarity allows individuals to successfully navigate social environments by combining sensory and emotional information to create complex representations of social situations [9–11].

5. Surgical technique

5.1 Preoperative planning and imaging

Preoperative planning for ATL resection is a meticulous process aimed at optimizing surgical outcomes and minimizing risks. A comprehensive evaluation of the patient's medical history, neurological status, and cognitive function is important. This includes a detailed review of previous imaging studies, neurological examinations, and neuropsychological evaluations to establish a baseline and identify potential risks. Collaboration between neurosurgeons, neurologists, radiologists, and neuropsychologists is very important. The team discusses the patient's condition, reviews imaging findings, and creates a surgical plan appropriate to the individual's anatomy and pathology. The surgical approach is carefully planned, taking into account the location of the lesion, its extent, and its proximity to critical brain structures. The goal is to maximize lesion resection while preserving basic functions such as language, memory, and motor skills. Informing the patient and family about the surgical procedure, possible risks, benefits, and expected results is a vital part of preoperative planning. This helps set realistic expectations and obtain informed consent.

Advanced imaging techniques are integral to the preoperative planning of ATL resection. These methods provide detailed anatomical and functional information that guides the surgical approach. MRI is the cornerstone of preoperative imaging for ATL resection. High-resolution structural MRI provides detailed imaging of the brain anatomy, allowing precise localization of the lesion. Functional MRI (fMRI) can be used to map critical functional areas such as language and motor areas, helping to avoid these areas during surgery. *Diffusion Tensor Imaging* It is a special form of MRI that maps white matter pathways in the brain. This technique is particularly useful for identifying and preserving important nerve pathways during ATL resection. DTI helps plan the surgical course to prevent disruption of critical connections. PET imaging provides metabolic information about the brain by identifying areas of abnormal metabolic activity. In epilepsy surgery cases, PET can help localize epileptogenic regions that may not be visible on structural MRI. This information is crucial for planning the extent of resection. *Electroencephalography (EEG) and Magnetoencephalography (MEG)* techniques are used to locate epileptic foci and map brain activity. While EEG provides temporal resolution of brain activity, MEG offers both temporal and spatial resolution. These methods are often used in conjunction with MRI to provide a comprehensive view of the brain's function and pathology. Intraoperative MRI or ultrasound can be used to provide real-time imaging during surgery, ensure accurate resection of the lesion, and minimize damage to surrounding tissues. These techniques help confirm the extent of resection and make any necessary adjustments during the procedure.

5.2 Surgical procedure

Performing ATL resection is a complex and delicate procedure that requires careful planning and precise execution. Below is a detailed description of each step, highlighting important information and key points to achieve a successful outcome [12].

- *Presurgery preparation*:

  Patient positioning: The patient is placed supine on the operating table with the head secured in a Mayfield head holder. The head is turned slightly to the contralateral side to provide the best exposure of the temporal region. Correct positioning is crucial to avoid pressure points and provide stable access to the surgical site. General anesthesia is applied to ensure that the patient is completely anesthetized and stable (**Figure 1**).

- *Incision and exposure*:

  Skin incision: A curvilinear incision is made starting just in front of the tragus, extending upwards and backward over the ear, and then curving downwards toward the mastoid process. This incision provides adequate visibility while minimizing cosmetic impact (**Figure 2**).

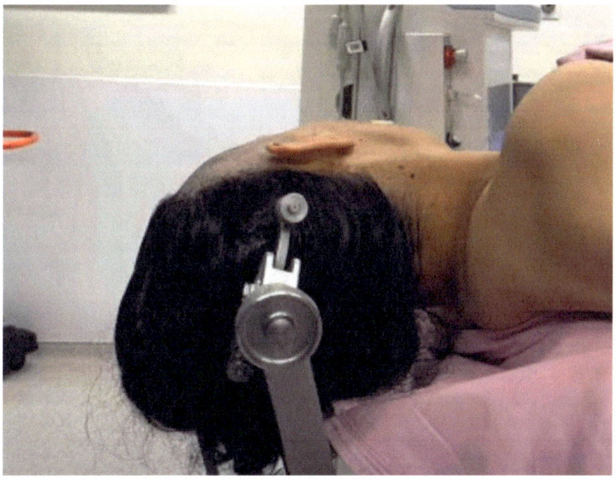

Figure 1.
The patient is placed in supine, secured in Mayfield had holder.

Soft tissue dissection: The temporalis muscle is carefully dissected and tilted forward to expose the temporal bone. Hemostasis is achieved using bipolar cautery to minimize bleeding. Craniotomy: Temporal craniotomy is performed using a high-speed drill to create burr holes, which are then ligated to remove the bony flap. The craniotomy should extend from the sphenoid process to the parietal bone, providing adequate exposure of the temporal lobe. Ensuring that the bone flap is large enough is crucial for adequate access and maneuverability.

- *Dural opening*:

Dural incision: A diagonal or curvilinear incision is made in the dura mater, which is then reflected to reveal the underlying brain tissue. It is important to handle the dura carefully to prevent tears and ensure a watertight seal afterward (**Figure 3**).

Hemostasis: Meticulous hemostasis is achieved by using bipolar cautery and hemostatic agents. This step is critical to maintaining a clear surgical field and preventing postoperative complications.

- *Cortical resection*:

Defining bookmarks: Important anatomical locations are identified, including the Sylvian fissure, superior temporal gyrus, and middle temporal gyrus. Correct identification of these landmarks is crucial to guiding the resection.

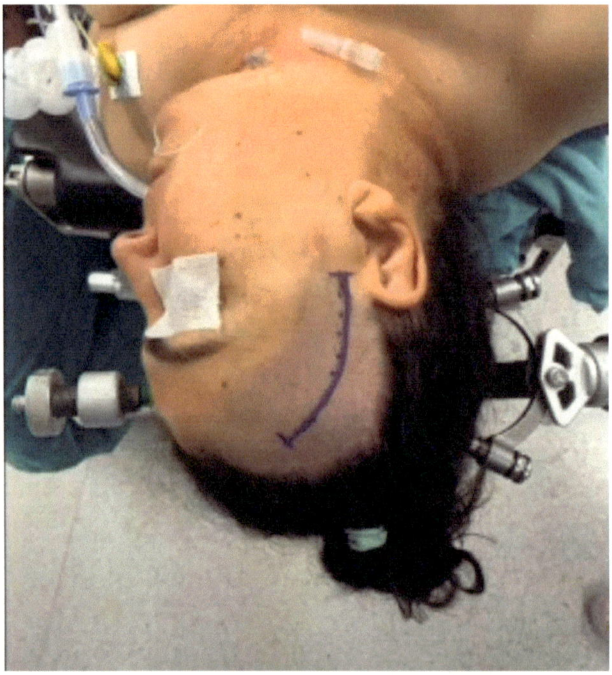

Figure 2.
A curvilinear incision, starting in front of the tragus, expanding upwords over the ear.

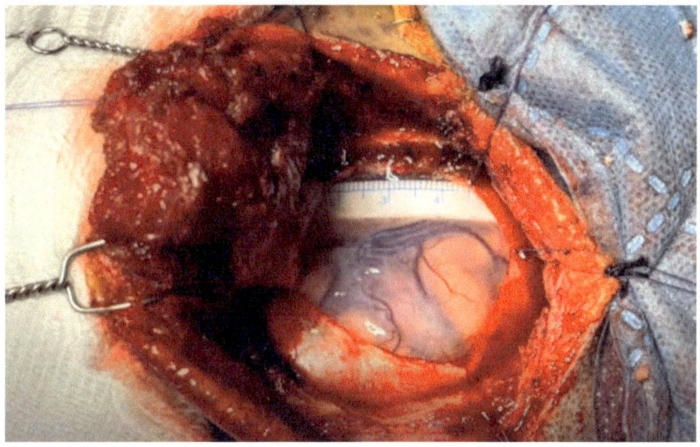

Figure 3.
A diagonal incission is made in dura matter, and important anatomical locations are identified, including Sylvian fissure, superior temporal gyrus and middle temporal gyros.

Cortical incision: A cortical incision is made parallel to the Sylvian fissure, extending from the temporal pole to the posterior edge of the resection area. The extent of resection typically varies from 4 to 6 cm from the temporal pole in the dominant hemisphere to 6–8 cm in the non-dominant hemisphere. Precise measurement and marking of resection margins is important to prevent damage to critical areas (**Figure 4**).

Subpial dissection: Subpial dissection is performed to remove the anterior temporal lobe. Suction and bipolar cautery are used to carefully dissect brain tissue while preserving the pia mater. This technique helps minimize bleeding and protects underlying structures. Gentle handling of brain tissue is crucial to avoid unnecessary trauma (**Figure 5**).

- *Resection of mesial structures*:

Hippocampus and amygdala: The anterior hippocampus and amygdala are identified and resected. This step is especially important for patients with

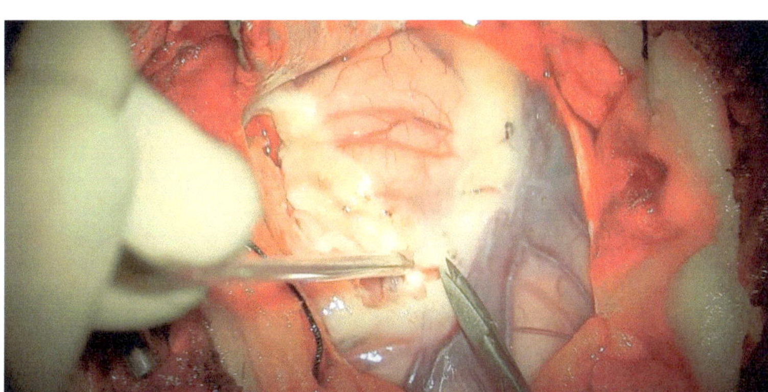

Figure 4.
A cortical incission is made parallel to sylvian fissure.

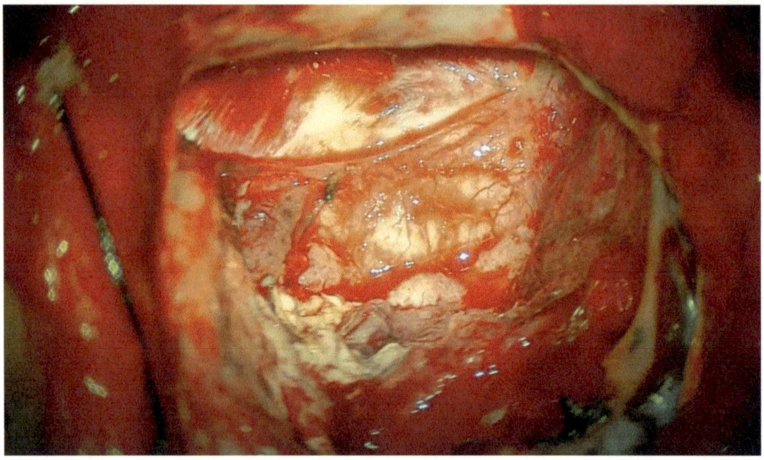

Figure 5.
Subpial dissection is performed to remove the anterior temporal lobe.

epilepsy, as these structures are often involved in seizure generation. A combination of suction, bipolar cautery, and microscissors is used to achieve a complete resection. Ensuring complete removal of the epileptogenic zone while preserving surrounding healthy tissue is a delicate balance.

Verification: Intraoperative navigation and imaging are used to confirm the extent of resection. This step ensures that the resection margins are clear of pathological tissue and helps prevent unnecessary removal of healthy brain tissue.

- *Hemostasis and closure*:

Hemostasis: Meticulous hemostasis is achieved by using bipolar cautery and hemostatic agents. It is important to examine the resection space for any residual bleeding to prevent postoperative hematoma formation.

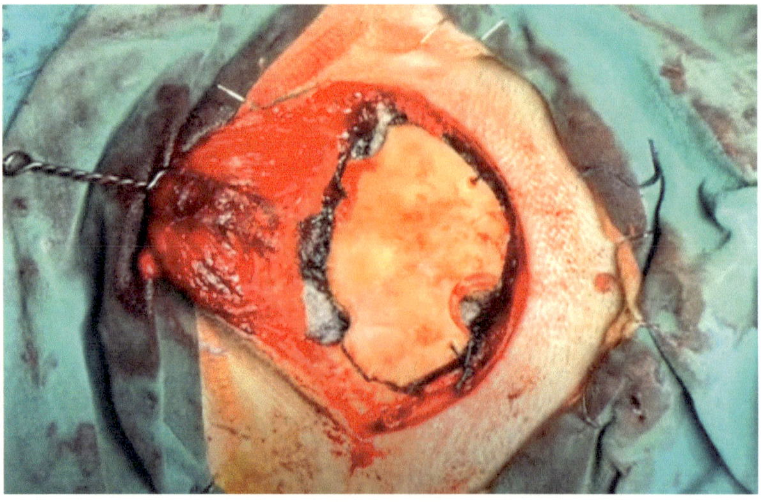

Figure 6.
The bone flap is replaced and fixed with plates after watertight dural closure.

Dural closure: The dura mater is sealed watertight using stitches or a dural substitute. It is crucial to provide a watertight seal to prevent cerebrospinal fluid leakage.

Bone flap replacement: The bone flap is replaced and fixed with plates and screws. Ensuring that the bone flap is stable and properly aligned is important for cosmetic and functional results (**Figure 6**).

Soft tissue and skin closure: Temporal muscle and soft tissues are brought closer together, and the skin incision is closed with stitches or staples. Proper closure techniques help minimize scarring and speed healing.

6. Consequences and complications

6.1 Success rates of anterior temporal lobe resection

Anterior temporal lobe resection is a highly effective surgical intervention, especially in patients with temporal lobe epilepsy refractory to medical treatment. The success rates of this procedure are well documented and show significant improvements in seizure control and overall patient outcomes. Approximately 60–70% of patients achieve complete seizure freedom following ATL resection (Engel Class I outcome). This high success rate highlights the effectiveness of the procedure in eliminating seizures for the majority of patients. An additional 20–30% of patients experience a significant reduction in seizure frequency. These patients may not be completely seizure-free, but they may still benefit from a significant reduction in seizure episodes, leading to improved daily functioning and quality of life. Long-term follow-up studies reveal that the benefits of ATL surgery persist over time. Many patients remain seizure-free or have reduced seizure frequency for years after surgery. For example, some studies report that up to 50% of patients remain seizure-free at 10 years after surgery. This long-term effectiveness highlights the durability of surgical outcomes.

6.2 Possible complications and management in anterior temporal lobe resection

Although anterior temporal lobe resection is highly effective in treating refractory temporal lobe epilepsy, it carries potential risks and complications. Understanding these complications and their management is crucial to optimizing patient outcomes and minimizing adverse effects.

Psychiatric disorders: Postoperative psychiatric disorders such as depression, anxiety, and psychosis are relatively common. These may occur due to the stress of surgery, changes in brain function, or pre-existing psychiatric conditions. The incidence of psychiatric complications is estimated to be around 7%. Preoperative psychiatric evaluation is important to identify patients at risk. Ongoing psychological support, both preoperatively and postoperatively, can help alleviate these problems. Postoperative psychiatric symptoms should be managed with appropriate medications and psychotherapy, such as antidepressants or antipsychotics. Close collaboration with a psychiatrist is often necessary to tailor treatment plans to individual patient needs [8, 13, 14].

Visual field defects: Visual field defects, especially superior quadrantanopia (loss of vision in the upper quadrant), may occur due to damage to the optic radiations during surgery. This complication occurs in approximately 6% of patients. Preoperative imaging, such as MRI, can help map optical radiations and guide the surgical approach to minimize risk. Postoperative visual field testing is recommended to assess the extent of any defects. Rehabilitation strategies such as visual field training and compensation techniques can help patients adapt to these changes. Regular follow-up with an ophthalmologist is also helpful [15].

Cognitive disorders: Cognitive impairments, especially in memory and language, may occur following ATL resection. These are more common in left-sided (dominant hemisphere) resections. Cognitive complications have been reported in approximately 5% of cases. Preoperative neuropsychological assessment helps identify patients at risk and establish a baseline for postoperative comparison. Cognitive rehabilitation after surgery, including memory training and speech therapy, may aid recovery. Continuous monitoring and support from neuropsychologists is useful in resolving emerging cognitive problems [8, 14, 16].

Hemiparesis and language disorders: Hemiparesis (weakness on one side of the body) and language disorders can result from accidental damage to motor or language areas. These complications are relatively rare, occurring in approximately 3% of patients. Intraoperative monitoring of motor and language functions using techniques such as electrocorticography (ECoG) and direct cortical stimulation may help prevent these complications. If deficits occur, postoperative physical therapy and speech therapy are crucial for rehabilitation. Early intervention and personalized rehabilitation programs can significantly improve outcomes.

Infections: Surgical site infections, meningitis, and bone flap osteomyelitis are potential complications. The infection rate is around 3%. Strict aseptic techniques and prophylactic antibiotics during surgery can reduce the risk of infection. If infections occur, early diagnosis and treatment with appropriate antibiotics are important. In cases of severe infection, surgical debridement may be necessary. Regular monitoring of the surgical site and education of the patient about signs of infection are also important [8, 14, 17].

Hemorrhage: Intraoperative or postoperative bleeding may occur and lead to hematoma formation. Bleeding is a serious but relatively rare complication, with an incidence of approximately 2%. Careful hemostasis during surgery is very important to prevent bleeding. It is important to monitor postoperatively for signs of bleeding, such as changes in neurological status or increased intracranial pressure. If bleeding occurs, immediate intervention, such as surgical evacuation of hematomas, is necessary. Blood transfusions and supportive care may also be necessary.

Cerebrospinal Fluid (CSF) leak: CSF leakage may occur from dural tears during surgery. This complication occurs in approximately 2% of patients. Ensuring that the dural closure is watertight during surgery is crucial to prevent CSF leaks. If a CSF leak occurs after surgery, conservative measures such as bed rest and head elevation may be sufficient. Persistent leaks may require surgical repair. Monitoring for signs of CSF leak, such as clear fluid drainage from the wound, is important for early diagnosis and management.

Cranial nerve deficiencies: Damage to cranial nerves, especially the optic and oculomotor nerves, may occur, resulting in visual and ocular motor disorders. The incidence of cranial nerve deficits is around 3%. Careful surgical techniques and intraoperative monitoring can help prevent these injuries. Postoperative management includes ophthalmological evaluation and corrective surgery or rehabilitation if necessary. Early diagnosis and intervention are crucial to minimizing long-term deficits.

Extra-axial fluid collections: Subdural or epidural fluid collections may develop after surgery. These collections occur in approximately 2% of patients. Liquid Monitoring with serial imaging such as CT or MRI is important to detect collections. Most fluid collections resolve spontaneously, but persistent or symptomatic collections may require surgical drainage. Close observation and timely intervention can prevent complications due to fluid accumulation.

Medical complications: General medical complications such as deep vein thrombosis (DVT), pulmonary embolism, and cardiac events may occur. The incidence of these complications is around 2%. Prophylactic measures, including anticoagulation therapy and early mobilization, are important to prevent DVT and pulmonary embolism. Prompt recognition and treatment of medical complications are crucial to the patient's recovery. Regular monitoring of vital signs and education of the patient regarding the signs and symptoms of medical complications are also important.

7. Conclusion

Anterior temporal lobe resection is a highly effective surgical intervention for patients with temporal lobe epilepsy refractory to medical treatment. The procedure offers significant benefits, including high rates of seizure freedom and significant improvements in quality of life. Success rates are supported by meticulous preoperative planning, advanced imaging techniques, and precise surgical execution.

While the procedure is generally safe, it is not without risks. Potential complications such as psychiatric disorders, visual field defects, cognitive impairments, and infections require careful treatment. Comprehensive preoperative evaluations, intraoperative monitoring, and careful postoperative care are necessary to minimize these risks and ensure optimal patient outcomes.

It is crucial for neurosurgery residents and healthcare professionals to understand the detailed steps of ATL resection, from patient positioning to postoperative care. Mastering this procedure can significantly improve the quality of life of patients suffering from refractory epilepsy, offering them the chance for a seizure-free future and improving overall well-being.

In summary, ATL resection remains a cornerstone in the surgical treatment of temporal lobe epilepsy, with a strong track record and a well-defined approach to managing potential complications. Thanks to continued advances in surgical techniques and patient care, the outcomes of ATL resection will continue to improve, offering hope and relief to many patients.

Acknowledgements

The author acknowledges the use of QuillBot Grammar Checker for language polishing of the manuscript.

Author details

Serdar Ercan
Department of Neurosurgery, Eskisehir City Hospital, Health Science University, Eskisehir, Turkey

*Address all correspondence to: drercan@gmail.com

References

[1] Ellis TL, Roper SN. Anterior temporal lobectomy: Indications and technique. In: Handbook of Stereotactic and Functional Neurosurgery. CRC Press; 2003. pp. 544-553

[2] Kuang Y et al. Comparison of therapeutic effects between selective amygdalohippocampectomy and anterior temporal lobectomy for the treatment of temporal lobe epilepsy: A meta-analysis. British Journal of Neurosurgery. 2014;**28**(3):374-377

[3] Matsuura M. Indication for anterior temporal lobectomy in patients with temporal lobe epilepsy and psychopathology. Epilepsia. 2000;**41**:39-42

[4] McIntosh A, Wilson SJ, Berkovic SF. Seizure outcome after temporal lobectomy: Current research practice and findings. Epilepsia. 2001;**42**(10):1288-1307

[5] Lindsay J, Ounsted C, Richards P. Long-term outcome in children with temporal lobe seizures, v: Indications and contra-indications for neurosurgery. Developmental Medicine & Child Neurology. 1984;**26**(1):25-32

[6] Ormond DR et al. Pediatric temporal lobe epilepsy surgery in Bonn and review of the literature. Neurosurgery. 2019;**84**(4):844-856

[7] Sinclair DB et al. Pediatric temporal lobectomy for epilepsy. Pediatric Neurosurgery. 2003;**38**(4):195-205

[8] Brotis AG et al. Complications after anterior temporal lobectomy for medically intractable epilepsy: A systematic review and meta-analysis. Stereotactic and Functional Neurosurgery. 2019;**97**(2):69-82

[9] Kiernan J. Anatomy of the temporal lobe. Epilepsy Research and Treatment. 2012;**2012**(1):176157

[10] Peuskens D et al. Anatomy of the anterior temporal lobe and the frontotemporal region demonstrated by fiber dissection. Neurosurgery. 2004;**55**(5):1174-1184

[11] Wen HT et al. Microsurgical anatomy of the temporal lobe: Part 1: Mesial temporal lobe anatomy and its vascular relationships as applied to amygdalohippocampectomy. Neurosurgery. 1999;**45**(3):549

[12] Schaller K, Cabrilo I. Anterior temporal lobectomy. Acta Neurochirurgica. 2016;**158**:161-166

[13] Blumer D et al. Psychiatric outcome of temporal lobectomy for epilepsy: Incidence and treatment of psychiatric complications. Epilepsia. 1998;**39**(5):478-486

[14] Popovic E et al. Temporal lobectomy for epilepsy—Complicationsin 200 patients. Journal of Clinical Neuroscience. 1995;**2**(3):238-244

[15] Cohen-Gadol AA et al. Prospective analysis of diplopia after anterior temporal lobectomy for mesial temporal lobe sclerosis. Journal of Neurosurgery. 2003;**99**(3):496-499

[16] Sasaki-Adams D, Hadar E. Temporal lobe epilepsy surgery: Surgical complications. In: Textbook of Epilepsy Surgery. CRC Press; 2008. pp. 1328-1339

[17] Georgiadis I, Kapsalaki EZ, Fountas KN. Temporal lobe resective surgery for medically intractable epilepsy: A review of complications and side effects. Epilepsy Research and Treatment. 2013;**2013**(1):752195

Chapter 10

Clinical Neurophysiology of Hippocampal Disorders: Oscillopathies in Cognitive, Affective, Behavioral, Movement, and Seizure Disorders

Nick Tsarouchas, Nicholas Tsarouchas and Constantin Tsarouchas

Abstract

The Hippocampus is a hub (local area network) integrated within smaller-to-larger scale limbocortical networks interacting through reciprocal excitatory and inhibitory connections. In biological systems built upon integrated recurrent positive and negative feedback loops, oscillations and oscillatory behaviors of neuronal assemblies emerge. Hippocampal and limbocortical oscillations encode network representations and memory regarding external and internal environment information, in the form of spatiotemporal mapping, motion and navigation, cognitive and affective processing, and motor and behavioral outputs. The limbocortical network (hippocampus, amygdala, hypothalamus, anterior thalamus, anterior cingulate cortex, medial prefrontal cortex, and orbitofrontal cortex) is a core network of long-range projections involved in multimodal sensory processing, spatiotemporal perception, short and long-term episodic memory, selective attention, working memory, reward expectation, cost/benefit assessment, decision making, motor planning and execution, emotional regulation, and social behaviors. Hippocampal and limbocortical disorders are thus crucially implicated in a range of disturbances of these large-scale oscillatory processes (oscillopathies) that underline the pathophysiology of cognitive, affective, behavioral, movement, and seizure disorders. In this study, we demonstrate the implications of hippocampal and limbocortical dysfunction in cognitive, emotional, and learning dysregulation, resulting in a wide spectrum of neurological, psychiatric, and behavioral disorders. We specifically focus on the clinical neurophysiology of dementia, schizophrenia, depression, anxiety, autistic spectrum disorders, attention-deficit hyperactivity disorder, post-traumatic stress disorder, functional neurological disorders, behavioral and movement disorders, seizures, and epilepsies, as manifestations of oscillatory imbalances (oscillopathies) in the function of hippocampal, limbocortical, and large-scale brain networks.

IntechOpen

Keywords: oscillopathies, dementia, cognitive impairment, depression, fear, anxiety, psychosis, schizophrenia, autistic spectrum disorders, attention-deficit hyperactivity disorders, functional neurological disorders, post-traumatic stress disorders, movement disorders, seizures, epilepsy, behavioral disorders, emotional dysregulation, hippocampus, limbic system, limbocortical network, default mode network, salience network, central executive network, memory, emotion, emotional regulation, learning, cognition, oscillations, neurophysiology, neurology

1. Introduction to hippocampal oscillations and oscillopathies

The hippocampus features a laminar and iterative architecture characterized by recurrent excitatory-inhibitory feedback loops [1]. This structural organization supports the interaction between hippocampal pyramidal cells and a highly sophisticated network of inhibitory interneurons, with distinct neurochemical, morphological, and functional properties. This interaction is critical in modulating the timing and synchronization of hippocampal neurons in the generation of theta oscillations [1]. The activity of excitatory principal cells, primarily pyramidal neurons, is regulated by a diverse array of GABAergic interneurons in the hippocampus. These include interneurons expressing Parvalbumin (PV), Somatostatin (SST), Cholecystokinin (CCK)/endocannabinoids, Vasoactive Intestinal Peptide (VIP), Neuropeptide-Y, Calretinin, Reelin, 5-HT3aR, NO, and others, which are crucial for various physiological processes like generation of oscillations, learning, and memory (**Figure 1**) [2].

Three main classes of hippocampal rhythms emerge in association with certain behavioral states [2, 3]: (1) theta (4–12 Hz) oscillations occurring during active awake

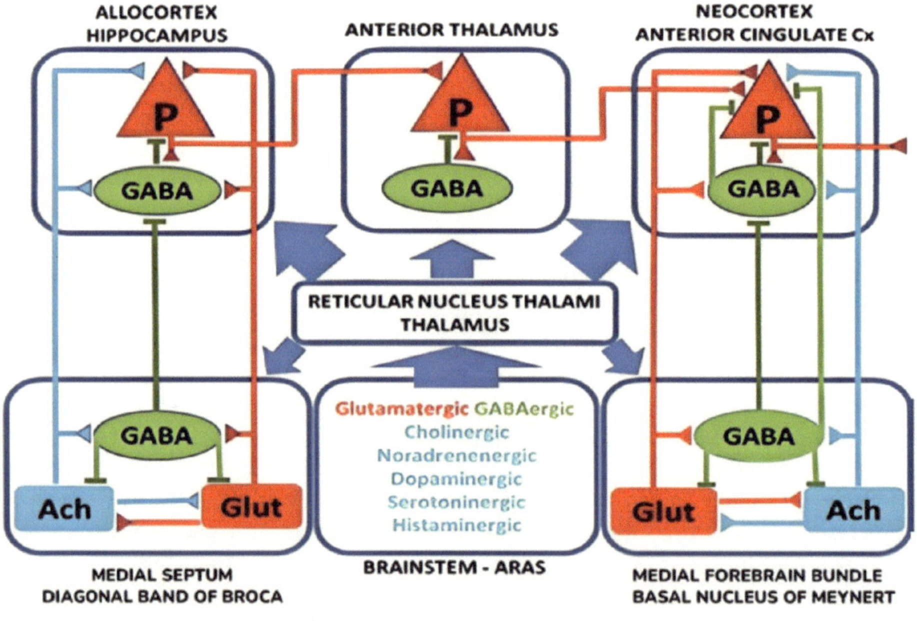

Figure 1.
The septal-hippocampal-thalamo-cortical axis. Overview of the complex interactive circuitry of excitatory, inhibitory, and modulatory components, underlying some of the structural and functional connectivity of the limbocortical networks with clinical implications for the pharmacological and neurosurgical/neurostimulation treatment strategies of epilepsy (modified from [1]).

behavior and REM sleep [4] (important for learning and memory [5]), (2) SPW-Rs with R-ripples (very fast oscillations or phase-modulations [FINO mechanism] [6]) between 150 and 300 Hz superimposed on slow irregularly occurring "sharp waves" (1–15 Hz) (during slow-wave sleep and periods of inactivity [7]) and high-frequency (20–150 Hz) gamma oscillations [PING mechanism] [6] that occur during many behaviors but are largest when theta rhythms are present [8] (theta-gamma phase coupling [9]). These three classes of rhythms play a unique role in coordinating interactions between the hippocampus (HPC) and multiple brain regions it communicates with (**Figure 1**), such as the septal nuclei (Medial Septum-Diagonal band of Broca: MS-DbB), the Anterior Nucleus of the Thalamus (ANT), the Anterior Cingulate Cortex (ACC), the medial Prefrontal Cortex (mPFC), the Amygdala (AMG), the Orbitofrontal Cortex (OFC), and the Hypothalamus (HPTH) [2, 10].

Hippocampal high-amplitude theta (4–12 Hz) oscillations of CA1 pyramidal cells are crucial in episodic memory formation through encoding of location, time, and context of events [11] during active exploration and voluntary movements or REM in sleep and arousal [5]. Sharp wave-ripple complexes emerge during slow-wave sleep and periods of inactivity [5]. Fast (8–12 Hz) theta oscillations (driven by atropine-resistant inputs on the distal dendrites) are associated with spatial navigation and movement, whereas slow (4–8 Hz) theta oscillations (driven by atropine-sensitive inputs on the somata, and chloride (Cl^-)-mediated inhibitory postsynaptic potentials) are associated with arousal and sensory stimulus salience [12, 13].

Although theta oscillations can be intrinsically generated from the interaction of excitatory and inhibitory hippocampal circuits [14], in vivo studies have shown that septal nuclei (MS-DbB) are important external drivers. They provide cholinergic, GABAergic, and glutamatergic inputs that induce and modulate hippocampal theta oscillations [15–17]. Septal nuclei send cholinergic (65%) and GABAergic fibers to CA1 and glutamatergic fibers to all parts of the hippocampus [18]. Elimination of the septal input seems to abolish theta oscillations in the septo-hippocampal axis (**Figure 1**) [19].

A modulatory cholinergic background input needs to interact with precisely timed excitatory (glutamatergic) and rhythmic inhibitory (GABAergic) inputs to generate theta oscillations [16, 20]. Septal cholinergic neurons target both hippocampal pyramidal and GABAergic interneurons, firing in a more irregular way, still phase-locked though to theta oscillations [21]. Rhythmic septal interneurons, which express parvalbumin and the hyperpolarization-activated cyclic nucleotide-gated (HCN) channels [18], act upon hippocampal inhibitory interneurons to exert a strong rhythmic disinhibition on pyramidal neurons [17, 18, 20, 22, 23]. Septal GABAergic neurons in burst-firing mode disinhibit hippocampal pyramidal neurons in a theta phase-locked manner (**Figure 1**) [20, 21, 24, 25].

Serotonergic projections from the Median Raphe Nucleus alter the firing pattern of septal neurons, resulting in desynchronization of theta oscillations in the hippocampus [26]. Serotonergic neurons in the median raphe nucleus (MRN) process reward and aversive information in opposite directions to dorsal raphe nucleus (DRN) serotonergic neurons (reward-seeking behavior). Extra-septal converging top-down (prefrontal cortex) and bottom-up (brainstem, ARAS, thalamus/basal ganglia) may play a crucial role in modulating hippocampal, limbic system, and large-scale vHPC-mPFC integrated oscillations. Robust wake-promoting actions of the locus coeruleus (LC)-noradrenergic system enhance arousal via action on β- and α1-receptors located within multiple subcortical structures, including the general regions of the medial septal area and the medial preoptic areas [27]. Activation of glutamate receptors or a decrease of GABAergic tone in the VTA leads to enhanced dopamine release and increased hippocampal theta power. High time-frequency cross-correlation was detected for the theta band between the VTA and hippocampus during active waking and REM sleep [28]. Thus, the RN, LC, and VTA are part of a broad brainstem-hippocampal network involved in the induction and regulation of HPC-PFC theta rhythm (where the MS-DbB acts as a central node for HPC drive, like the medial forebrain bundle/NBM acts as a central node for mPFC drive) (**Figure 1**). The pedunculopontine and laterodorsal tegmental (cholinergic) nuclei, the raphe (serotonergic) nuclei, the locus coeruleus (noradrenergic) nuclei, and the ventral tegmental (dopaminergic) area regulate theta rhythm synchronization between HPC-mPFC during awake (sensorimotor) and sleep (REM) activity (**Figure 1**) [24, 26–28].

Sharp wave-ripples (a single high-amplitude 1–15 Hz wave followed by fast 100–250 Hz oscillations in the pyramidal cell layer [29]) are caused by highly synchronous excitation of the hippocampus. They occur during awake immobility, consummatory behaviors, and slow-wave sleep, and are associated with memory consolidation and replays [29]. When the HPC neurons fire synchronously during SPW-Rs, the majority of the MS neurons are inhibited [30]. On the other hand, when MS-driven theta oscillations dominate in the septo-hippocampal axis, SPW-Rs do not occur [29]. There seems to exist a flip-flop mechanism influenced by the aforementioned brainstem structures. Optogenetic activation of the MS cholinergic neurons enhances theta oscillations and suppresses occurrence of SPW-Rs in the HPC suggesting that the MS-DbB cholinergic inputs to the HPC control the switch of these two mutually exclusive states [31]. The hippocampal-to-septal feedback projections via GABAergic neurons also contribute to the theta oscillations in the septo-hippocampal axis (**Figure 1**) [32].

In humans, faster theta oscillations (~8 Hz) seem to be more prevalent in the posterior hippocampus and slower theta oscillations (~3 Hz) seem to be more prevalent in the anterior hippocampus [33]. Theta-gamma phase/amplitude coupling was shown also in humans, thought to support memory and learning [34]. The hippocampus is involved via theta oscillations in learning and memory [35–38]. Hippocampal theta activity is involved in forming new episodic memories, especially in encoding of location and time or the context of events [11]. During these active states, gamma oscillations are prominent in the entorhinal-hippocampal network during a variety of memory tasks in different species and participate in memory formation [39–42].

We focus on their relationship of theta oscillations to locomotion, memory, and spatiotemporal navigation [12, 43, 44]. Theta oscillations may represent a timing mechanism where firing of hippocampal pyramidal neurons is phase-locked to the theta cycle when excitation by MS-DbB glutamatergic neurons coincides with maximal sustained excitation by cholinergic inputs, and minimal periodic perisomatic inhibition [45–49]. This timing mechanism (based on the sampling frequency of theta oscillations) may facilitate sensory processing and memory encoding into a time series of movement sequences and planned trajectories for spatiotemporal navigation [44].

2. Limbocortical network oscillations and oscillopathies

Highly integrated brain regions through reciprocal excitatory and inhibitory feedback loops, such as the medial prefrontal cortex (mPFC), anterior cingulate cortex (ACC), hippocampus (HPC), amygdala (AMG), and hypothalamus (HPTH) [collectively limbocortical network], play crucial roles in the regulation of affective and visceral functions and undergo marked changes in their activity caused by stress-induced mental disease [9, 50–52]. The extensive HPC-AMG-ACC-mPFC circuit is a core network formed by long-range projections in which the ventral HPC (vHPC) and the mPFC transfer sensory and contextual information to the basolateral amygdala (BLA) [53, 54] and the BLA, in turn, transfer information of negative valence back to the mPFC and vHPC [55–58]. The mPFC is involved in sensory processing, motor planning, emotional regulation, reward, attention, working memory, decision-making, long and short-term memory, and social behaviors [59].

The mPFC is important for working memory, as well as executive functions including decision-making, goal-oriented behaviors, and attentional selection of task-relevant information [60]. The mPFC receives direct projections from ventral CA1 and subiculum subfields of the hippocampus [61, 62], and these synapses are plastic [63]. The hippocampus is thought to activate mPFC during behaviors in which the functions of mPFC are involved. For example, the hippocampus may encode the memory of a circumstance associated with a particular goal-directed behavior. When a similar circumstance arises later, the hippocampus may retrieve its memory and communicate that to the prefrontal cortex, so that behavior can be adjusted from the prefrontal cortex to achieve the desired goal.

Recent studies support the hypothesis that rhythm synchronization processes facilitate functional interactions between the hippocampus and mPFC during behaviors requiring both regions. Coherent oscillations in the hippocampus and mPFC are believed to mediate memory operations in humans [64, 65] and other species [62, 66]. Increased theta-slow gamma coupling between the hippocampus and medial prefrontal cortex (mPFC) suggests that enhancement of theta-slow gamma coupling reflects a compensatory mechanism to maintain spatial working memory performance in the setting of increased difficulty. Epochs of high hippocampal theta-prefrontal slow gamma coupling are associated with increased synchronization of neurons within the mPFC [9]. Such diverse sets of functions are sustained by a dense pattern of reciprocal connectivity with other cortices, thalamus, subcortical, and brainstem regions. A recent study in mice found that the mPFC can be differentiated from other cortices based on more complex ganglio/thalamocortical and limbocortical connectivity patterns. The mPFC has the highest proportion of feedback projections (**Figure 1**) [67].

The hippocampus is thus integrated via small-to-large-scale limbocortical networks with the prefrontal cortex through reciprocal excitatory and inhibitory connections (positive and negative feedback loops). Septo-hippocampal axis theta oscillations (4–12 Hz) act as a carrier wave frequency (part of a pacemaker system stemming from the brainstem/ARAS all the way to the thalamus) of large-scale synchronization processes across extensive limbocortical and ganglio/thalamocortical networks. The modulations induced through theta/gamma coupling encode the fine contextual information of place, time, people, events, through episodic memories and representations, complex cognitive/emotional processes, and resultant motor/behavioral outputs. Inevitably, hippocampal disorders are crucially implicated in a range of disturbances of small and large-scale oscillatory processes (oscillopathies) that underline cognitive, emotional, behavioral, movement, and seizure disorders. Limbocortical and ganglio/thalamocortical networks (with reciprocal connectivity across different levels of neural organization) interwoven through hierarchical multimodular organization account for large-scale oscillations and their derangements (oscillopathies) (**Figure 1**) [2, 68–71].

The pedunculopontine (PPTN) and laterodorsal tegmental (LDTN) nuclei, the raphe (RN) nuclei, the locus coeruleus (LC) nuclei, and the ventral tegmental area

(VTA) are brainstem structures that through widespread neurotransmitter/receptor systems (cholinergic, serotonergic, noradrenergic, dopaminergic) short-cut through multiple limbocortical/thalamocortical circuitries and feedback loops in order to regulate theta rhythm synchronization in long-range interactions between HPC-mPFC during awake (sensorimotor) and sleep (REM) activities [26–28]. Their dysfunction in any direction can result in long-range oscillopathies and large-scale brain network imbalances.

3. Hippocampal oscillopathies in psychosis and schizophrenia

Psychosis is usually associated with impaired sensorimotor gating (prepulse inhibition startle, latent inhibition, auditory sensory gating) and cognitive dysfunctions (impaired social interaction and working memory deficits). Psychotic symptoms seem to originate from two pathophysiological processes: (1) enhanced gamma oscillations related to glutamate (glutamatergic hypothesis) and (2) hyperactive mesolimbic and mesocortical dopamine systems (dopaminergic hypothesis). High dopamine in ventral tegmental area (VTA) causes positive symptoms of schizophrenia, while low dopamine receptor activation in the prefrontal cortex seems to be associated with negative symptoms of schizophrenia (**Figure 2**) [72].

The glutamatergic and dopaminergic hypotheses of psychosis in schizophrenia can be explained by the hyperactive hippocampus [73] and ventral tegmental area pathways [74]. Psychotic symptoms are thus caused by hyperactivity of midbrain

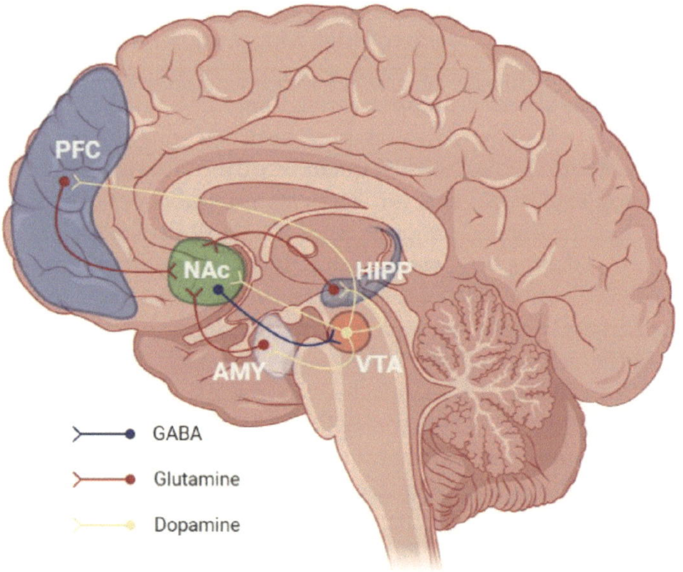

Figure 2.
Diagram showing some of the key components of the mesocorticolimbic ("reward") circuit. Includes dopaminergic, glutaminergic and GABA-ergic pathways between the ventral tegmental area, nucleus accumbens, prefrontal cortex, amygdala and hippocampus. Dopaminergic brain pathways: the mesocortical connects the ventral tegmental area (VTA) with the prefrontal cortex; the mesolimbic pathway connects the VTA with the nucleus accumbens; the nigrostriatal connects the substantia nigra with the dorsal striatum; the tuberoinfundibular connects the hypothalamus with the pituitary. Mesocorticolimbic Circuit.png, Created: 4 November 2020 by GeorgeVKach - Own work CC BY - SA 4.0. https://en.wikipedia.org/wiki/Dopaminergic_pathways#/media/File:Mesocorticolimbic_Circuit.png.

dopaminergic neurons, which is positively modulated by pyramidal neurons in the ventral hippocampus via the nucleus accumbens and the ventral pallidum (**Figure 2**) [73]. Brain imaging studies of schizophrenia patients suggest hyperactivity of the anterior hippocampus (enhanced gamma oscillations) leading to hyperactivity of dopaminergic neurons in the ventral tegmental area via the pathway from ventral hippocampus to nucleus accumbens to ventral pallidum to ventral tegmental area [73, 74]. The septal nuclei and the diagonal band of Broca critically modulate the activity of the ventral hippocampus (regulate theta and gamma band oscillations along the septo-hippocampal axis) and thus may also be involved in sensorimotor and auditory sensory gating deficits [15–19].

Decreased dopamine release in the prefrontal cortex, and excessive dopamine release in the mesolimbic pathway have been associated with psychosis in schizophrenia and bipolar disorder [75, 76]. Excessive activity in midbrain VTA can induce symptoms of psychosis [72, 77], while amphetamine (a dopamine reuptake inhibitor) induces psychotic-like symptoms and blockers of dopamine D_2 receptors (neuroleptics like haloperidol and chlorpromazine) alleviate positive symptoms of psychosis [75, 76].

Psychoactive drugs (Phencyclidine, Ketamine, Amphetamine, or MDMA) enhance gamma oscillations in the hippocampus and can induce "schizophrenia" phenotypes in rats. NMDA receptor blockers by inhibiting NMDA receptors on parvalbumin-positive GABAergic interneurons can induce abnormal gamma oscillations with psychosis. The enhanced gamma oscillations mediated by GABAergic neurons in septal nuclei can be abolished by ablation of septal GABAergic neurons (by orexin-saporin). The enhanced gamma oscillations mediated by GABAergic neurons in septal nuclei can be normalized by inactivation of the medial septum by muscimol infusion or deep brain burst stimulation of the septum at 100 Hz or abolished by ablation of septal GABAergic neurons by orexin-saporin [12].

Typical antipsychotics (from high-potency Fluphenazine, Haloperidol, Pimozide, (Trifluo)perazine, Thiothixene, Perphenazine, Clopenthixol, to low-potency Promethazine, Prochlorperazine, and Chlorpromazine, the last ones with additional anticholinergic and antihistaminergic effects) are not very selective and can block dopamine receptors in the mesocortical, tuberoinfundibular, and nigrostriatal pathways, resulting in extrapyramidal side effects (involuntary movement disorders of dystonia, akathisia, parkinsonism, tardive dyskinesia) along with gynecomastia, impotence, weight gain, and metabolic syndrome [78].

Atypical antipsychotics (from low to higher D_2 potency and strong anti-$5HT_{2A}$ effect like Clozapine, Brexpiprazole, Quetiapine, Ziprasidone, Olanzapine, to highest anti-D_2 potency Risperidone, and even partial D_2 agonist effects of Aripiprazole and Cariprazine) act effectively against $5\text{-}HT_{2A}$ receptors (different alleles of which have been associated with schizophrenia and depression), in addition to H_1, $\alpha_1/_2$-adrenergic and muscarinic antagonism with lower extrapyramidal side effects or prolactin secretion [79–81]. Higher concentrations of $5\text{-}HT_{2A}$ receptors have been found in cortical and subcortical areas, and in particular in the right caudate nucleus [79].

In schizophrenia, there is a reported imbalance in the interaction between large-scale brain networks (SN, DMN, and FPN), with the SN having dysfunctional connectivity with both DMN and FPN networks, potentially contributing to difficulties in appropriately filtering salient stimuli, resulting in cognitive and affective dysregulation, with sensory or auditory gating deficits. This dysregulation might manifest as cognitive deficits (impaired attention and executive function), affective symptoms (inappropriate emotional responses and mood disturbances), inability to filter out irrelevant stimuli, and focus attention on relevant ones (sensory overload, hallucinations, and cognitive disorganization) [71, 82].

4. Hippocampal oscillopathies in fear and anxiety

Fear is an adaptive component of transient responses to internal and external aversive events such as potentially threatening stimuli. Anxiety is an emotional state characterized by an unpleasant sense of heightened alertness even without actual exposure to danger [68]. During exposure of animals to anxiogenic stimuli, local field potential (LFP) recordings from the ventral hippocampus (vHPC) and the medial prefrontal cortex (mPFC) were highly coherent in power and phase at all frequencies, with peaks in both theta (4–12 Hz) and gamma (30–100 Hz) frequency ranges. mPFC-vHPC coherence was even higher at most frequencies than coherence between the two hippocampi, while coherence between the dorsal hippocampus (dHPC) and mPFC was only high for frequencies below 4 Hz, and low at gamma frequencies [83, 84]. Theta-frequency activity in the vHPC and mPFC was highly correlated at baseline, and this correlation increased in anxiogenic environments. Increases in mPFC theta power predicted avoidance of the aversive situations, and were larger in serotonin 1A-receptor knockout mice (a genetic model of increased anxiety behavior). This provides evidence that such synchronization is a general mechanism by which the hippocampus communicates with downstream target structures that influence anxiety (**Figure 1**) [85].

Theta oscillations arise in the septo-hippocampal axis in anxious environments or when confronted with novelty. The anxiety is represented as synchronization of the ventral HPC with the mPFC and the AMG [85]. Inactivation or lesion of the medial septum disrupts theta oscillations in the hippocampus and decreases anxiety behaviors in rats [86, 87]. During the acquisition phase of fear conditioning or REM-sleep periods after fear conditioning, and during retrieval phases where the same conditioned stimulus is applied, there is an increase and lasting effect of HPC-mPFC-BLA theta (4–12 Hz) and gamma (20–100 Hz) oscillations [68, 88, 89].

Dysregulation of emotions and increased anxiety are hallmarks of stress-induced mental disorders in both animal models and human patients. Through different behavioral paradigms to estimate the levels of emotional valence and anxiety, a number of studies with genetic and pharmacological approaches have suggested that the HPC-mPFC-AMG regions are a hub network related to fear and anxiety-like behavior [89, 90]. Electrophysiological studies confirm the importance of theta-range (4–12 Hz) oscillations in LFP signals of the HPC-mPFC-AMG circuit related to emotional behavior as potential substrates for temporal circuit coordination and long-term plasticity in neuronal networks [90, 91].

Similar observations to the animal brain recordings are extrapolated in humans through functional neuroimaging of large-scale brain networks (Triple Network Model). Overactivity in the Anterior Insula (AI)-dorsal Anterior Cingulate Cortex (dACC) AI-dACC network is associated with affective disorders of anxiety and neuroticism [71]. Elevated AI activity has been found in response to facial emotional expressions, particularly in individuals with high levels of anxiety, neuroticism, and risk avoidance [91]. People with high levels of anxiety may interpret relatively safe situations as threatening. Hence, AI overactivation leads to excessive sensitivity and anxiety arousal, with generalization and over-mobilization of stress reactions in non-threatening situations (**Figure 3**) [92].

DOI: http://dx.doi.org/10.5772/intechopen.1011136

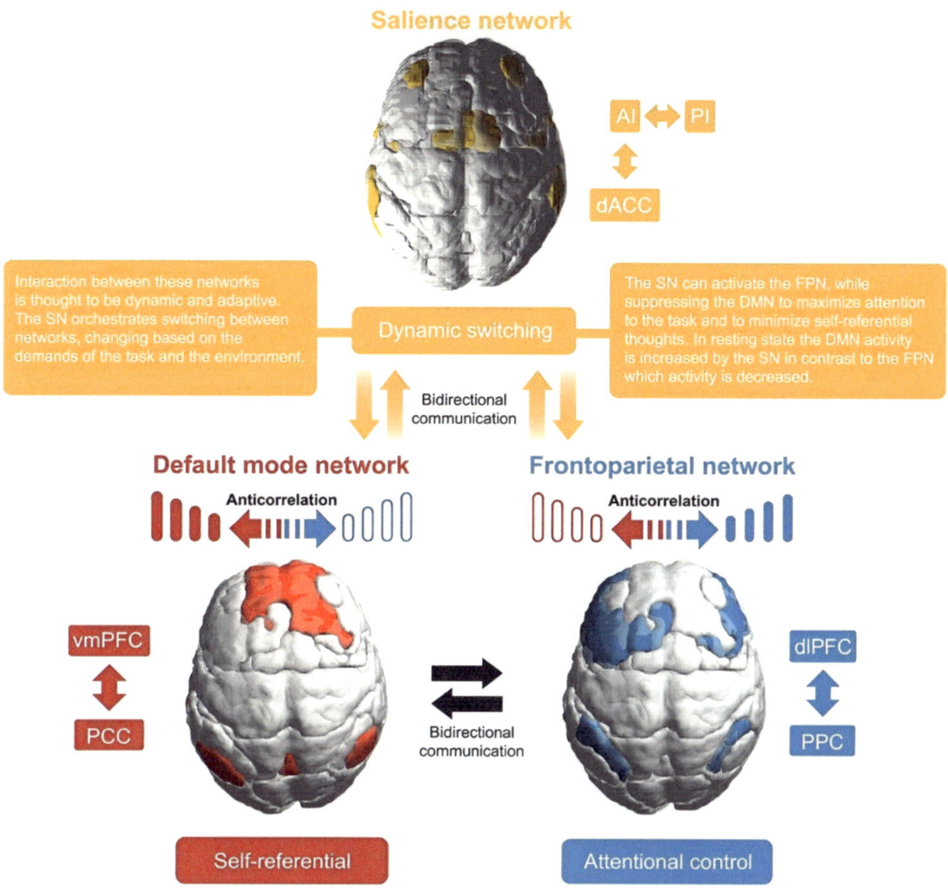

Figure 3.
The role of the salience network orchestrating the dynamic switching and balance between the default-mode and central executive (frontoparietal) networks – dysfunctions and imbalances among these three large-scale brain networks can result in various cognitive, affective and behavioral deficits. Reproduced under CC BY 4.0. licence from Schimmelpfennig et al. [71].

In anxiety disorders, heightened sensitivity within the SN results in increased perception of threats and heightened emotional responses, leading to an overactive response to potential threats or stressors. The disrupted connectivity between the SN and other networks like the DMN and CEN/FPN can lead to difficulties in appropriately filtering and prioritizing stimuli, resulting in cognitive biases toward negative or threatening information. The inability to switch effectively between the DMN and CEN/FPN may lead to persistent negative thinking, rumination, and impaired executive function. This imbalance in network coordination can contribute to cognitive and affective dysregulation in anxiety disorders. As the SN integrates emotional and physiological states, its dysfunction can result in inappropriate emotional responses, heightened anxiety, and difficulties in emotional regulation (**Figure 3**) [71].

Anti-anxiety medications (anxiolytics) are drugs used for the treatment of anxiety disorders, which may be mediated by neurotransmitters like norepinephrine, serotonin, dopamine, and gamma-aminobutyric acid (GABA) in the CNS.

Anti-anxiety medications are classified into six types according to their mode of action: antidepressants, benzodiazepines, azapirones, antiepileptics, antipsychotics, and beta blockers [93].

5. Hippocampal oscillopathies in autistic spectrum and attention-deficit hyperactivity disorders

Autism Spectrum Disorder (ASD) is a group of developmental disorders manifesting qualitative abnormalities in social interactions and behavioral patterns, as well as a limited and repetitive repertoire of interests and activities. ASD affects how people interact socially and behave when in uncertainty [71]. fMRI studies have shown that brain regions, like the anterior insula (AI) and anterior cingulate cortex (ACC), are less active in people with autism during social tasks (difficulties in processing social information) compared to those without autism. A theory proposed by Uddin and Menon [94] suggests that ASD may stem from problems in communication between sensory and limbic areas and the insula, involved in processing sensory information and emotions. The brain's salience network (SN), which determines the importance of social stimuli in our environment, might underestimate the importance of social cues in people with autism. This could help explain why individuals with ASD often struggle with social interactions. Changes in the functional connectivity among the salience (dAIC), default mode network (DMN), and frontoparietal network (FPN) correlate with the severity of ASD symptoms [71]. People with ASD may also have difficulty adjusting their expectations when faced with new or uncertain situations. Because of their rigid expectations, they have an attentional bias toward anticipated stimuli and tend to suppress unanticipated stimuli, which can make it harder to adapt to changes in dynamic real-world contexts. This could lead to a preference for familiar routines and difficulty dealing with unexpected situations. In summary, ASD may involve a combination of social communication issues and difficulty in contextualizing sensory input, especially in social situations or when faced with uncertainty (**Figure 3**) [94, 95].

Attention-Deficit/Hyperactivity Disorder (ADD/ADHD) is the most common neurodevelopmental disorder occurring in childhood, characterized by developmentally excessive levels of inattention, impulsivity, and hyperactivity. In ADHD, there may be a dysfunction in the Salience Network (SN) responsible for detecting and filtering out relevant stimuli and determining which sensory information is important. This may lead to challenges in focusing on important tasks and an increased likelihood of being distracted by irrelevant stimuli. In ADHD, there may also be a dysfunction of the DMN being overly active during tasks that require attention, leading to difficulties in maintaining focus and a tendency to drift off [96]. The Frontoparietal Network (FPN) is involved in executive functions, such as working memory, attention, and problem-solving. An imbalance in the FPN in ADHD could manifest as difficulties in planning, organizing, and executing tasks, contributing to the hallmark symptoms of inattention and hyperactivity [97].

Studies have shown that functional connectivity within the DMN and SN is disrupted in individuals with ADHD. These networks do not appropriately switch between tasks, leading to persistent attention deficits. The hyperactivity of the DMN during tasks that require focus, combined with a dysregulated SN, contributes to the inability to sustain attention and increased distractibility seen in ADHD. The findings highlight the importance of neural network balance for proper cognitive function and suggest that treatments aimed at restoring this balance could be beneficial for managing ADHD symptoms (**Figure 3**) [97].

A range of behavioral therapies (CBT parent-child-school), dietary interventions, physical activities (exercise, yoga), psychological interventions (social skills, support groups), lifestyle modifications (sleep hygiene, time management), educational interventions, mindfulness and meditation, neurobiofeedback, and complementary therapies are available for managing ADHD. When all conservative measures have been exhausted, medications used for ADHD include, as first line, methylphenidate-based stimulants and, as second line, amphetamine-based stimulants. If stimulants are ineffective or have significant side effects, then selective norepinephrine reuptake inhibitor (atomoxetine), α2-adrenergic agonists (guanfacine, clonidine), and antidepressants (off-label bupropion, TCAs (desipramine, nortriptyline)) may be used. Rarely, and only in specific cases with other comorbidities, drugs like modafinil, venlafaxine, aripiprazole, and risperidone may be used [98].

6. Hippocampal oscillopathies in depression

Depression is a mental state of low mood and aversion to activity. Nearly 3 in 10 people will experience depression at some point in their life. Depression affects a person's thoughts, behavior, feelings, and sense of well-being. Depressed people often experience loss of motivation or interest in, or reduced pleasure or joy from, experiences that would normally bring them pleasure or joy. They feel sad, irritable, empty and/or hopeless, with significant changes in appetite (eating much less or more than usual) and/or weight (notable loss or gain unrelated to dieting), sleeping too little or too much, decreased energy or increased tiredness or fatigue, increase in purposeless physical activity or slowed movements or speech (severe enough to be observable by others), feeling worthless or excessively guilty, having difficulty thinking or concentrating, forgetfulness and/or difficulty making minor decisions, having thoughts of death, suicidal ideation, or suicide attempts. It is normal to experience moments of sadness, at times low mood, or the blues as part of the human experience. A diagnosis of depression requires that the above symptoms occur for most of the day, nearly every day, for more than 2 weeks, along with a clear change in day-to-day functioning [99].

Recent studies have suggested that there are oscillatory disturbances in the limbocortical networks of depressed patients and rodent models of depression. The oscillatory disturbances in the septo-hippocampal axis, related to symptoms of depression, could be used as biomarkers of response to treatment with antidepressants [12]. Furthermore, the symptoms of depression have been alleviated by restoring the abnormal oscillations in patients [100]. Clinical studies have reported altered patterns of electroencephalogram (EEG) oscillatory signals in depressed patients, such as altered power and functional coupling in the alpha (8–13 Hz) and gamma (30–100 Hz) bands in the frontal cortex [101, 102]. Similarly, in PTSD patients, resting electrical signals in the PFC show decreased alpha power-mediated inhibition and increased gamma power, suggesting hypofunction in the PFC [103]. Accumulated evidence from these studies implies that small-to-large-scale oscillopathies represent a pathophysiological biomarker of mood disorders (**Figure 4**) [101, 105].

A model of depression with olfactory bulbectomy is based on degeneration of cholinergic neurons in the medial septum (MS) [106]. Early studies investigating the role of the medial septum as a center of reward and pleasure implied that

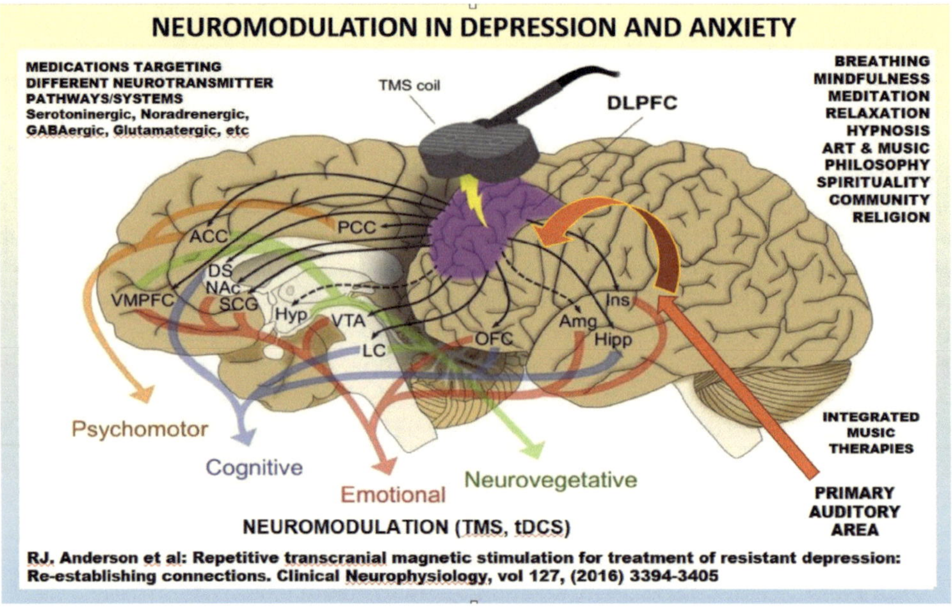

Figure 4.
Transcranial magnetic stimulation (TMS) and complementary approaches targeting major brain centers and functions in the treatment of depression. Adapted from Anderson et al. [104], with modifications to emphasize the diverse physical (e.g. TMS, tDCS), chemical (e.g. psychoactive medications, drugs, trace elements), biological (e.g. breathing control, sleep hygiene, proper nutrition, light therapy), cognitive (e.g. mindfulness, relaxation, hypnosis, mental activities and exercises, cognitive–behavioral therapies), emotional (e.g. psychotherapies, emotion-focused, attachment-based and dialectical behavioral therapies, interpersonal, rewarding, graceful, compassionate, psychodrama and role-play therapies, reflective journaling), sensory-perceptual-kinaesthetic (e.g. art and music therapies, physical activities and exercises, dancing, yoga, acupuncture, aromatherapy, massage), psychosocial (e.g. community-based, group-specific and systemic therapies such as Hellinger therapy), and metaphysical (e.g. philosophy, religion, meditation, spirituality) factors that contribute to neuromodulation and neuroplasticity. These interventions can act synergistically to influence cognitive, limbic, psychomotor and autonomic functions and potentially restore the balance of large-scale brain networks, including the central executive, default mode, salience, and attention networks.

stimulation of the septal-hippocampal axis might be effective for improving symptoms of depression [12]. Deep brain stimulation (DBS) has thus been considered for patients with depression resistant to pharmacological treatments. DBS of the medial forebrain bundle (MFB) has been employed for patients with treatment-resistant depression [107]. The antidepressive effects of MFB stimulation may be mediated by co-activation of the septal-hippocampal axis, as the rewarding effects of the medial forebrain bundle encourage rats to repeat self-stimulation and septal lesions attenuate this effect. Positive feelings induced by MS electrical stimulation have been reported in earlier studies of depression, epilepsy, schizophrenia, and refractory pain patients [12, 108].

Systemic administration of an antidepressant drug (Reboxetine, a norepinephrine reuptake inhibitor) increased theta power and gamma power in the HPC and increased theta phase-locking of septal-hippocampal activities [109]. Antidepressants nowadays include selective serotonin reuptake inhibitors (SSRIs), serotonin-norepinephrine reuptake inhibitors (SNRIs), tricyclic antidepressants (TCA), and monoamine oxidase inhibitor (MAOI). SSRIs (Citalopram, Escitalopram, Fluoxetine, Fluvoxamine, Paroxetine, Sertraline) can also be used in all types of anxiety disorders, while SNRIs (Desvenlafaxine, Duloxetine, Levomilnacipran,

Milnacipran, Venlafaxine) are used for depression and/or generalized anxiety disorder (GAD). Both of them are considered as first-line anti-anxiety medications. TCAs (Imipramine, Clomipramine, Doxepin, Amitriptyline, Nortriptyline, and Desipramine) and TeCAs (Mirtazapine) are second-line treatment, as they can cause significant adverse effects. Benzodiazepines (Alprazolam, Bromazepam, Chlordiazepoxide, Clonazepam, Diazepam, Lorazepam, Oxazepam, Temazepam, and Triazolam) are effective in emergent and short-term treatment of anxiety disorders due to their fast onset but carry the risk of dependence. Buspirone is an azapirone indicated for GAD, which has a much slower onset but with the advantage of less sedating and withdrawal effects [110].

The accumulation of mental stress loads is a primary risk factor for psychiatric disorders such as generalized anxiety disorder (GAD), major depressive disorder (MDD), and post-traumatic stress disorder (PTSD) [111].

Increased activity of key SN structures (AI and ACC) and the amygdala was shown in response to negative stimuli in depressed individuals [112]. Meta-analysis of bipolar disorder patients with rs-fMRI and analysis of effective connectivity have shown abnormal functional integration within and among the three core brain networks (SN, DMN, and FPN) [113]. Altered connectivity patterns both within networks (FPN, SN) and between (DMN-SN, DMN-FPN) were dependent on the mood and type of bipolar disorder [113]. Compared to the depression stage, patients with the euthymic stage expressed a hyperconnectivity among the FPN and reduced connectivity between SN-FPN and SN-DMN (**Figure 3**) [71].

The findings underscore the importance of targeting the SN and its connectivity with other networks in first-line therapeutic interventions, before the use of antidepressant medications [110]. This could include techniques such as cognitive-behavioral therapy (CBT), mindfulness-based interventions, and neuromodulation therapies like transcranial magnetic stimulation (TMS) to normalize network activity and improve symptoms (**Figure 4**). Behavioral modification/activation with physical exercise and engaging in interpersonal and social rewarding tasks (social interaction, community life, group therapy) might help shift the balance toward activation of the central executive network and off the default mode network, hence improving depression [100, 114].

7. Hippocampal oscillopathies in dementia

Alzheimer's disease (AD) is a chronic neurodegenerative disease (2/3 of dementia cases worldwide) characterized by deposition of extracellular beta amyloid (neuritic plaques), pyramidal cells, cortical intracellular neurofibrillary tangles, and neuronal loss in both cortical and subcortical regions. Neuronal loss is significant in the hippocampus, in the frontal, parietal, and anterior temporal lobes, in the amygdala, and olfactory system. In the cerebrospinal fluid of AD patients, the $A\beta_{1-42}$ amino acid form of Aβ amyloid peptide and the phosphorylated tau protein are specific biomarkers for AD and correlate with disease severity [99].

A large reduction in brain choline acetyltransferase is noted in AD due to the loss of cholinergic neurons in the basal forebrain cholinergic nuclei. There are also significant losses in noradrenergic, serotonergic, and glutamatergic systems. In particular, losses in the glutamatergic pathways projecting to and from the hippocampus lead to functional isolation of the hippocampus, thus the inability to form long-term memories in AD. The human cholinergic systems in the basal forebrain bundle (BFB)

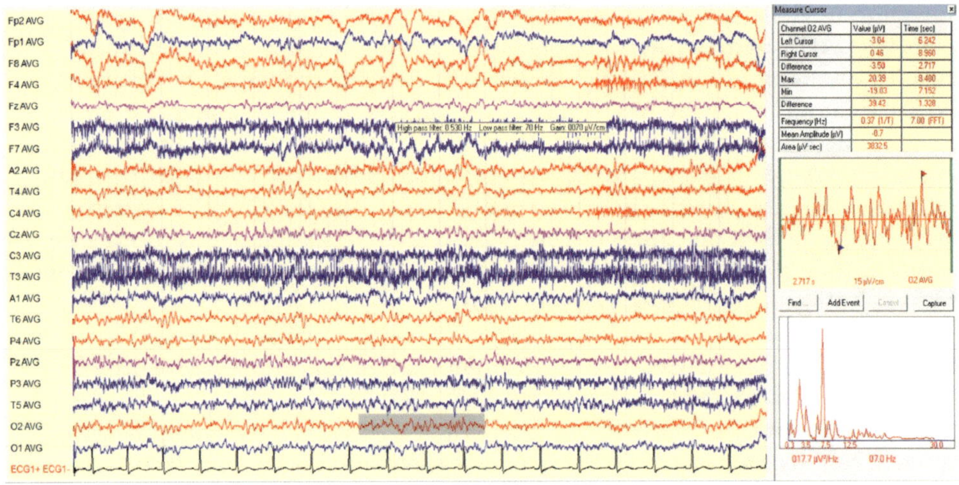

Figure 5.
EEG resting state in a dementia patient, please note in the right lower corner the spectrogram indicating a reduction in the background alpha band power and an increase in theta and delta band power.

comprise neurons in the septal and diagonal complex (Group Ch1 of the medial septum [10% of cells] and the diagonal band of Broca groups Ch2 and Ch3) that drive the hippocampus and neurons in the basal nucleus (nucleus basalis) of Meynert (the largest group of cholinergic cells in the basal forebrain (around 90%), Ch4, with approx. 210,000 cholinergic cells per hemisphere) that drives the cingulate gyrus and the prefrontal cortex (**Figure 1**) [115].

Electroencephalography (EEG) has emerged as a non-invasive dynamic investigation for assessing oscillatory disturbances in the brain of AD patients [116–120]. Large-scale oscillopathies in AD involve a decrease of high-frequency oscillations (alpha/beta/gamma band), increased delta and theta power, and decreased alpha and beta/gamma power across different topographies, graph theory models, and resting states (**Figure 5**). Smaller-scale hippocampal oscillopathies in AD involve disruptions of theta oscillations, gamma oscillations, and theta-gamma cross-frequency phase-amplitude coupling in the hippocampus and the entorhinal cortex [14, 121]. Hippocampal oscillopathies seem to underlie the cognitive dysfunction in AD patients as these oscillations are crucial for memory encoding and retrieval. The theta and gamma disruptions in AD are partially due to dysfunctions of SST- and PV-positive interneuron circuits in the HPC, respectively [122]. In addition, these oscillatory disturbances can originate from dysfunctions of the MS in AD because HPC gamma oscillations are generated and modulated by the medial septum cholinergic tone [19, 20, 24, 31].

The number of cholinergic neurons of the basal forebrain bundle (BFB) and medial septum (MS) was severely decreased in post-mortem brains of AD patients, resulting in decreased cholinergic innervation to the HPC [115, 123]. Amyloid beta peptide injection into the MS caused degeneration of MS cholinergic neurons, disrupted rhythmic activities of MS GABAergic neurons, decreased power of theta oscillations in the HPC, and induced memory deficit in rats [124]. Therefore, cognitive dysfunctions in AD could be improved by restoring theta and gamma oscillations in the septo-hippocampal and MFB-neocortical axes via DBS. Electrical stimulation of the fornix via DBS increased cholinergic input in the HPC and enhanced memory while decreasing amyloid beta deposition in the brain of an AD rat model [125]. Stimulation of the BFB/NBM may also increase cholinergic input and activation of the neocortex [126, 127]. Optogenetic gamma stimulation of PV-positive neurons in the MS improved spatial memory in an AD mouse model [128]. The septo-hippocampal theta rhythm stimulation improved novel object recognition and spatial learning in chronic epileptic models [129] and a traumatic brain injury model in rodents [130]. Theta oscillations in the septo-hippocampal axis can also be induced by Vagal Nerve Stimulation (VNS) with less invasive stimulation [131].

Enhancing cholinergic tone by Tacrine (an acetylcholinesterase [AChE] inhibitor) improved impaired theta and gamma oscillations in the HPC of an AD mouse model [132]. In humans, Donepezil, a non-competitive, non-selective, reversible AChE inhibitor with a long half-life, improves cognition and daily functioning in moderate to severe AD, without essentially modifying the disease process [106]. Rivastigmine is a pseudo-irreversible inhibitor of AChE with fewer side effects. Galantamine is an AChE inhibitor and a positive allosteric modulator of nicotinic receptors; it may enhance the signal mediated by nicotinic receptors and has fewer and milder side effects. AChE inhibitors induce a global improvement in cognitive performance, although the response is variable among patients, depending also on tolerance (gastrointestinal side effects). Based on the decreased cholinergic tone in AD, muscarinic receptor agonists and nicotinic receptor agonists or allosteric modulators (such as Galantamine) may have distinct advantages with fewer side effects [115].

Glutamate is a key excitatory transmitter in cortico-subcortical projections and in corticocortical fibers. It is likely that the pathophysiology of AD involves a chronic excitotoxic effect due to dysregulated glutamatergic transmission, which may be further enhanced by amyloid peptides. In addition, the activation of glutamatergic transmission through NMDA receptors enhances the production of phosphorylated tau. Memantine is a noncompetitive NMDA receptor antagonist that has relatively strong voltage-dependency and rapid unblocking kinetics (similar to the stabilizing action of Mg^{2+} blocking the NMDA receptor channel only under resting conditions). As it does not interfere with normal glutamatergic transmission but blocks increased transmission in chronic conditions, Memantine significantly slows down the rate of cognitive and functional decline and has a positive synergistic effect with AChE inhibitors such as Donepezil, reducing the burden of side effects [115].

8. Hippocampal oscillopathies in seizures, movement, and behavioral disorders

The lifetime prevalence of seizures (the risk of having a non-febrile epileptic seizure at some point in an average lifetime) is estimated between 2% and 5%. Around 70–80% of people with seizures will achieve remission, the longer seizures occur for, the poorer the prognosis (or the patient dies) [133]. Epilepsy is defined by at least two unprovoked (or reflex) seizures occurring more than 24 hours apart, increasing the risk of further seizures over the following 12 months to more than 60%. Epilepsy can be outgrown as an age-dependent self-limited developmental process or resolve for those who have remained seizure-free for 10 years, with no seizure medication for the last 5 years. Excessive or hypersynchronous activity of populations of neurons (epileptogenicity) is an inherent or acquired property of the underlying neuronal networks that any brain could manifest under certain conditions (sleep deprivation, emotional dysregulation, extreme fatigue and exhaustion, alcohol and drug (toxic) exposure, flashing/strobe lights, overbreathing, overheating, brain hypoxia, infection, dehydration, electrolyte disturbances, metabolic derangements, diabetes, etc.) [133].

The age epidemiology of epilepsy, movement, and behavioral disorders shows a remarkable bimodal distribution, more common in the young (<20 years of age) and in the elderly (>60 years of age). The incidence of epilepsy is highest in the first year of life and in early childhood, with a relative decrease in adolescence, reaching its lowest between 20 and 40, and steadily increasing after age 50 [134]. At birth, the average baby's brain is about 25% of the size of the average adult brain. It doubles in size in the first year of life and keeps growing to about 80% of adult size by age 3 and 90% by age 5. Throughout childhood and into early adolescence, the brain undergoes significant development, characterized by the growth, branching, and myelination of neuronal processes, as well as the apoptosis (programmed cell death) of certain

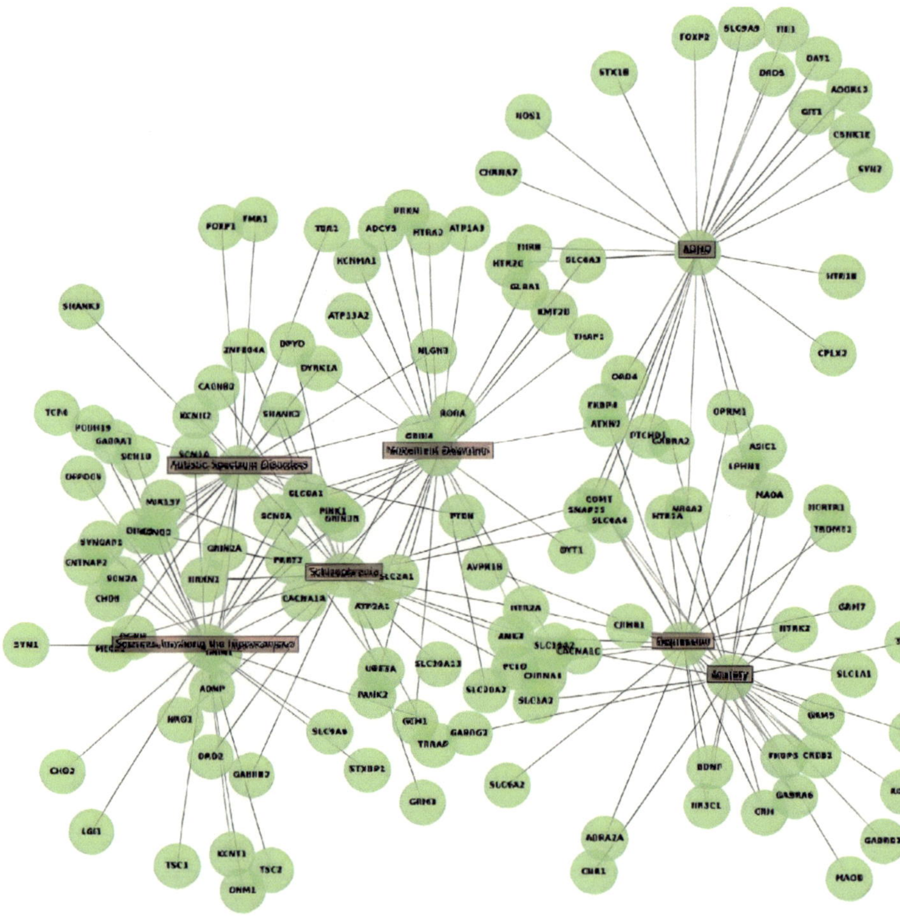

Figure 6.
Graph-theoretical network representation of the 100 most common genes linking hippocampal and limbocortical oscillopathies with various seizure disorders, movement disorders, neuropsychiatric and behavioral disorders. Nodes correspond to individual genes, while edges denote their associations with disorder categories (epilepsy and seizures, schizophrenia, autism spectrum and movement disorders, attention-deficit/hyperactivity disorders, anxiety and depression). Edge weights (represented by length) reflect the relative degree of gene involvement across conditions, thereby illustrating the polygenic architecture, pleiotropic effects, and developmental trajectories underlying the heterogeneous and complex phenotypic outcomes.

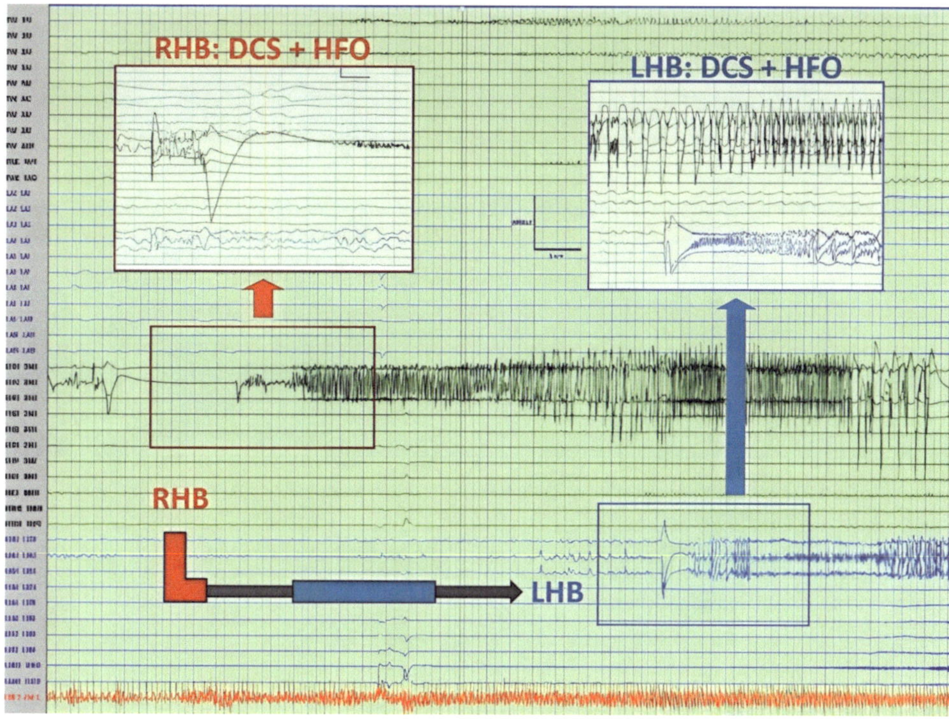

Figure 7.
Human intracranial EEG recordings of bilateral hippocampi to demonstrate baseline (DC) shifts and high-frequency oscillations (HFOs) as surrogate markers of the ictal onset zone. In this patient, they always started from the most atrophic and sclerotic (burnt out) right hippocampus and subsequently spread to the left hippocampus. Resection of the right hippocampus in this case conferred seizure freedom and confirmed the epileptogenic zone.

neurons. Simultaneously, synapses proliferate, grow, and are pruned, undergoing continuous plasticity changes [135]. These processes collectively contribute to the brain's "rewiring" for improved impulse control [136] during the teenage years, gradually forming a complex and dynamic neuronal network, with ongoing structural and functional connectivity changes through the first 20–25 years of life [135]. Early-life epilepsy, movement, and behavioral disorders are often rooted in genetic factors and abnormal brain development, particularly related to the rapid or aberrant growth of neural connectivity (**Figure 6**). Many idiopathic (genetic) focal or generalized epilepsies can improve, become self-limited, or even be outgrown after the age of 20–25 [134].

Seizures start somewhere locally in the brain from aberrant [excessive or hypersynchronous] electrical activity of a population of neurons and use the same neuronal machinery (that generates brain oscillations during normal brain function) to propagate. By using the intrinsic functional connectivity of brain networks, seizures can spread and generalize, entraining large-scale brain networks for seizure output. Thus, a wide range of aetiopathogenic microscale mechanisms of seizure-onset converge through large-scale brain networks into common pathways of seizure evolution and phenotypic expression (clinical manifestation) (**Figure 7**) [1].

In focal limbocortical and mesial temporal lobe epilepsies, there is either decreased inhibition and/or increased excitation and/or structural and functional

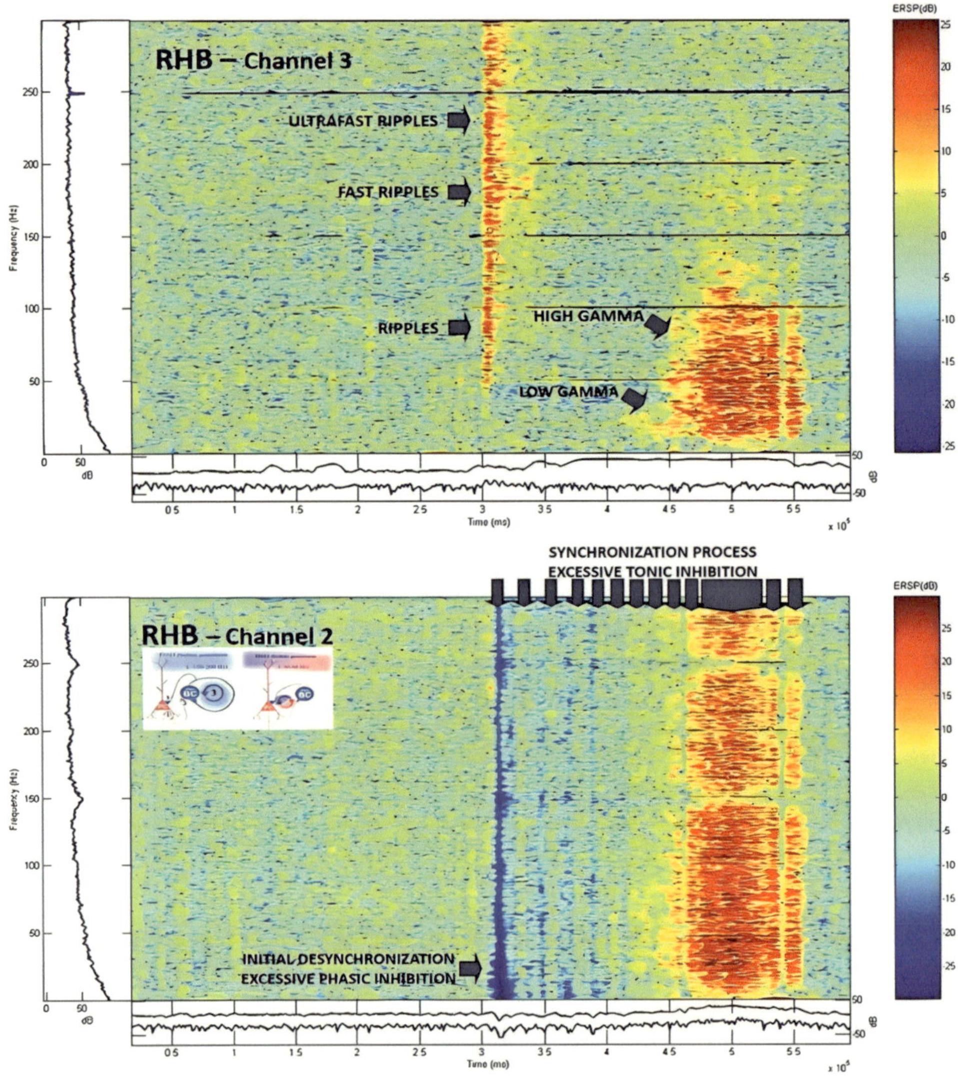

Figure 8.
Time–frequency analysis of human hippocampal intracranial EEG recordings, with power represented on the colour scale. Within the right posterior hippocampus (Channel 3 Spectrogram), an initial phase of hyperexcitation is evident, characterized by high-frequency ripple synchronization (ripples and fast ripples). This is followed by excessive inhibitory feedback and a brief period of background attenuation (broadband suppression) reflecting desynchronization or phase-resetting of neuronal oscillators in the right middle hippocampus (Channel 2 spectrogram). Subsequently, recurrent excitation–inhibition oscillatory cycles (synchronization process) emerge, ultimately giving rise to a sustained paroxysmal depolarization shift marked by pathological low/high gamma, ripple, and fast ripple oscillations. The inset illustrates the interaction of hippocampal pyramidal neurons with parvalbumin-positive basket interneurons, which generate high-frequency gamma oscillations through the pyramidal–interneuron gamma (PING) mechanism and ripple-frequency phase-modulations via the feedback-inhibition–network oscillation (FINO) mechanism, reproduced from [1] and [6].

connectivity changes in the hippocampal network that can alter the dynamic interaction of excitatory and inhibitory network components and result in increased network synchronization (**Figure 8**) [1, 137]. The following fundamental mechanisms in different combinations can alter this dynamic interaction of excitatory and inhibitory network components, resulting in focal-onset seizures:

Receptor/channel/process	Associated genes
Sodium channels (Nav)	SCN1A, SCN2A, SCN3A, SCN4A, SCN5A, SCN7A, SCN8A, SCN9A, SCN10A, SCN11A, SCN12A
Potassium channels (Kv)	KCNQ2, KCNQ3, KCNQ4, KCNQ5, KCNB1, KCNB2, KCNT1, KCNJ10, KCNJ11, KCNH2
Potassium channel regulation	KCNC1, KCTD7
Calcium channels (Cav)	CACNA1A, CACNA1H, CACNB2, CACNB4, CACNA2D1, CACNG2, CACNG3, CACNG5
GABA receptors (GABAergic signaling)	GABRA1, GABRA2, GABRA3, GABRA4, GABRA6, GABRB1, GABRB2, GABRB3, GABRG2, GABRD, GABRQ, GABBR1, GABBR2, GABBR3
Glutamate receptors (AMPA/Kainate/NMDA)	GRIN1, GRIN2A, GRIN2B, GRIN2C, GRIN2D, GRIN3A, GRIN3B, GRIA2, GRIA3, GRIK1, GRIK2, GRIK3, GRIK4, GRIK5
Nicotinic Acetylcholine receptors	CHRNA2, CHRNA3, CHRNA4, CHRNA5, CHRNA6, CHRNA7
Muscarinic ACh receptors	CHRM1, CHRM2, CHRM3
Glycine receptors	GLRA1, GLRB
Cl^-/HCN/ATPase channels	CLCN2 [Cl^-], HCN1, HCN2, ATP1A2, ATP1A3 [Na/K ATPase]
Neurotransmitter release vesicle/synaptic function	STXBP1, SYN1, SYN2, SYNGAP1, PRRT2 [SNARE], MECP2 [regulates chromatin/gene expression], BSN [cytoskeleton], CDKL5 [development]
Neurotrophin signaling/ neuronal survival	NTRK1, NTRK2, NTRK3, FOXG1 [regulates GABAergic circuits]
mTOR signaling pathway	MTOR, DEPDC5, TSC1/TSC2, PIK3CA
Transporter functions	SLC1A1 [glutamate], SLC2A1 [glucose], SLC12A5 [KCC2], SLC9A6 [NHE6]
Magnesium homeostasis	TRPM6, TRPM7 [Tropomyosin]
Miscellaneous	LGI1 [Regulates Kv1.1 and AMPA-R], GNAS [G-protein], UBE3A [Ubiquitin Protein Ligase E3A], CSTB [Cystatin B], CHD2 [chromatin remodeling], RELN [Reelin/neurodevelopment], CDKL5 [neurodevelopment]

Table 1.
This table groups more than 100 most common genes by their involvement in specific ion channels, neurotransmitter receptors, or key pathways/processes that are commonly implicated in the development of hippocampal seizures.

i. Decreased inhibition due to deficient GABA-A receptor complex subunits/ ligand-gated Cl^- ion channel function [e.g. GABRG2, GABRA1] or presynaptic GABA-B receptor complex [e.g. GABBR2] or Voltage-Gated Cl^- Channels [e.g. CLCN2], presynaptic [e.g. Kv1.1/1.2/1.3, Kv3.1/3.2, BK, SK, Kir2.x, TREK-1, TASK-1, TASK-3] and postsynaptic K^+ channels [e.g. KCNQ2, KCNJ10, Kv4.2, Kv2.1], aberrant structural and functional connectivity with deficient feedforward and feed-backward GABAergic inhibition or defective activation/function of GABAergic neurons (**Table 1**) [1, 137].

ii. Increased excitation or increased network synchronization due to alterations or mutations in the chloride [e.g. GABRG2, GABRA1, CLCN2] and potassium [e.g. KCNQ2, KCNJ10] or the sodium [e.g. SCN1A, SCN2A] and calcium [e.g. CACNA1H, CACNB2] channel subunits or the molecules that regulate their function. Such abnormalities may decrease or increase the membrane permeability and conductance of chloride and potassium or sodium and calcium ions forming the chloride-mediated and potassium-mediated hyperpolarizing currents (IPSPs) that counterbalance the sodium-mediated and calcium-mediated depolarizing currents (EPSPs). The overall network balances and imbalances in inhibitory and excitatory components critically modulate the seizure-threshold (**Table 1**) [1, 137].

iii. A lower seizure-threshold may also result from inappropriate activation of fast or long-acting glutamatergic channels. AMPA/Kainate [coupled to Na^+/K^+ currents], NMDA [coupled to Na^+/K^+/Ca^{+2} currents], and metabotropic [late-onset/prolonged postsynaptic phosphorylation and gene expression via a Ca^{+2}-driven second-messenger intracellular system] Glutamate receptors are coupled by means of different postsynaptic membrane mechanisms to several depolarizing channels. Mutations or dysregulation of glutamate receptors [e.g. GRIN2A, GRIA2] or alterations in glutamate transporters (e.g. SLC1A1) can impair the reuptake of glutamate (elevated extracellular levels), and enhance excitatory neurotransmission, resulting in hyperexcitability and increased risk for seizures. Normal NMDA receptor function is associated with learning and memory, whereas increased activation has been observed in several animal models of focal epilepsy, such as kindling, kainic acid, pilocarpine, etc. (**Table 1**) [1, 137].

iv. Reduced intracellular Ca^{+2}-buffering proteins (parvalbumin and calbindin) increase the vulnerability of neurons to cellular stress, injury, and death in status epilepticus, febrile convulsions, brain hypoxia, and other metabolic, toxic, ischemic, infectious, autoimmune, and inflammatory insults. Interindividual differences in the Ca^{+2}-binding proteins may explain the variable susceptibility of different patients with advancing age to epileptogenesis via the premature loss of critical interneurons, a process that alters inhibitory controls of local neuronal networks in favor of excitation [1, 137].

v. Widespread electrical fields emerging from synchronous activation of many pyramidal neurons in laminar hippocampal structures or local changes in ionic concentrations of extracellular K^+ and intracellular Ca^{+2} or increased neuronal coupling due to more permanent changes in functional gap junctions may further increase the excitability of neuronal assemblies by non-synaptic interactions (ephaptic phenomena), predisposing to focal-onset seizures and status [1].

vi. Abnormal synaptic plasticity (alterations in long-term potentiation or depression) can disrupt normal learning and memory processes and can contribute to hyperexcitability and seizure generation. In long-term potentiation (LTP), synaptic connections are strengthened through high-frequency stimulation (crucial for learning and memory formation, e.g. in CA1 area, it supports the formation and storage of spatial and episodic memories). In long-term depression (LTD), synaptic connections are weakened through low-frequency stimulation (crucial for synaptic pruning and memory extinction, to avoid overload with unnecessary or outdated information). An abnormal increase in LTP due to excessive activation of NMDA receptors or intracellular Ca^{+2} or upregulation of proteins involved in synaptic strengthening (e.g. CaMKII) or high-frequency stimulation due to recurrent seizures could lead to excessive strengthening of synapses, causing excessive neuronal firing, hypersynchronous neural circuits, and larger-scale network hyperexcitability. In impaired LTD due to a reduction in the activity of phosphatases like PP1 or calcineurin, synaptic connections that should be weakened or pruned remain strong, also contributing to hyperexcitability. An imbalance between long-term potentiation (LTP) and long-term depression (LTD) disrupts memory processes, leading to impaired formation of new memories and reduced ability to filter out irrelevant information. This disruption contributes to confusion, cognitive deficits, and—through recurrent seizures such as those seen in temporal lobe epilepsy—progressive memory impairment, particularly of episodic memory, and accelerated network degeneration, possibly resulting in cognitive impairment and even dementia. Although most current antiepileptic drugs are classified primarily as anti-seizure medications that raise the seizure threshold, seizure reduction and control indirectly support synaptic plasticity, stabilise receptor function, and reduce aberrant excitatory drive, thereby facilitating long-term homeostatic adaptations that exert additional disease-modifying effects on epileptogenesis [138].

vii. Disruptions or dysregulation in the balance between excitatory and inhibitory hippocampal circuits (loss of inhibitory interneurons or aberrant network connections) can lead to enhanced excitability and increased seizure propensity. In the dentate gyrus, loss or dysfunction of Granule cells can contribute to hippocampal atrophy/sclerosis and temporal lobe epilepsy. The Mossy cells of the hilar polymorphic region of the dentate gyrus receive feedforward input from the Entorhinal Cortex and feedback activation from CA3 and appear to activate GABAergic neurons and gate-control the inhibitory tone of the network. They may be susceptible to seizure-related neuronal death. The loss of Mossy cells results in impairment of GABAergic interneuron activation, synaptic reorganization, and changes in network plasticity, with formation of newly sprouted circuits of excitatory and inhibitory cells in an attempt to restore inhibition. However, with epilepsy progression, the sprouted synaptic contacts also create recurrent excitatory collateral circuitries that permanently alter the balance between excitatory and inhibitory tone in the hippocampal network [1]. Intractable focal or generalized epilepsies are frequently accompanied by abnormalities in limbocortical networks, particularly in the hippocampal formation. Hippocampal atrophy and sclerosis are common lesions associated with neuronal loss and gliosis, particularly affecting the hilar polymorphic region and CA1 pyramidal regions, with relative sparing of the CA2 pyramidal region and intermediate severity lesions in the CA3 pyramidal region and dentate granule neurons. Loss of pyramidal cells in CA1 and CA3 regions or alterations in their function can also lead to aberrant excitation. About 2/3 of patients with intractable temporal-lobe epilepsy have marked hippocampal sclerosis, while animal models with >100 brief convulsions or epileptic status showed similar changes, suggesting that epileptogenesis or hippocampal/limbic system kindling can be a self-perpetuating process [1].

viii. Neuroinflammation—Autoimmune inflammatory processes in the mesial temporal lobe result in release of pro-inflammatory cytokines such as IL-1β (modulate glutamate receptors and decrease GABAergic inhibition), inflammation-induced activation of astrocytes (release of glutamate), and activation of microglia (release pro-inflammatory factors that can modulate ion channel activity and synaptic transmission), thereby enhancing neuronal excitability in the mesial temporal lobe and the risk for seizures (autoimmune epilepsy) [139].

Receptor/channel/target	Resulting dysfunction predisposing to seizures
NMDA receptor (anti-NMDAR)	Receptor internalization reduces NMDA receptor function or dysfunction in the GluN2B and GluN1 subunits of the NMDAR alter synaptic plasticity, leading to seizures
Anti-GluN2B/Anti-GluN1 Subunits	
Anti-mGluR5 antibodies	
VGKC complex (anti-LGI1)	Disruption of LGI1—K^+ channel interaction
VGKC complex (anti-CASPR2)	CASPR2 Ab impairs K^+ channel function, synaptic dysfunction
GAD65 (glutamic acid decarboxylase)	Reduces GABA synthesis, leading to decreased inhibition
Anti-GAD67 antibodies	Reduces GABA synthesis, leading to decreased inhibition
AMPA receptor (anti-AMPAR 1/2)	Altered excitatory synaptic transmission, receptor dysfunction
GABA(B) receptor (anti-GABABR)	Impaired inhibitory signaling/B2 subunit reduces inhibition
Anti-GABA(A) receptor/δ-subunit	Reduced GABAergic/inhibitory signaling
Glycine receptor (anti-GlyR)	Disruption of glycine receptor function decreases inhibition
Anti-Hu antibodies (ANNA-1)	Paraneoplastic/neuronal damage, especially in hippocampus
Anti-Ri antibodies (ANNA-2)	Paraneoplastic limbic encephalitis, neuronal dysfunction
Anti-Ma2 antibodies	Neuronal dysfunction and disrupted synaptic transmission
Anti-Yo antibodies	Contribute to hippocampal hyperexcitability
Anti-Tr (DNER) antibodies	Affect brainstem/cerebellar function, potentially TLE
Anti-DPPX antibodies	Disrupt K^+ channels, increasing neuronal excitability
Anti-Neurexin-3α Antibodies	Impair synaptic adhesion and function
Anti-IgLON5 antibodies	Can cause brainstem/limbic system dysfunction
Anti-Contactin-2 antibodies	Disrupt axonal conduction and synaptic function
Anti-MOG antibodies	Primarily affect myelin, but also hippocampal excitability
Anti-AQP4 antibodies	Neuromyelitis optica, secondary hippocampal hyperexcitability

Table 2.
Most common autoimmune inflammatory processes affecting the mesial temporal lobe that can lead to enhanced neuronal excitability and increased risk for seizures, organized by specific antibodies against receptor/channel/targets and the resulting dysfunctions (a review from Graus et al. [140]).

For example, antibodies against NMDA receptors lead to a reduction in receptor density and subsequent dysregulation of excitatory synaptic transmission. VGKC complex antibodies can disrupt K^+ channel function, LGI-1 disrupts synaptic proteins associated with the regulation of AMPA receptors, and CASPR2 antibodies disrupt the Kv1 K^+ channels. GAD65 antibodies against Glutamic Acid Decarboxylase (GAD) can impair GABA synthesis and reduce GABAergic inhibition. Autoantibodies against AMPA receptors can alter excitatory synaptic transmission. GABA(B) receptor antibodies impair inhibitory signaling, resulting in an imbalance between excitation and inhibition. Glycine receptor antibodies disrupt inhibitory neurotransmission. Anti-Hu and other anti-neuronal antibodies lead to neuronal damage and dysfunction, particularly in the hippocampus (paraneoplastic limbic encephalitis) (**Table 2**) [141].

ix. Genetic mutations and hippocampal epileptic and neuropsychiatric syndromes

Genetic mutations in various genes associated with epilepsy (e.g. SCN1A, KCNQ2, DEPDC5, etc.) can lead to structural and functional abnormalities in the hippocampus which can directly impact neuronal excitability and predispose to seizures. Genetic mutations that disrupt the normal functioning of ion channels, neurotransmitter systems, or synaptic structures in the hippocampus can precipitate this spectrum of disorders. For instance, mutations in the SCN1A gene, which encodes a sodium channel, are well-known for causing Dravet syndrome, a condition marked by severe epilepsy, movement abnormalities, and behavioral challenges such as cognitive impairment and autistic traits. Similarly, mutations in the KCNQ2 gene, which affects potassium channels, are linked to early-onset epileptic encephalopathies with significant motor and cognitive deficits. The DEPDC5 gene (regulation of the mTOR signaling pathway), associated with familial focal epilepsy, underscores the genetic connection between focal seizures, often originating in the hippocampus, and broader neuropsychiatric manifestations. These few examples, among thousands of others, highlight how genetic mutations affecting brain development, structural and functional connectivity, or excitability of neurons and neuronal networks can lead to a constellation of clinical symptoms involving seizures, motor disturbances, neuropsychiatric disorders, and behavioral changes, particularly when they impact the hippocampal region (**Table 1**) [142].

The network diagram of **Figure 6** shows the 100 most common genes linking hippocampal oscillopathies with various seizure disorders (focal and generalized epileptic syndromes or epileptic encephalopathies), movement and motor control disorders (myoclonus, dystonias, dyskinesias, choreoathetosis, etc.), and neuropsychiatric and behavioral disorders (autism, schizophrenia, depression, anxiety, attention-deficit-hyperactivity disorder, intellectual disability, learning difficulties, etc.). The seizures can, in turn, influence motor functions, leading to movement disorders, and can affect mood and cognition, resulting in behavioral disturbances (**Figure 6**) [143].

x. Developmental and structural abnormalities of the hippocampus, such as hippocampal sclerosis, malformations, or dysplasias, can disrupt normal hippocampal structure and function. Febrile seizures (FS), commonly seen up to 5 years of age, may affect the development of the hippocampus and may be the precursor of mesial temporal sclerosis and epilepsy later in life. Certain mutations in the SCN1A gene, encoding the voltage-gated sodium channel NaV1.1, may predispose to FS (due to a decrease in the Na^+ current density, mainly affecting inhibitory neuronal transmission), or β_1 subunit of the SCN1B gene (usually associated with loss of function) or the SCN2A (encodes the neuronal sodium channel NaV1.2) or the GABRG2 (GABA-A receptor subunit $\gamma 2$) [144].

Human intracranial brain recordings for epilepsy surgery purposes give us a unique insight into the electrophysiological dynamics of the hippocampal network, especially in regard to seizure disorders. We have described in detail the mechanisms of seizure generation (epileptogenesis) in our previous monograph (Clinical Neurophysiology of Epileptogenic Networks) [1]. In **Figures 7–9**, we present a typical example of a hippocampal seizure. An initial wave of hyperexcitation as a result of stochastic resonance in a population of hippocampal neurons from the right anterior hippocampus (high-frequency synchronization with ripples/fast ripples, Channel 3 Spectrogram) is followed by excessive feedback inhibition and a brief period of attenuation (desynchronization or phase-resetting of unit oscillators) of the right middle hippocampus (Channel 2 Spectrogram) which, in turn, goes through recurrent excitation-inhibition oscillatory cycles (synchronization process) before a sustained paroxysmal depolarization shift develops with pathological low/high gamma, ripple, and fast ripple oscillations [1].

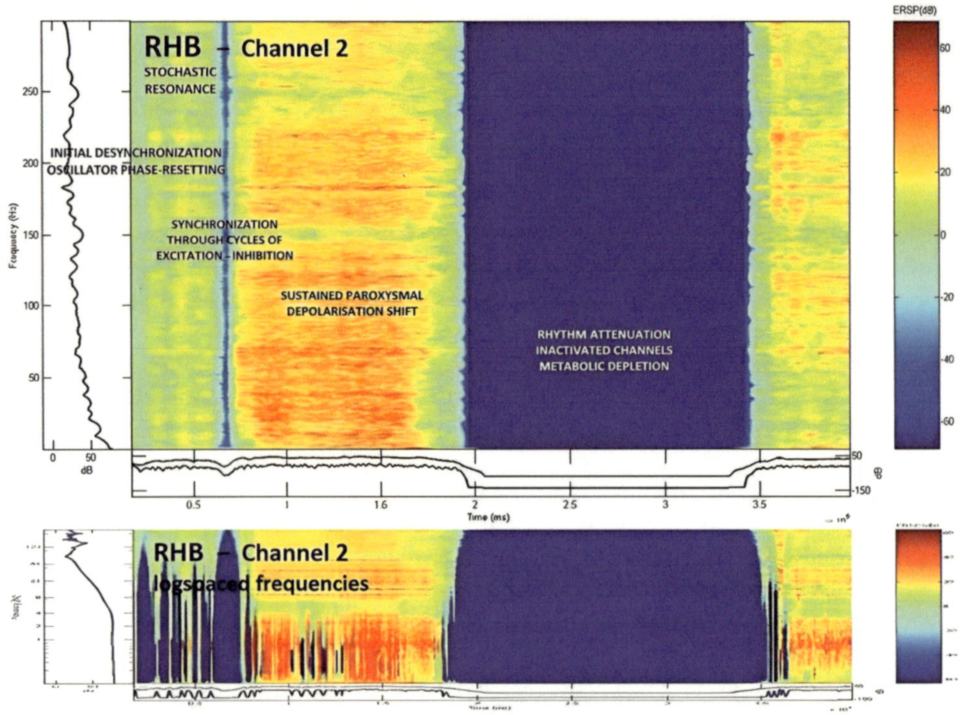

Figure 9.
Seizure onset in the right hippocampus was preceded by a brief broadband attenuation, consistent with desynchronization or phase resetting of unit oscillators. This was followed by an initial phase of network resynchronization, characterized by recurrent cycles of depolarization and repolarization, which then evolved into a sustained broadband paroxysmal depolarization shift. The ictal episode lasted approximately 2 minutes and 15 seconds and terminated with a prolonged postictal period marked by broadband suppression of background rhythms for an additional ~2.5 minutes. The upper spectrogram displays power in 1 Hz frequency bins from 1–300 Hz using a nonorthogonal 3-cycle wavelet decomposition, while the lower spectrogram presents log-spaced frequencies (pseudo-orthogonal decomposition), highlighting that the dominant power was concentrated <4 Hz, though more sustained over time between 12–64 Hz (beta and low/high gamma) frequency ranges.

Focal hippocampal seizures (mesial Temporal Lobe Epilepsy/mTLE) manifest with a variable combination of auras, sensory, motor, limbic, or autonomic phenomena, with or without loss of awareness, with secondary unilateral or bilateral propagation and generalization. They can occur at any age. Patients usually have a normal perinatal history and development. They generally have a normal neurological examination and are cognitively intact. A childhood history of febrile seizures is an important precursor for the development of mTLE. Follow-up neuroimaging on these patients often reveals hippocampal sclerosis and/or hippocampal volume loss (atrophy). Other risk factors include head trauma, birth trauma, childhood CNS infection, posterior cerebral artery territory infarcts, tumors, and a range of acquired structural, ischemic/vascular, inflammatory, infectious, metabolic, autoimmune, neoplastic, degenerative, epigenetic, etc. focal pathologies, which could result in localized or more widespread focal (within the same or both hemispheres) epileptogenic networks.

On the other hand, focal/multi-focal or generalized symptomatic epilepsies are usually associated with more apparent or striking focal or generalized brain dysfunction, injury or developmental abnormality, manifesting from early life. People with symptomatic epilepsies have neurological or cognitive deficits and a higher chance of intellectual disability, cerebral palsy, Lennox-Gastaut syndrome, and other neurodevelopmental conditions/problems.

In regard to the treatment of hippocampal oscillopathies associated with seizure disorders, we need to identify focal lesions or more widespread abnormalities of structural and/or functional connectivity (focal cortical dysplasias, developmental dysplasias/malformations, previous or perinatal brain injuries, hypoxic or metabolic and toxic insults, ischaemic or vascular lesions and malformations, tumors, space-occupying lesions, infiltrative, (para)neoplastic, inflammatory, infective/postinfective, autoimmune, vasculitic, (epi)genetic, neurodegenerative, etc.) and modify the local and global, structural and/or functional connectivity and network excitability. Nowadays, as a result of widespread applications of epilepsy surgery with direct intracranial EEG recordings, focal neocortical and allocortical/limbocortical epileptogenic networks have been more thoroughly studied and better understood [1].

After the age of 40, most adult-onset epilepsies in individuals with otherwise normal brain development and no prior seizure history are attributed to cumulative, often subtle, acquired insults and progressive local network alterations. These may include ischemic, toxic, cerebrovascular, traumatic, inflammatory, autoimmune, paraneoplastic, and/or degenerative processes. Such factors can alter or disrupt structural and functional connectivity, impair inhibitory control, or accelerate synaptic pruning, coinciding with age-related decline in memory and learning. The incidence of both epilepsy and movement disorders thus rises with advancing age (>60 years); however, seizure severity often diminishes in late life, as ongoing neurodegeneration contributes to connectivity degradation and breakdown of neuronal networks.

In order to modify and optimize the local and global functional connectivity and control the network excitability, a strategic approach involving antiepileptic medications is employed [1]. These anti-seizure medications are commonly utilized either as monotherapy or in carefully selected combinations (polytherapy) to achieve desired therapeutic outcomes. Specifically, medications can be categorized into the following five groups based on their primary effects: Groups I, II, III, and V modulate and suppress intrinsic local and global network excitability, while Group IV drugs enhance local and global network inhibition:

i. Fast voltage-gated Na^+-channel blockers: Carbamazepine also increases dopamine turnover, reduces glutamate release, and indirectly enhances GABA transmission, Oxcarbazepine also inhibits the release of glutamate, Eslicarbazepine (active metabolite of oxcarbazepine) more selectively inhibits high-frequency firing in the epileptic focus and also inhibits T-type Ca^{+2} channels. Lamotrigine stabilizes presynaptic neuronal membranes and inhibits presynaptic glutamate/aspartate release, acts also on L-type Ca^{+2}-channels, and inhibits reuptake of serotonin, dopamine, and noradrenaline. Cenobamate also acts as positive allosteric modulator of GABA-A receptors. Valproate acts also on Ca^{+2} and K^+ channels and has anti-NMDA and indirect GABAergic effects. Zonisamide acts also on T-type Ca^{+2}-channels. Lacosamide is a slow voltage-gated Na^+-channel blocker. Phenytoin is a pure Na^+ channel blocker.

ii. SVPA2 receptor inhibitors: Levetiracetam acts also on N-Type Ca^{+2}-channels, inhibits high-voltage-gated calcium currents, modulates inhibitory (GABA) and excitatory (NMDA, AMPA) postsynaptic ligand-gated receptors, Brivaracetam (20× higher affinity for SVP2A) also inhibits sodium channels and modulates synaptic GABA.

iii. AMPA glutamate receptor antagonists: Perampanel and Topiramate act also on GABA-A receptors.

iv. GABA-A receptor agonists (increase the frequency and duration of Cl^--channel opening): Clobazam, Clonazepam, Midazolam, Lorazepam, Diazepam, Phenobarbital, Primidone—Stiripentol elevates the levels of GABA and acts as a positive allosteric modulator of GABA-A receptors, etc.

v. Miscellaneous: Cannabidiol acts on CB1/CB2 receptors as an agonist at 5-HT_{1A} receptors and as an antagonist to GPR55, interacts with TRPV1, modulates intracellular Ca^{+2}, and inhibits adenosine reuptake. Fenfluramine increases the release of serotonin and inhibits its reuptake (SERT) and indirectly affects glutamatergic and GABAergic systems. Acetazolamide carbonic anhydrase inhibitor causes mild acidosis that reduces neuronal excitability. Gabapentin and Pregabalin act as presynaptic voltage-dependent Ca^{+2} channel inhibitors, and dose-dependent inducers of L-glutamic acid decarboxylase that enhance GABA synthesis. Rufinamide prolongs the inactive state of voltage-gated Na^+ channels and inhibits mGluR5 subtype receptors at high concentrations.

Alternative approaches to modifying the local and global, structural, and functional network connectivity and excitability are by means of neurosurgery (with resection or thermocoagulation of highly epileptogenic lesions/zones and disruption or disconnection of epileptogenic networks, etc.) and neurostimulation (vagus nerve, electrical/magnetic or optogenetic cortical stimulation or deep brain stimulation of the thalamus [anterior, centromedian, subthalamic nuclei]/basal ganglia, hippocampus, etc.) [1, 145].

There are currently five approaches to neurostimulation: (1) Deep Brain Stimulation (DBS), (2) Responsive Neural Stimulation (RNS), and indirect neurostimulation like Vagus Nerve Stimulation (VNS) [131], or non-invasive brain stimulation like transcranial magnetic stimulation (repetitive or theta-burst TMS) and transcranial direct DC current stimulation (tDCS). DBS is an open-loop neurostimulator that provides continuous periodic electrical stimulation, while RNS is a closed-loop neurostimulator that automatically analyzes electrocortical activity to detect and rapidly deliver electrical stimulation to terminate seizures [146]. TMS can be used for functional mapping or excitability studies in epilepsy or for patients with drug-resistance/intolerance in depression and other conditions (**Figure 4**) [104, 111].

Fisher has anticipated possible benefits of medial septum-diagonal band of Broca (MS-DbB) stimulation based on septum stimulation in animal models of epilepsy, depression, or dementia, and clinical studies on septum stimulation in schizophrenia and pain patients [108]. A few clinical studies have been conducted to study antiepileptic effects of stimulation of the cerebellum and the nucleus accumbens (NAc). Stimulation of the anterior nucleus of the thalamus [145], the centromedian nucleus of the thalamus, and the hippocampus, has been found to be effective in reducing seizures in drug-resistant epilepsy patients [147].

9. Epilogue

We have systematically investigated the clinical neurophysiology of hippocampal disorders and the broader limbocortical networks, with a particular focus on hippocampal oscillopathies as fundamental mechanisms underlying cognitive, affective, behavioral, and seizure disorders. This approach builds on our previous efforts to understand the pathophysiology of seizures and epilepsy, from the molecular and cellular levels to the scale of neuronal networks, using mathematical models, simulations with complex artificial neuronal networks, and artificial intelligence (AI). Our ultimate goal is to develop optimization algorithms for pharmacological, neurostimulation, and neurosurgical treatment strategies for oscillopathy-related disorders.

The implications of this work are profound, not only for the advancement of AI—which increasingly relies on realistic simulations of biological neuronal networks—but also for deepening our understanding of how cognitive, emotional, behavioral, movement, and seizure disorders arise. For the first time, our approach enables the prediction and simulation of the effects of channel or receptor mutations, as well as specific drug interventions, from the level of individual neurons to the scale of entire neuronal networks. This breakthrough paves the way for precision medicine in neurodiagnostics and pharmacogenetics, facilitating the development of novel drugs and optimizing therapeutic strategies for conditions such as epilepsy, movement disorders, dementia, schizophrenia, depression, anxiety, and various behavioral and functional neurological disorders. Additionally, it holds promise for developing more effective neurostimulation and neurosurgical treatment strategies [1].

Author details

Nick Tsarouchas[1,2], Nicholas Tsarouchas[3]* and Constantin Tsarouchas[4]

1 East Kent University Hospitals NHS Foundation Trust, UK

2 King's College Hospital London, UK

3 Department of Clinical Neurosciences, University of Cambridge, UK

4 Department of Science, Langton Star Centre SLBS, UK

*Address all correspondence to: nicholas.tsarouchas.medic@gmail.com

References

[1] Tsarouchas N. Clinical neurophysiology of epileptogenic networks. In: Neurophysiology—Networks, Plasticity, Pathophysiology and Behavior. IntechOpen; 2022. DOI: 10.5772/intechopen.104952

[2] Buzsaki G, Leung LW, Vanderwolf CH. Cellular bases of hippocampal EEG in the behaving rat. Brain Research. 1983;**287**:139-171

[3] Colgin LL. Oscillations and hippocampal-prefrontal synchrony. Current Opinion in Neurobiology. 2011;**21**(3):467-474

[4] Vanderwolf CH. Hippocampal electrical activity and voluntary movement in the rat. Electroencephalography and Clinical Neurophysiology. 1969;**26**:407-418

[5] Buzsaki G. Theta rhythm of navigation: Link between path integration and landmark navigation, episodic and semantic memory. Hippocampus. 2005;**15**:827-840

[6] Schlingloff D, Káli S, Freund TF, Hájos N, Gulyás AI. Mechanisms of sharp wave initiation and ripple generation. Journal of Neuroscience. 2014;**34**(34):11385-11398

[7] Buzsaki G. Hippocampal sharp waves: Their origin and significance. Brain Research. 1986;**398**:242-252

[8] Bragin A, Jando G, Nadasdy Z, Hetke J, et al. Gamma (40-100 Hz) oscillation in the hippocampus of the behaving rat. The Journal of Neuroscience. 1995;**15**(1 Pt 1):47-60

[9] Tamura M, Spellman TJ, et al. Hippocampal-prefrontal theta-gamma coupling during performance of a spatial working memory task. Nature Communications. 2017;**8**:2182

[10] Colgin LL. Rhythms of the hippocampal network. Nature Reviews. Neuroscience. 2016;**17**(4):239-249

[11] Lisman J, Buzsáki G, et al. Viewpoints: How the hippocampus contributes to memory, navigation and cognition. Nature Neuroscience. 2017;**20**(11):1434-1447

[12] Takeuchi Y et al. The medial septum as a potential target for treating brain disorders associated with oscillopathies. Frontiers in Neural Circuits. 2021;**15**:701080

[13] Buzsáki G. Theta oscillations in the hippocampus. Neuron. 2002;**33**(3):325-340

[14] Goutagny R, Jackson J, Williams S. Self-generated theta oscillations in the hippocampus. Nature Neuroscience. 2009;**12**(12):1491-1493

[15] Petsche H et al. The significance of the rabbit's septum as a relay station between the midbrain and the hippocampus. I. The control of hippocampus arousal activity by the septum cells. Electroencephalography and Clinical Neurophysiology. 1962;**14**:202-211

[16] Desikan S, Koser DE, et al. Target selectivity of septal cholinergic neurons in the medial and lateral entorhinal cortex. Proceedings of the National Academy of Sciences of the United States of America. 2018;**115**:E2644-E2652

[17] Unal G et al. Spatio-temporal specialization of GABAergic

septo-hippocampal neurons for rhythmic network activity. Brain Structure & Function. 2018;**223**(5):2409-2432

[18] Hangya B et al. GABAergic neurons of the medial septum lead the hippocampal network during theta activity. Journal of Neuroscience. 2009;**29**(25):8094-8102

[19] Partlo LA, Sainsbury RS. Influence of medial septal and entorhinal cortex lesions on theta activity recorded from the hippocampus and median raphe nucleus. Physiology & Behavior. 1996;**59**(4-5):887-895

[20] Smythe JW, Colom LV, Bland BH. The extrinsic modulation of hippocampal theta depends on the coactivation of cholinergic and GABA-ergic medial septal inputs. Neuroscience & Biobehavioral Reviews. 1992;**16**(3):289-308

[21] King C, Recce M, O'Keefe J. The rhythmicity of cells of the medial septum/diagonal band of Broca in the awake freely moving rat: Relationships with behaviour and hippocampal theta. The European Journal of Neuroscience. 1998;**10**(2):464-477

[22] Freund TF. GABAergic septal and serotonergic median raphe afferents preferentially innervate inhibitory interneurons in the hippocampus and dentate gyrus. Epilepsy Research. Supplement. 1992;7:79-91

[23] Tóth K, Freund TF, Miles R. Disinhibition of rat hippocampal pyramidal cells by GABAergic afferents from the septum. The Journal of Physiology. 1997;**500**:463-474

[24] Yoder RM, Pang KC. Involvement of GABAergic and cholinergic medial septal neurons in hippocampal theta rhythm. Hippocampus. 2005;**15**(3):381-392

[25] Borhegyi Z, Varga V, Szilágyi N, et al. Phase segregation of medial septal GABAergic neurons during hippocampal theta activity. The Journal of Neuroscience. 2004;**24**(39):8470-8479

[26] Leranth C, Vertes RP. Median raphe serotonergic innervation of medial septum/diagonal band of broca (MSDB) parvalbumin-containing neurons: Possible involvement of the MSDB in the desynchronization of the hippocampal EEG. The Journal of Comparative Neurology. 1999;**410**(4):586-598

[27] Broncel A, Bocian R, Kłos-Wojtczak P, Konopacki J. Effects of locus coeruleus activation and inactivation on hippocampal formation theta rhythm in anesthetized rats. Brain Research Bulletin. 2020;**162**:180-190. ISSN: 0361-9230

[28] Orzeł-Gryglewska J, Matulewicz P, et al. Brainstem system of hippocampal theta induction: The role of the ventral tegmental area. Synapse. 2015;**69**(11):553-575

[29] Buzsáki G. Hippocampal sharp wave-ripple: A cognitive biomarker for episodic memory and planning. Hippocampus. 2015;**25**(10):1073-1188

[30] Dragoi G et al. Interactions between hippocampus and medial septum during sharp waves and theta oscillation in the behaving rat. The Journal of Neuroscience. 1999;**19**(14):6191-6199

[31] Vandecasteele M, Varga V, Berényi A, et al. Optogenetic activation of septal cholinergic neurons suppresses sharp wave ripples and enhances theta oscillations in the hippocampus. Proceedings of the National Academy of Sciences of the United States of America. 2014;**111**(37):13535-13540

[32] Kang D, Ding M, Topchiy I, Kocsis B. Reciprocal interactions between medial septum and hippocampus in Theta generation: Granger causality decomposition of mixed spike-field recordings. Frontiers in Neuroanatomy. 2017;**11**:120

[33] Goyal A, Miller J, Qasim SE, et al. Functionally distinct high and low theta oscillations in the human hippocampus. Nature Communications. 2020;**11**:2469

[34] Vivekananda U, Bush D, Bisby JA, et al. Theta power and theta-gamma coupling support long-term spatial memory retrieval. Hippocampus. 2021;**31**(2):213-220

[35] Wang Y, Romani S, Lustig B, Leonardo A, et al. Theta sequences are essential for internally generated hippocampal firing fields. Nature Neuroscience. 2015;**18**(2):282-288

[36] Aronov D, Nevers R, Tank DW. Mapping of a non-spatial dimension by the hippocampal-entorhinal circuit. Nature. 2017;**543**(7647):719-722

[37] Korotkova T, Ponomarenko A, Monaghan CK, Poulter SL, et al. Reconciling the different faces of hippocampal theta: The role of theta oscillations in cognitive, emotional and innate behaviors. Neuroscience and Biobehavioral Reviews. 2018;**85**:65-80

[38] Mastrogiuseppe M, Bertelsen N, et al. The spatiotemporal organization of episodic memory and its disruption in a neurodevelopmental disorder. Scientific Reports. 2019;**9**:18447

[39] Buzsáki G, Draguhn A. Neuronal oscillations in cortical networks. Science. 2004;**304**(5679):1926-1929

[40] Montgomery SM, Buzsáki G. Gamma oscillations dynamically couple hippocampal CA3 and CA1 regions during memory task performance. Proceedings of the National Academy of Sciences of the United States of America. 2007;**104**(36):14495-14500

[41] Sederberg PB, Schulze-Bonhage A, et al. Hippocampal and neocortical gamma oscillations predict memory formation in humans. Cerebral Cortex. 2007;**17**(5):1190-1196

[42] López-Madrona VJ et al. Different theta frameworks coexist in the rat hippocampus and are coordinated during memory-guided and novelty tasks. eLife. 2020;**9**:e57313

[43] Cherubini E, Miles R. The CA3 region of the hippocampus: How is it? What is it for? How does it do it? Frontiers in Cellular Neuroscience. 2015;**9**:19

[44] Nuñez A, Buño W. The Theta rhythm of the hippocampus: From neuronal and circuit mechanisms to behavior. Frontiers in Cellular Neuroscience. 2021;**15**:649262

[45] Núñez A, García-Austt E, et al. Synaptic contributions to theta rhythm genesis in rat CA1-CA3 hippocampal pyramidal neurons in vivo. Brain Research. 1990b;**533**:176-179

[46] Freund TF, Buzsáki G. Interneurons of the hippocampus. Hippocampus. 1996;**6**(4):347-470

[47] Csicsvari J, Hirase H, Czurko A, Mamiya A, Buzsaki G. Fast network oscillations in the hippocampal CA1 region of the behaving rat. The Journal of Neuroscience. 1999;**19**:RC20

[48] Klausberger T, Somogyi P. Neuronal diversity and temporal dynamics: The unity of hippocampal circuit operations. Science. 2008;**321**(5885):53-57

[49] Müller C, Remy S. Septo-hippocampal interaction. Cell and Tissue Research. 2018;**373**(3):565-575

[50] Tovote P, Fadok JP, Lüthi A. Neuronal circuits for fear and anxiety. Nature Reviews. Neuroscience. 2015;**16**(6):317-331

[51] Drysdale AT et al. Resting-state connectivity biomarkers define neurophysiological subtypes of depression. Nature Medicine. 2017;**23**(1):28-38

[52] Çalışkan G, Stork O. Hippocampal network oscillations at the interplay between innate anxiety and learned fear. Psychopharmacology. 2019;**236**(1):321-338

[53] Orsini CA et al. Hippocampal and prefrontal projections to the basal amygdala mediate contextual regulation of fear after extinction. The Journal of Neuroscience. 2011;**31**(47):17269-17277

[54] Ciocchi S, Passecker J, et al. Brain computation. Selective information routing by ventral hippocampal CA1 projection neurons. Science. 2015;**348**(6234):560-563

[55] Ishikawa A, Nakamura S. Convergence and interaction of hippocampal and amygdalar projections within the prefrontal cortex in the rat. The Journal of Neuroscience. 2003;**23**(31):9987-9995

[56] Senn V, Wolff SB, Herry C, Grenier F, et al. Long-range connectivity defines behavioral specificity of amygdala neurons. Neuron. 2014;**81**(2):428-437

[57] Hartley CA, Phelps EA. Changing fear: The neurocircuitry of emotion regulation. Neuropsychopharmacology. 2010;**35**(1):136-146

[58] Burgos-Robles A, Kimchi EY, Izadmehr, et al. Amygdala inputs to prefrontal cortex guide behavior amid conflicting cues of reward and punishment. Nature Neuroscience. 2017;**20**(6):824-835

[59] Le Merre P, Ährlund-Richter S, Carlén M. The mouse prefrontal cortex: Unity in diversity. Neuron. 2021;**109**(12):1925-1944

[60] Miller EK, Cohen JD. An integrative theory of prefrontal cortex function. Annual Review of Neuroscience. 2001;**24**:167-202

[61] Jay TM, Witter MP. Distribution of hippocampal CA1 and subicular efferents in the prefrontal cortex of the rat studied by means of anterograde transport of Phaseolus vulgaris-leucoagglutinin. The Journal of Comparative Neurology. 1991;**313**:574-586

[62] Hoover WB, Vertes RP. Anatomical analysis of afferent projections to the medial prefrontal cortex in the rat. Brain Structure & Function. 2007;**212**:149-179

[63] Laroche S et al. Long-term potentiation in the prefrontal cortex following stimulation of the hippocampal CA1/subicular region. Neuroscience Letters. 1990;**114**:184-190

[64] Anderson KL et al. Theta oscillations mediate interaction between prefrontal cortex and medial temporal lobe in human memory. Cerebral Cortex. 2010;**20**:1604-1612

[65] Sederberg PB, Schulze-Bonhage A, Madsen JR, Bromfield EB, et al. Gamma oscillations distinguish true from false memories. Psychological Science. 2007;**18**:927-932

[66] Nieuwenhuis IL, Takashima A. The role of the ventromedial prefrontal

cortex in memory consolidation. Behavioural Brain Research. 2011;**218**:325-334

[67] Harris JA, Mihalas S, Hirokawa KE, et al. Hierarchical organization of cortical and thalamic connectivity. Nature. 2019;**575**:195-202

[68] Okonogi T, Sasaki T. Theta-range oscillations in stress-induced mental disorders as an oscillotherapeutic target. Frontiers in Behavioral Neuroscience. 2021;**15**:698753

[69] Sigurdsson T, Duvarci S. Hippocampal-prefrontal interactions in cognition, behavior and psychiatric disease. Frontiers in Systems Neuroscience. 2016;**9**:190

[70] Mocellin P, Mikulovic S. The role of the medial septum-associated networks in controlling locomotion and motivation to move. Frontiers in Neural Circuits. 2021;**15**:699798

[71] Schimmelpfennig J, Topczewski J, Zajkowski W, Jankowiak-Siuda K. The role of the salience network in cognitive and affective deficits. Frontiers in Human Neuroscience. 2023;**17**:1133367

[72] Powell SB. Models of neurodevelopmental abnormalities in schizophrenia. Current Topics in Behavioral Neurosciences. 2010;**4**:435-481

[73] Kätzel D, Wolff AR, et al. Hippocampal hyperactivity as a druggable circuit-level origin of aberrant salience in schizophrenia. Frontiers in Pharmacology. 2020;**11**:486811

[74] Sonnenschein SF, Gomes FV, Grace AA. Dysregulation of midbrain dopamine system and the pathophysiology of schizophrenia. Frontiers in Psychiatry. 2020;**11**:613

[75] Pickar D et al. Neurochemical and neural mechanisms of positive and negative symptoms in schizophrenia. Modern Problems of Pharmacopsychiatry. 1990;**24**:124-151

[76] Liemburg EJ et al. Antipsychotic medication and prefrontal cortex activation: A review of neuroimaging findings. European Neuropsychopharmacology. 2012;**22**(6):387-400

[77] Wang X, Li Z, Kuai S, Wang X, et al. Correlation between desynchrony of hippocampal neural activity and hyperlocomotion in the model mice of schizophrenia and therapeutic effects of aripiprazole. CNS Neuroscience & Therapeutics. 2024;**30**(5):e14739

[78] Preskorn SH. A roadmap to key pharmacologic principles in using antipsychotics. Primary Care Companion to the Journal of Clinical Psychiatry. 2007;**9**(6):444-454

[79] McDonald C, Murphy KC. The new genetics of schizophrenia. The Psychiatric Clinics of North America. 2003;**26**(1):41-63

[80] Schmidt CJ, Sorensen SM, Kehne JH, Carr AA, Palfreyman MG. The role of 5-HT2A receptors in antipsychotic activity. Life Sciences. 1995;**56**(25):2209-2222

[81] Shayegan DK, Stahl SM. Atypical antipsychotics: Matching receptor profile to individual patient's clinical profile. CNS Spectrums. 2004;**9**(S11):6-14

[82] Menon V, Palaniyappan L, Supekar K. Integrative brain network and salience models of psychopathology and cognitive dysfunction in schizophrenia. Biological Psychiatry. 15 Jul 2023;**94**(2):108-120

[83] Sirota A, Buzsáki G. Interaction between neocortical and hippocampal networks via slow oscillations. Thalamus & Related Systems. 2005;**3**(4):245-259

[84] Gloveli T, Dugladze T, et al. Orthogonal arrangement of rhythm-generating microcircuits in the hippocampus. Proceedings of the National Academy of Sciences of the United States of America. 2005;**102**(37):13295-13300

[85] Adhikari A et al. Synchronized activity between the ventral hippocampus and the medial prefrontal cortex during anxiety. Neuron. 2010;**65**(2):257-269

[86] Menard J, Treit D. Lateral and medial septal lesions reduce anxiety in the plus-maze and probe-burying tests. Physiology & Behavior. 1996;**60**(3):845-853

[87] Jacinto LR et al. Stress affects theta activity in limbic networks and impairs novelty-induced exploration and familiarization. Frontiers in Behavioral Neuroscience. 2013;**7**:127

[88] Buzsaki G, Watson BO. Brain rhythms and neural syntax: Implications for efficient coding of cognitive content and neuropsychiatric disease. Dialog. Clinical Neuroscience. 2012;**14**:345-367

[89] Shin L, Liberzon I. The neurocircuitry of fear, stress, and anxiety disorders. Neuropsychopharmacology. 2010;**35**:169-191

[90] Karalis N, Dejean C, Chaudun F, Khoder S, et al. 4-Hz oscillations synchronize prefrontal-amygdala circuits during fear behavior. Nature Neuroscience. 2016;**19**(4):605-612

[91] Stein MB, Simmons AN, et al. Increased amygdala and insula activation during emotion processing in anxiety-prone subjects. The American Journal of Psychiatry. 2007;**164**(2):318-327

[92] Menon V, Uddin LQ. Saliency, switching, attention and control: A network model of insula function. Brain Structure & Function. 2010;**214**(5-6):655-667

[93] Cassano GB, Baldini Rossi N, Pini S. Psychopharmacology of anxiety disorders. Dialogues in Clinical Neuroscience. 2002;**4**(3):271-285

[94] Menon V. The triple network model, insight and large-scale brain organization in autism. Biological Psychiatry. 2018;**84**:236-238

[95] Harikumar A et al. A review of the default mode network in autism Spectrum disorders and attention deficit hyperactivity disorder. Brain Connectivity. 2021;**11**(4):253-263

[96] Saad JF et al. Intrinsic functional connectivity in the default mode network differentiates the combined and inattentive attention deficit hyperactivity disorder types. Frontiers in Human Neuroscience. 2022;**16**:859538

[97] Castellanos FX, Proal E. Large-scale brain systems in ADHD: Beyond the prefrontal-striatal model. Trends in Cognitive Sciences. 2012;**16**(1):17-26

[98] Drechsler R, Brem S, Brandeis D, Grünblatt E, et al. ADHD: Current concepts and treatments in children and adolescents. Neuropediatrics. 2020;**51**(5):315-335

[99] American Psychiatric Association. The Diagnostic and Statistical Manual of Mental Disorders (DSM-5). Washington, DC: American Psychiatric Publishing, Inc.; 2013

[100] Noda Y et al. Enhanced theta-gamma coupling associated with hippocampal volume increase following high-frequency left prefrontal repetitive transcranial magnetic stimulation in patients with major depression. International Journal of Psychophysiology. 2018;**133**:169-174

[101] Fitzgerald PJ, Watson BO. Gamma oscillations as a biomarker for major depression: An emerging topic. Translational Psychiatry. 2018;**8**:177

[102] Iosifescu DV. Electroencephalography-derived biomarkers of antidepressant response. Harvard Review of Psychiatry. 2011;**19**(3):144-154

[103] Clancy KJ et al. Posttraumatic stress disorder is associated with α dysrhythmia across the visual cortex and the default mode network. eNeuro. 2020;**7**(4):ENEURO.0053-20.2020

[104] Anderson RJ et al. Repetitive transcranial magnetic stimulation for treatment resistant depression: Re-establishing connections. Clinical Neurophysiology. 2016;**127**(11):3394-3405

[105] Liu X, Liu S, et al. Altered gamma oscillations and beta–gamma coupling in drug-naive first-episode major depressive disorder: Association with sleep and cognitive disturbance. Journal of Affective Disorders. 2022;**316**:99-108

[106] Yamamoto Y, Fukunaga K. Donepezil rescues the medial septum cholinergic neurons via nicotinic ACh receptor stimulation in olfactory bulbectomized mice. Advances in Alzheimer's Disease. 2013;**2**:161-170

[107] Dandekar MP et al. Deep brain stimulation for treatment-resistant depression: An integrative review of preclinical and clinical findings and translational implications. Molecular Psychiatry. 2018;**23**(5):1094-1112

[108] Fisher RS. Stimulation of the medial septum should benefit patients with temporal lobe epilepsy. Medical Hypotheses. 2015;**84**:543-550

[109] Hajós M et al. Norepinephrine but not serotonin reuptake inhibitors enhance theta and gamma activity of the septo-hippocampal system. Neuropsychopharmacology. 2003;**28**(5):857-864

[110] Jennings L. Antidepressants. In: Grossberg G, Kinsella L, editors. Clinical Psychopharmacology for Neurologists. Cham: Springer; 2018

[111] Arnsten AF. Stress weakens prefrontal networks: Molecular insults to higher cognition. Nature Neuroscience. 2015;**18**(10):1376-1385

[112] Hamilton JP, Gotlib IH. Neural substrates of increased memory sensitivity for negative stimuli in major depression. Biological Psychiatry. 2008;**63**(12):1155-1162

[113] Zhang Z, Bo Q, Li F, Zhao L, et al. Altered effective connectivity among core brain networks in patients with bipolar disorder. Journal of Psychiatric Research. 2022;**152**:296-304

[114] Beck JS. Cognitive Behavior Therapy: Basics and Beyond. 2nd ed. New York: The Guilford Press; 2011. pp. 19-20

[115] Michael-Titus SA, Revest P, Shortland P. 14—Dementia. In: Michael-Titus A, Revest P, Shortland P, editors. The Nervous System. 2nd ed. Churchill Livingstone; 2010. pp. 251-266

[116] Triggiani AI et al. Classification of healthy subjects and Alzheimer's disease

patients with dementia from cortical sources of resting state EEG rhythms: A study using artificial neural networks. Frontiers in Neuroscience. 2017;**10**:604

[117] Babiloni C et al. Classification of single normal and Alzheimer's disease individuals from cortical sources of resting state EEG rhythms. Frontiers in Neuroscience. 2016;**10**:47

[118] Traikapi A, Konstantinou N. Gamma oscillations in Alzheimer's disease and their potential therapeutic role. Frontiers in Systems Neuroscience. 2021;**15**:782399

[119] Babiloni C et al. Measures of resting state EEG rhythms for clinical trials in Alzheimer's disease: Recommendations of an expert panel. Alzheimer's & Dementia. 2021;**17**(9):1528-1553

[120] Del Percio C et al. What a single electroencephalographic (EEG) channel can tell us about Alzheimer's disease patients with mild cognitive impairment. Clinical EEG and Neuroscience. 2023;**54**(1):21-35

[121] Wang S et al. Early-stage dysfunction of hippocampal theta and gamma oscillations and its modulation of neural network in a transgenic 5xFAD mouse model. Neurobiology of Aging. 2020;**94**:121-129

[122] Chung H et al. Dissociation of somatostatin and parvalbumin interneurons circuit dysfunctions underlying hippocampal theta and gamma oscillations impaired by amyloid β oligomers in vivo. Brain Structure & Function. 2020;**225**:935-954

[123] Hampel H et al. The cholinergic system in the pathophysiology and treatment of Alzheimer's disease. Brain. 2018;**141**:1917-1933

[124] Colom LV et al. Medial septal β-amyloid 1-40 injections alter septo-hippocampal anatomy and function. Neurobiology of Aging. 2010;**31**:46-57

[125] Leplus A et al. Chronic fornix deep brain stimulation in a transgenic Alzheimer's rat model reduces amyloid burden, inflammation, and neuronal loss. Brain Structure & Function. 2019;**224**:363-372

[126] Nazmuddin M et al. Electrical stimulation of the nucleus basalis of meynert: A systematic review of preclinical and clinical data. Scientific Reports. 2021;**11**:11751

[127] Jiao L et al. The role of the nucleus basalis of Meynert in neuromodulation therapy: A systematic review from the perspective of neural network oscillations. Frontiers in Aging Neuroscience. 2024;**16**:1376764

[128] Etter G et al. Optogenetic gamma stimulation rescues memory impairments in an Alzheimer's disease mouse model. Nature Communications. 2019;**10**:5322, 1-11

[129] Wang Y et al. Deep brain stimulation in the medial septum attenuates temporal lobe epilepsy via entrainment of hippocampal theta rhythm. CNS Neuroscience and Therapeutics. 2021;**27**:577-586

[130] Lee DJ et al. Septohippocampal neuromodulation improves cognition after traumatic brain injury. Journal of Neurotrauma. 2015;**32**:1822-1832

[131] Broncel A et al. Medial septal cholinergic mediation of hippocampal theta rhythm induced by vagal nerve stimulation. PLoS ONE. 2018;**13**:e0206532. DOI: 10.1371/journal.pone.0206532

[132] Kumari E et al. Tacrine accelerates spatial long-term memory via improving impaired neural oscillations and modulating GAD isomers including neuro-receptors in the hippocampus of APP/PS1 AD mice. Brain Research Bulletin. 2020;**161**:166-176

[133] Beghi E. The epidemiology of epilepsy. Neuroepidemiology. 2020;**54**(2):185-191

[134] Beghi E, Giussani G. Aging and the epidemiology of epilepsy. Neuroepidemiology. 2018;**51**(3-4): 216-223

[135] Tau GZ, Peterson BS. Normal development of brain circuits. Neuropsychopharmacology. 2010;**35**(1):147-168

[136] Shakeshaft A et al. BIOJUME consortium. Trait impulsivity in juvenile myoclonic epilepsy. Annals of Clinical Translational Neurology. 2021;**8**(1):138-152

[137] Noebels JL, Avoli M, Rogawski MA, Olsen RW, Delgado-Escueta AV, editors. Jasper's Basic Mechanisms of the Epilepsies. 4th ed (Contemporary Neurology Series 80). USA: Oxford University Press. ISBN-10: 0199746540 | ISBN-13: 978-0199746545

[138] Beck H, Blumcke T, Scheid P. Synaptic plasticity and temporal lobe epilepsy: Insights from animal models. Journal of Neuroscience. 2002;**111**(2):193-204

[139] Li W, Wu J, Zeng Y, Zheng W. Neuroinflammation in epileptogenesis: From pathophysiology to therapeutic strategies. Frontiers in Immunology. 2023;**14**:1269241

[140] Graus F, Dalmau J, et al. A clinical approach to diagnosis of autoimmune encephalitis. Lancet Neurology. 2016;**15**(4):391-404. DOI: 10.1016/S1474-4422(15)00401-9. Epub 2016 Feb 20

[141] Bien CG et al. Pathogenesis, diagnosis, and treatment of autoimmune epilepsy. Nature Reviews Neurology. 2012

[142] Steriade C, Bauer J, Bien CG. Autoimmune encephalitis-associated epilepsy. Nature Reviews Neurology. 2025;**21**:312-326

[143] Peall KJ, Owen MJ, Hall J. Rare genetic brain disorders with overlapping neurological and psychiatric phenotypes. Nature Reviews. Neurology. 2024;**20**(1):7-21

[144] Yi Y, Zhong C, Wei-wei H. The long-term neurodevelopmental outcomes of febrile seizures and underlying mechanisms. Frontiers in Cell and Development Biology. 2023;**11**:1186050

[145] Fisher R et al. Electrical stimulation of the anterior nucleus of thalamus for treatment of refractory epilepsy. Epilepsia. 2010;**51**(5):899-908

[146] Foutz TJ, Wong M. Brain stimulation treatments in epilepsy: Basic mechanisms and clinical advances. Biomedical Journal. 2022;**45**(1):27-37

[147] Kokkinos V, Sisterson ND, Wozny TA, Richardson RM. Association of closed-loop brain stimulation neurophysiological features with seizure control among patients with focal epilepsy. JAMA Neurology. 2019;**76**(7):800-808